FRONTIERS IN TRANSPLANTOLOGY

Edited by **Hesham Abdeldayem, Ahmed F. El-Kased** and **Ahmed El-Shaarawy**

Frontiers in Transplantology
http://dx.doi.org/10.5772/61412
Edited by Hesham Abdeldayem, Ahmed F. El-Kased and Ahmed El-Shaarawy

Contributors
Maria Jose Herrero, Juan Eduardo Megías, Virginia Bosó, Jesús Ruiz, Luis Rojas, Ignacio Sánchez-Lázaro, Luis Almenar, Julio Hernández, Jose Luis Poveda, Amparo Pastor, Amparo Solé, Rafael López-Andújar, Salvador F. Aliño, Francisco Marco-Jimenez, Cesar David Vera Donoso, Ximo García-Domínguez, Jose S. Vicente, Luís García-Valero, Cristina Baleriola, William Rawlinson, Hesham Abdeldayem, Ahmed El-Kased, Ahmed Elshaarawy, Essam Hammad, Naglaa Allam, Omkolsoum Al-Haddad, Gihan Sobhi, Masayuki Tasaki, Kazuhide Saito, Yuki Nakagawa, Yoshihiko Tomita, Kota Takahashi, Jayan Nagendran, Nader Aboelnazar, Sayed Himmat, Darren Freed, Sagar Kadakia, Vishnu Ambur, Yoshiya Toyoda, Sharven Taghavi, Akira Shiose, Markus Selzner, Nicolas Goldaracena, Andrew Barbas, Juan Echeverri, Moritz Kaths, Wei-Chen Lee, Ahmed Zidan, Emica Shimozono, Cristina Caruy, Adilson Cardoso, Derli Servian, Ilka Boin, Julio Wiederkehr, Carole Guillonneau, Laetitia Boucault, Séverine Bézie, Jason Ossart

Published by InTech
Janeza Trdine 9, 51000 Rijeka, Croatia

Publishing Process Manager Iva Simcic
Technical Editor SPi Global
Cover InTech Design team

First published September, 2016
Printed in Croatia

Additional hard copies can be obtained from orders@intechopen.com

Frontiers in Transplantology, Edited by Hesham Abdeldayem, Ahmed F. El-Kased and Ahmed El-Shaarawy
p. cm.
Print ISBN 978-953-51-2523-5
Online ISBN 978-953-51-2524-2

For EU product safety concerns:
IN TECH d.o.o., Prolaz Marije Krucifikse Kozulić 3, 51000 Rijeka, Croatia,
info@intechopen.com or visit our website at intechopen.com.

Meet the editors

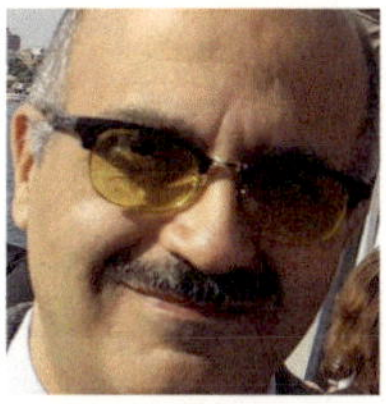

Hesham Abdeldayem is a professor of Surgery and Vice Dean of Postgraduate Studies and Research at the National Liver Institute, Menoufia University, Egypt. Professor Abdeldayem graduated from Kasr Elaini School of Medicine in 1987 where he was appointed as a resident of General Surgery and assistant lecturer of Microbiology. He joined the National Liver Institute in 1993. He has several publications in the fields of hepato-pancreato-biliary surgery and liver transplantation. He was appointed as a member of InTech's Editorial Advisory Board and associate editor of Frontiers in Surgery.

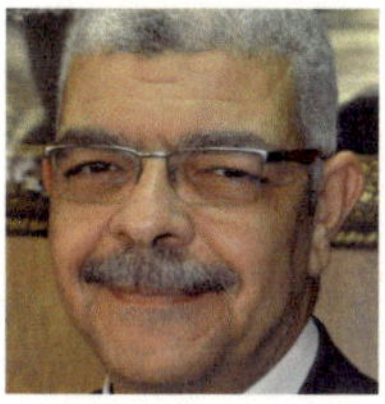

Professor Ahmed F. El-Kased graduated from Cairo University Medical School in 1989 and trained at the Cairo University National Cancer Institute. He was formerly the director of the Menoufia University Hospitals (2009–2010), head of the Surgery Department (2011–2013), and Dean of the Medical Faculty (2013–2015). He currently holds the position of University Vice President for Postgraduate Affairs and Research.

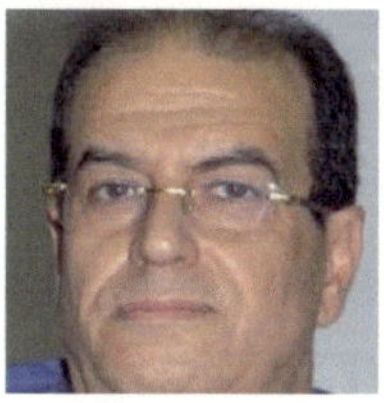

Ahmed El-Shaarawy is a professor of Clinical Pathology and Dean of the National Liver Institute, Menoufia University, Egypt. Professor El-Shaarawy was graduated from the School of Medicine, Benha University, in 1981, where he was appointed as a resident of Clinical Pathology, then he moved to the National Liver Institute in 1988 as an assistant lecturer in Clinical Pathology. After that, Prof. El-Shaarawy was promoted as a lecturer, assistant professor, and lastly, professor of Clinical Pathology. He shared in many research projects and publications in the fields of clinical pathology, liver diseases, liver transplantation, and stem cells.

Contents

Preface

The outstanding advances and new discoveries in organ transplantation science have resulted in remarkable changes in this field. The aim of our book is to present some of these advances. This book is addressed to researchers, practicing physicians, and surgeons in the field of organ transplantation, as well as the medical students, residents, and fellows. The topics covered include the religious concepts in organ transplantation, embryonic organ transplantation, tolerance, normothermic graft perfusion, pharmacogenetics of immunosuppressors, viral transmission in organ transplantation, pediatric and split-liver transplantation, portopulmonary hypertension, mechanical circulatory support, ex vivo lung perfusion, and ABO-incompatible kidney transplantation.

We wish to thank all our distinguished authors for their cooperation and desire to share their precious experience with the medical community. On their behalf, we wish to express hope that this publication will facilitate access to the latest scientific achievements in the field of organ transplantation. We are particularly thankful to Ms. Iva Simcic and her colleagues at InTech, for their expertise and support in bringing this edition to completion.

Prof. Hesham Abdeldayem
Prof. Ahmed F. El-Kased
Prof. Ahmed El-Shaarawy
Menoufia University
Egypt

Section 1

Introduction

Chapter 1

Religious Concepts in Organ Transplantation

Hesham Abdeldayem, Ahmed Farag El-Kased,
Ahmed Elshaarawy, Essam Salah Hammad,
OmKolsoum Al-Haddad, Gihan Sobhi and
Naglaa Allam

Additional information is available at the end of the chapter

http://dx.doi.org/10.5772/62401

Abstract

Beside cultural, social, and educational issues, religious beliefs are assumed to play a significant role on the attitude towards organ transplantation much more often than clinicians believe. At the same time, health-care providers may lack sufficient knowledge on religious issues pertaining to transplantation.

This chapter aims to provide an overview on the different religious concepts on organ transplantation. Such knowledge among transplant physicians and surgeons, donor coordinators, and intensivists may provide a background to deal with religious concerns towards organ and tissue donation professionally and appropriately and to increase the transplant numbers.

Keywords: deceased donor, faith, living donor, religion, transplantation

1. Introduction

One of the most touching forms of human compassion is related to the transplantation of human organs from a mother to a son, from a father to daughter, from a brother to a sister, from a friend to a friend, and from a stranger to a stranger.

Organ donation, from both living and deceased donors, is considered by most religions as an expression of the believer's altruism, generosity, duty, charity, and cooperation as long as the following conditions are fulfilled [1]:

1. The procedure occurs in the context of respect for the dignity of the dead person.
2. Organs from deceased donors are removed only after certain death has be confirmed.
3. Live organ donation does not impede the life of the donor.
4. Organ donations are given as a free gift without reward.
5. Commercialization and/or considering organs as items for trade or exchange are prohibited.

However, there are different schools of thought, between different religions and within each religion, regarding the issue of transplantation of human organs. In fact, religious concerns are considered by many as an important reason that explains why many individuals decline deceased and live organ donation and/or the willingness to accept a transplant.

2. Concerns around brain death

There are concerns and uncertainty regarding the issue of brain death. For example, some Muslim scholars, Orthodox Jews, Catholic theologians, and Buddhist scholars do not accept the concept of brain death [2].

3. Religiosity and willingness to donate

Religious views have been identified as a factor influencing the willingness to donate, with religion tending to be cited as a barrier to donation. Those who are described as being more religious may be less likely to support donation, believing that their religions oppose donation. In fact, most of the negative attitudes towards organ transplantation may be due to the uncertainty about the religious stance rather than the interpretations of religious teachings. The conservativeness of religious belief, rather than religiosity itself, may be the underlying factor against donation [3].

Negative attitudes are also related to how the individual interprets his or her relationship with God at the times of sickness. The response to illness is that it is God's will and they have to accept. Therefore, organ donation may conflict with the belief that one should respect God's will [4].

4. Body integrity

The importance of body integrity is much related to religious and cultural beliefs. The belief of being resurrected in the afterlife and the need for own organs after death is an obstacle against organ donation. Showing respect to the deceased individual may be also a barrier against donation. Dissecting the body is commonly perceived as a violation, believing that the deceased person could still feel pain [5].

http://dx.doi.org/10.5772/62401

5. Funeral

The expectation that the process of organ donation will delay funeral and prevent it from proceeding in the traditional way may also be a factor explaining negative attitudes against deceased organ donation [6].

6. Interplay of religious and cultural beliefs

There are striking differences between countries as to the willingness to donate. Besides the religious factors, some of the differences could be attributed to different infrastructure, law, and consent systems. At the same time, the interplay between religious and cultural beliefs is also an important factor. Barriers to organ donation that are perceived as religious may actually reflect cultural attitudes that transcend religion [7].

7. Directed donation and religion

This is defined as organ donation directed to a group of recipients determined by the presence or absence of a particular characteristic, such as ethnicity, religion, age, or gender. Most transplant centers emphasize unconditional altruism as the fundamental principle of deceased organ transplantation and do not allow directed deceased donation [8].

8. Attitudes of different religions towards organ transplantation

8.1. Christianity and organ donation

The predominantly Christian countries of Europe and America have higher rates of organ donation [9]. However, there is no conclusive evidence regarding the role of the Christian religion as regards to its influence on the willingness to organ donation. It is the strength of religious belief and the interpretation of individual relationship to God, rather than the teachings of the faith, that will influence the attitudes towards organ donation [10].

Christians believe in eternal life and that nothing that may happen to the body, before or after death, would impair the relationship with God. "In eternity we will neither have nor need our earthly bodies: former things will pass away, all things will be made new" (Revelation 21: 4–5).

The cross (**Figure 1**), a central Christian symbol, is about Jesus giving for the salvation of the world. The Christian faith is based upon the revelation of God in the life of Jesus Christ. John 3:16 says, "God so loved the world that God gave his only son. Jesus sent his twelve disciples out with the imperative to heal disease and illness: "Heal the sick…freely ye have received, freely give" (Matthew 10:8). Healing and saving life is a great gift.

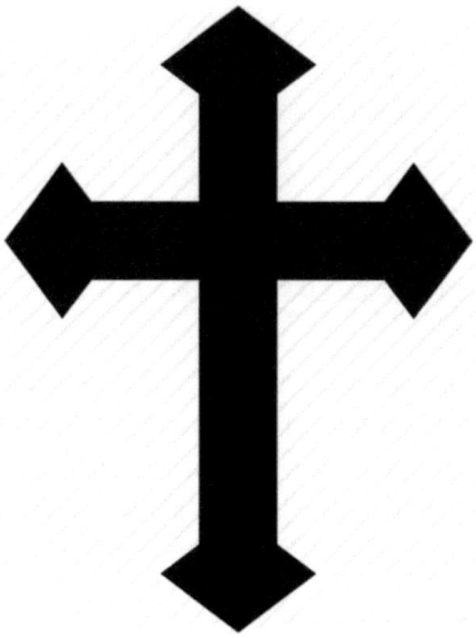

Figure 1. The cross, the central Christian symbol.

On this basis, organ donation to save other lives is considered to be the ultimate humanitarian act, and with this understanding, donating organs for transplantation is acceptable in terms of moral Christian law. On the contrary, organ donation is not morally allowed if the donor or his proxy has not given formal and clear consent. At the same time, it is not acceptable to cause death or mutilation of a human being to delay the death of another person [10].

8.1.1. Catholicism and organ donation

Roman Catholicism is the largest Christian denomination in Europe. Almost half of the European Union population consider themselves Catholic. It has been noticed that countries with a higher proportion of Catholics have higher rates of deceased organ donation [9]. Many Catholics view organ donation as an act of charity and love. In fact, Catholicism is one of many factors that predict willingness to organ donation, and making a causal link between Catholicism and donation is difficult [10].

The Vatican considers both organ donation and transplantation morally acceptable and encourages organ donation [11]. In 1956, Pope Pius XII [12] (**Figure 2**) declared that: "A person may will to dispose his body and destine it to ends that are useful, morally irreproachable and even noble, among them is the desire to aid the sick and suffering…this decision should not be condemned but positively justified." In August 2000, Pope John Paul II (**Figure 3**) told attendees at the International Congress on Transplants in Rome that "Transplants are a great step forward in science" and stated that "the Catholic Church would promote the fact that there is a need for organ donors and that Christians should accept this as a 'challenge to their generosity and fraternal love' so long as ethical principles are followed." Lately, in October 2014, Pope Francis described the act of organ donation as "a testimony of love for our neighbor".

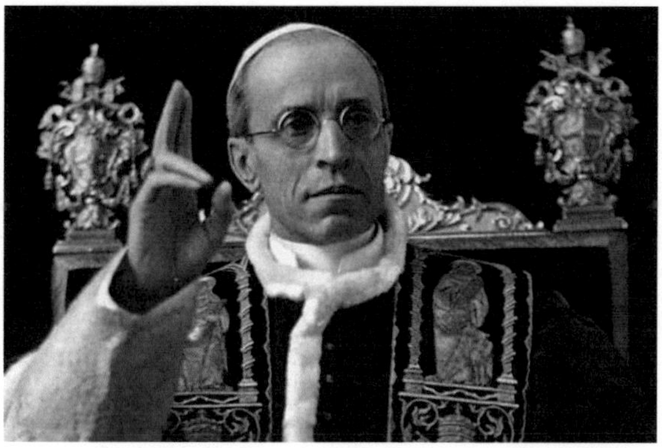

Figure 2. Pope Pius XII.

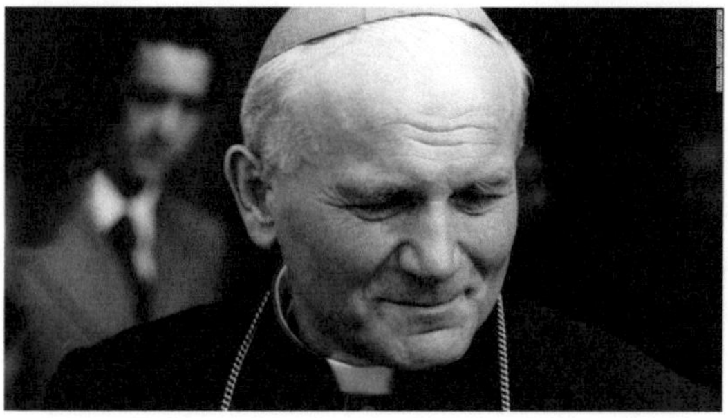

Figure 3. Pope John Paul II.

8.1.2. Orthodox Christian Church

In the Orthodox Church tradition, organ donation could be considered as an act of charity. If the donor is living, the decision to donate an organ should be made in consultation with the spiritual father and the medical professionals. Deceased organ donation is also an act of charity that helps to make possible a sick patient to live a longer and better life. Organ donation is acceptable only if the deceased donor had willed such donation or if the relatives permit. The body of the donor should be treated respectfully. Organ transplantation should never be commercialized nor taken place without clear consent. The death of the donor should never be hastened to recover organs for transplantation [13].

8.1.3. Protestantism

Because of the many different Protestant denominations, a generalized statement on their views regarding organ donation and transplantation cannot be made. The Protestant faith shares a common belief in the New Testament (Luke 6:38: "Give to others and God will give to you.") and respects individual conscience and the right to make decisions regarding the person's own body. It is generally not believed that resurrection requires making the body whole again. Most Protestant Churches encourage the spirit of generosity of organ and tissue donation [14].

Churches, such as African Methodist Episcopal (AME) and African Methodist Episcopal Zion (AME Zion), Assembly of God, Brethren, Christian Church (Disciples of Christ), Church of the Nazarene, Episcopal, Evangelical Covenant Church, Evangelical Lutheran Church in America, Lutheran Missouri Synod, Mormon (Church of Jesus Christ of Latter-day Saints), Presbyterians, Unitarian Universalist, United Church of Christ, and United Methodist Church, are highly supportive of donation. They encourage their members to consider the possibility of organ donation as an act of Christian love. However, the decision to donate is left to each individual [15, 16].

On the contrary, Churches, such as, Unitarian Universalism, Southern Baptist Convention, Society of Friends (Quakers), Pentecostals, Mennonite, Moravians, Christian Science, and Amish, have no official position on organ donation and consider that there are no spiritual or theological beliefs that would prevent an individual from donating. They believe that the decision to donate is up to the individual and/or his or her family [15, 16].

8.1.4. Jehovah's Witnesses

Jehovah's Witnesses are a non-Trinitarian Christian denomination. They are distinct from the mainstream Christianity. The issue of transplantation is compounded by their refusal of blood transfusion. This includes full blood, platelets, and plasma. On the contrary, dialysis, plasma exchange, albumin, clotting factors, and erythropoietin infusions are all allowed [17].

Jehovah's Witnesses are often assumed to oppose organ donation because of their belief against blood transfusion. However, this merely means that all blood must be removed from the organs and tissues before being transplanted (Office of Public Information for Jehovah's Witnesses, October 20, 2005). Some have argued that consent to rescue transfusion should be a prerequisite for transplant listing [18].

Organ transplantation was not allowed for Jehovah's Witnesses until recently. The religious guidance from the 1960s stated that those who submit to human organ transplantation are living off the flesh of other humans. That is cannibalistic. Jehovah God does not grant permission for humans to perpetuate their lives by cannibalistically taking into their bodies' human flesh. This view was only revised in the 1980s, and the decision for or against transplantation is regarded as an individual choice under the assumption that no blood is transfused. Small series of kidney and pancreas transplants in Jehovah's Witnesses have been described. Early postoperative deaths in anemic cases have been reported [19].

8.2. Islam and organ donation

When a Muslim dies, it is a religious requirement that the body is ritually washed and draped and the corpse is buried. Cremation is not allowed in Islam. Washing and shrouding is carried out by respected persons of the same sex as the deceased, who is experienced in the rules of Muslim burial. All clothes are removed and the body is covered. Private parts are covered with a sheet and never exposed during the wash [20]. Muslims are buried in such a way that the face of the deceased faces Mecca. The arms and legs should be straightened and the mouth and eyes are closed. Muslims believe in the Day of Judgment and the afterlife. It is a religious recommendation that an ill person, whether a relative or a stranger, be visited. This is considered a form of worship. It is traditional for Muslims to be buried as quickly as possible. Violating the human body, whether living or dead, is forbidden in Islam [21].

Muslim laws (Shari'ah) are derived from Koran and Hadith (practices and sayings of the prophet Mohammed). Islam recognizes no intermediary between humans and God, such as a clergy. High-ranking Muslim jurists (Ulamas) help Muslims on the interpretation of the Koran and the Hadith. Organ transplantation has not been dealt with in the Koran or the Hadith, and there is a difference of opinion among the Ulamas. The majority of Islamic scholars have concluded that organ donation as treatment for otherwise lethal disease is a good and faithful thing [22].

Islam considers that life is sacred and it must be preserved by all possible means, and one of the basic rules in Islam is the saving of human life. This is a fundamental aim of Islam. Many Muslim scholars consider organ donation as an expression of the believer's altruism, generosity, duty, charity, cooperation, etc. [23].

Although, in Islam, violating the human body, whether living or dead, is greatly forbidden, this prohibition may be waived in the cases of necessity, such as saving a human's life. The fundamental Islamic rule that "necessities permit the prohibited" (al-darurat tubih al-mahzurat) will support donation of both living and deceased human organs by saving a life of another because the benefit outweighs the cost that has to be paid [24].

The following are some verses that have been used to support organ donation:

1. "Whosoever saves the life of one person it would be as if he saved the life of all mankind." Holy Qur'an, chapter 5 vs. 32 (**Figure 4**).

مِنْ أَجْلِ ذَٰلِكَ كَتَبْنَا عَلَىٰ بَنِىٓ إِسْرَٰٓءِيلَ أَنَّهُۥ مَن قَتَلَ نَفْسًۢا
بِغَيْرِ نَفْسٍ أَوْ فَسَادٍ فِى ٱلْأَرْضِ فَكَأَنَّمَا قَتَلَ ٱلنَّاسَ
جَمِيعًا وَمَنْ أَحْيَاهَا فَكَأَنَّمَآ أَحْيَا ٱلنَّاسَ جَمِيعًا ۚ وَلَقَدْ
جَآءَتْهُمْ رُسُلُنَا بِٱلْبَيِّنَٰتِ ثُمَّ إِنَّ كَثِيرًا مِّنْهُم بَعْدَ ذَٰلِكَ فِى
ٱلْأَرْضِ لَمُسْرِفُونَ ﴿٣٢﴾

Figure 4. Holy Qur'an, chapter 5 vs. 32: "Whosoever saves the life of one person it would be as if he saved the life of all mankind."

2. "Whosoever helps another will be granted help from Allah."—Prophet Mohammed (PBUH)

Most of the major academies of the Muslim world support organ transplantation as a means of alleviating pain or saving lives and encourage Muslims to donate organs for transplantation [25]. These include the following:

1. Al-Azhar Academy of Egypt,
2. The Organization of Islamic Conference (representing all Muslim countries).
3. The Grand Ulamas Council of Saudi Arabia, and
4. The Iranian Religious Authority.

In 1952, the supreme head of the Islamic School of Jurisprudence in Egypt stated that if anything was of "good" for mankind, then "necessity allows what is prohibited." Such rulings allow transplants of organs as long as the following conditions are satisfied [24]:

1. This is the only form of treatment available.
2. The likelihood of success of the transplant is high.
3. The consent of the donor is obtained.
4. The death of the donor has been fully confirmed, in the case of deceased donors.
5. There is no imminent danger to the life of the donor, in the case of living donors.
6. The recipient has been informed of the operation and its implications.

The Islamic Jurisprudence Assembly Council in Saudi Arabia approved deceased and live donations in 1988. Similar rulings are in place in, among other countries, Egypt, Iran, and Pakistan [25].

Islam, as all religions, is not monolithic. Some of Muslim scholars are less approving of organ donation. Various reasons are given for the skepticism. These include the following [26]:

1. The thought that the human body is entrusted to man and man is not allowed to interfere with.
2. The human body has a special honor, and violating the human body, whether living or dead, is greatly forbidden. This is supported by the words of the Prophet Mohammed (PBUH): "The breaking of a bone of a dead person is equal in sin to doing this while he was alive."
3. The concept and definition of brain stem death is still controversial.

It is also important to mention that religious concerns play a role even among Muslim physicians.

8.3. Judaism and organ donation

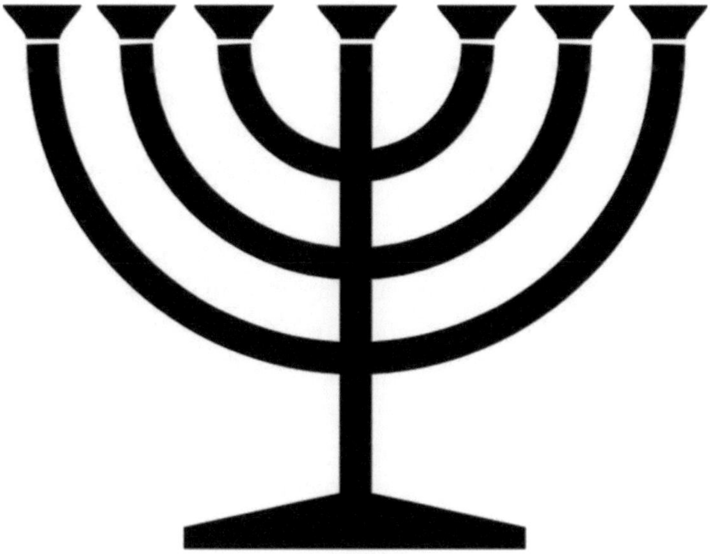

Figure 5. The seven-branched menorah, a traditional symbol of Judaism.

Judaism religion stresses on the honor and respect of the dead (kavod hamet). According to Solomon, the following three Jewish principles should be followed in the treatment of the body after death [27]:

1. Respect and dignity to a cadaver,
2. Not benefiting from a corpse, and
3. Immediate burial.

At the same time, many Jewish scholars disagree to accept the concept of brain death. In fact, Halachic guidance, which is so important in Judaism faith, is not settled to whether the Jewish law considers a person dead or not when the whole brain dies or when the heart stops beating. A Goses, a Halachic term describing a person who is critically ill and likely to die within 3 days, must not be interfered with in order not to hasten death. Therefore, there may be reluctance to medically interfere with a dying patient for the purpose of preparing for organ donation [28].

On the contrary, saving a life is a fundamental value in Judaism (pikuach nefesh). Many Jewish scholars state that the urge to save lives overrides the above-mentioned concerns. In fact, Jewish law mandates that, to save a life, one may violate almost all commandments (except for the prohibitions of murder, idolatry, and illicit sexual relations). This guidance has been used to support the concept organ donation, as it results in saving lives [29].

The Jewish principles of saving a life (pikauch nefesh) and the respect to the dead (kavod hamed), therefore, may come into conflict with one another considering the organ donation [29].

Rabbi Elliott N. Dorff, a professor of Jewish theology at the American Jewish University (formerly the University of Judaism) in California, an author and a bioethicist, wrote: "Saving lives by organ donation could override the rules concerning treatment of a dead body. Transplantation neither desecrates nor disrespects the dead body, and the delay in burial to facilitate organ donation is respectful to the decedent. Organ donation honors the deceased as it would save a life" [30].

At the same time, the Conservative Movement's Committee on Jewish Laws and Standards argued that deceased organ donation for transplantation represents not only an act of generosity but are also a "commanded obligation," which could save a human life. "Do not stand idly by your neighbor's blood" (Leviticus 19:16), which directs we use any resource possible to save a life [29, 30].

Another question is whether or not a kidney transplantation is truly life saving, so long survival on dialysis is possible, and whether corneal transplantation, which is not life saving, is justified. Some Jewish scholars argue that blindness is nearly similar to death, and corneal transplantation is Halachicly acceptable [28].

The important question is whether or not the Jewish law considers someone dead when the whole brain dies or when the heart stops beating. There are scholars on both sides of the question. For this reason, uniquely, the donor card issued by the Halachic Organ Donor Society provides two options, i.e., donation after brain death and/or after cardiac arrest [31].

Disagreements between rabbinic authorities and physicians on the concept of brain death were only settled in 2008, when a new Organ Transplant Law in Israel was approved. However, refusal to the acceptance of brain death remains, and not all rabbinic authorities approve it [30].

8.4. Buddhism

Organ donation rates, in the predominantly Buddhist countries of Southeast Asia particularly in Thailand, Cambodia, Singapore, and Vietnam, are low. Beside the religious barriers, cultural barriers to donation also exist due to a lack of acceptance of brain death [32].

Central to the faith of Buddhism is the idea that all of life is suffering (dukkha). This suffering can be overcome by an eightfold path of virtues. Buddhism considers everything on earth transitory and believes in rebirth. In Buddhism tradition, the time of death is very important and should be treated with great respect. The concept of brain death is doubted, and according to some Buddhism traditions, the spiritual "consciousness" will remain in the body for days after cessation of breathing. The departure of this spirit is the actual moment of death. Until then, the body must remain undisturbed. Disturbance of this process may adversely affect the individual's next rebirth. In other words, the moment of death is defined according to criteria very different from those of modern Western medicine [33].

http://dx.doi.org/10.5772/62401

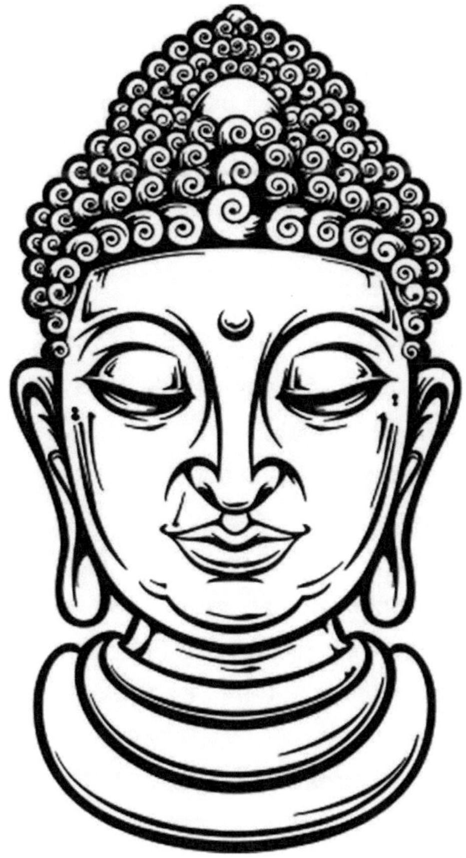

Figure 6. Drawing of Buddha face.

The above-mentioned considerations are in conflict with generosity (dāna) or selfless giving. Dāna is central to Buddhism faith. It entails the wish to relieve suffering; therefore, there may be circumstances where organ donation may be seen as an act of generosity [34]. Buddha (**Figure 6**) said to his monks, when he discovered a sick monk, "Whoever would care for me, let him care for those who are sick" [Mahavagga VIII.26.1-8 (Kucchivikara-vatthu—The Monk with Dysentery, translated from the Pali by Thanissaro Bhikkhu)] [35]. Reverend Gyomay, President and Founder of the Buddhist Temple of Chicago said, "We honor those people who donate their bodies and organs to the advancement of medical science and to saving lives."

Overall, it is probably a mixture of beliefs within the East Asian tradition rather than the true Buddhist beliefs that influence the attitudes towards organ donation and transplantation [33].

8.5. Hinduism

Hinduism is the predominant religion in South Asia with approximately 1 billion followers. Hindus believe in the transmigration of the soul and that the deeds of an individual in the present life will eventually determine its fate in the next life. In the Hindu faith, life is an ongoing process of rebirth after death. The law of Karma determines the way the soul will go in the next life. The Bhagavad Gita, a narrative framework of a dialogue between Pandava prince Arjuna and his guide and charioteer Lord Krishna (**Figure 7**), describes the mortal body and the immortal soul like the relation of clothes to a body: "vasamsi jirnani yatha vihaya navani grhnati naro 'parani tatha sarirani vihaya jirnany anyani samyati navandi dehi.'" "As a person puts on new garments giving up the old ones the soul accepts new material body giving up the old one" (Bhagavad Gita chapter 2:22). The physical integrity of the dead body is not seen as crucial to reincarnation of the soul [36].

KṚISHṆA COMFORTS ARJUNA

(A page from the *Bhagavad-Gîtâ* in Devanâgarî)

॥ श्रीभगवानुवाच ॥
अशोच्यानन्वशोचस्त्वं प्रज्ञावादांश्च भाषसे ।
गतासूनगतासूंश्च नानुशोचन्ति पण्डिताः ॥ ११ ॥
न त्वेवाहं जातु नासं न त्वं नेमे जनाधिपाः ।
न चैव न भविष्यामः सर्वे वयमतः परम् ॥ १२ ॥
देहिनोऽस्मिन्यथा देहे कौमारं यौवनं जरा ।
तथा देहान्तरप्राप्तिर् धीरस्तत्र न मुह्यति ॥ १३ ॥
मात्रास्पर्शास्तु कौन्तेय शीतोष्णसुखदुःखदाः ।
आगमापायिनोऽनित्यास् तांस्तितिक्षस्व भारत ॥ १४ ॥
यं हि न व्यथयन्त्येते पुरुषं पुरुषर्षभ ।
समदुःखसुखं धीरं सोऽमृतत्वाय कल्पते ॥ १५ ॥
नासतो विद्यते भावो नाभावो विद्यते सतः ।
उभयोरपि दृष्टोऽन्तस् त्वनयोस्तत्त्वदर्शिभिः ॥ १६ ॥
अविनाशि तु तद्विद्धि येन सर्वमिदं ततम् ।
विनाशमव्ययस्यास्य न कश्चित्कर्तुमर्हति ॥ १७ ॥
अन्तवन्त इमे देहा नित्यस्योक्ताः शरीरिणः ।
अनाशिनोऽप्रमेयस्य तस्माद्युध्यस्व भारत ॥ १८ ॥
य एनं वेत्ति हन्तारं यश्चैनं मन्यते हतम् ।
उभौ तौ न विजानीतो नायं हन्ति न हन्यते ॥ १९ ॥

Figure 7. A page from Bhagavad Gita: "Those who are faithful do not grieve for the dead or for the living. Neither I, you, nor the princes of the earth shall ever cease to be. Anyone confirmed in this belief will not be disturbed by anything that may come to."

An important tenet of Hinduism is to help those who are suffering. Daan is the original word in Sanskrit for donation meaning selfless giving. Daan ranks third among the list of 10 Niyamas (virtuous acts). Of all the things that are is possible to donate, to donate your own body is infinitely more worthwhile. The important issue for a Hindu is that which sustains life should be accepted and promoted as Dharma (righteous living) [37].

The Hindu faith perhaps represents less of a barrier to donation than cultural factors concerning family approval and death rituals. Hindu religion does not prohibit living or cadaveric donation to alleviate suffering. The use of body parts to benefit others is embedded in Hindi mythology [37]. The best known and widely worshipped deities in the Hindu pantheon is "Ganesha," who is pictured with an elephant head and may represent the earliest depiction of xenotransplantation (**Figure 8**).

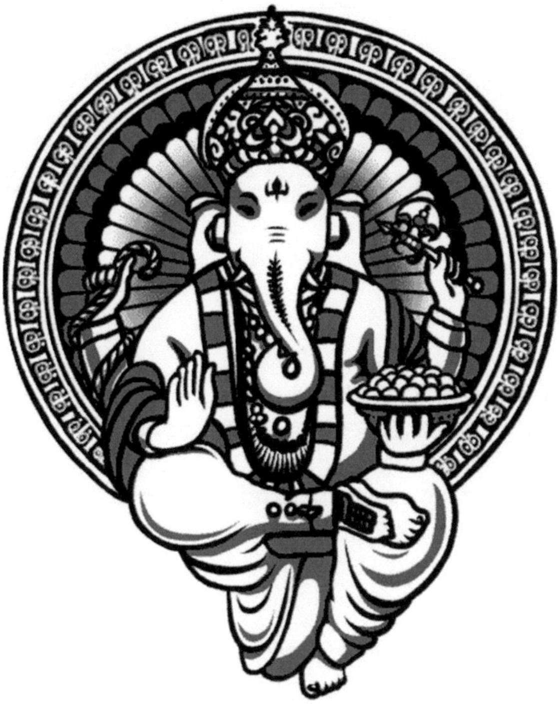

Figure 8. The Hindu God, Ganesha.

8.6. Sikhism

Sikhism is a monotheistic religion. It was founded in 15th century in India by Guru Nanak Dev Ji (1469–1538). The word "Sikh" means learner [19]. There are no ordained priests in Sikhism. Gurdwara (the Sikh temple) (**Figure 9**) is in the care of a granthi (reader) who is appointed by the community. Sikhs think that faith is practiced by coping with life's everyday problems. Sikhism stresses the importance of good deeds. Sikhs believe in life after death and a continuous rebirth. Sikhs are cremated and the physical body is not crucial to the cycle of rebirth. The soul is eternal and the body is just a flesh. Sikhism, as Hinduism, perhaps represents less of a barrier to donation than cultural factors concerning family approval and death rituals [38].

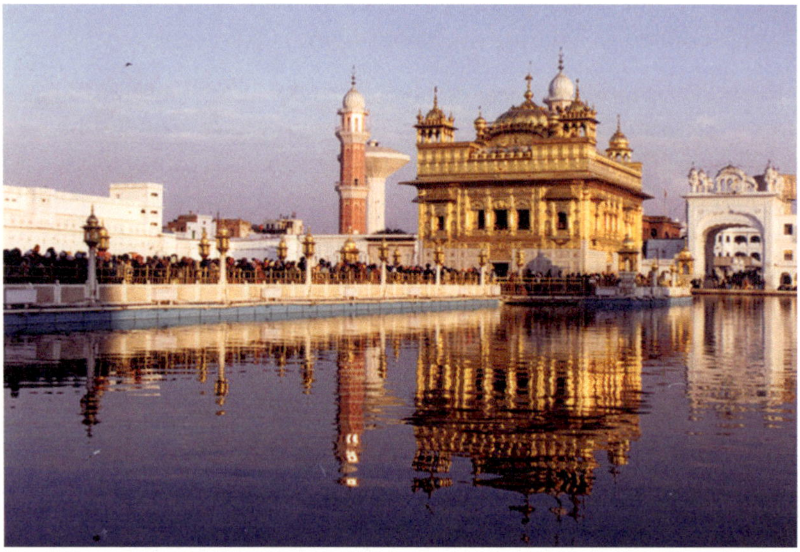

Figure 9. The golden Gurdwara in Amritsar.

8.7. Confucianism

Confucianism is a Chinese philosophical tradition developed from the lessons of the Chinese philosopher Confucius (K◉ng Fūz◉, 551–478 BC) (**Figure 10**). Confucianism is prevalent in the Mainland China, Taiwan, Hong Kong, Singapore, and Korea. The key principle in Confucianism is the Filial piety, which is the basis of Jen (humaneness). Children should be obedient to their parents when young, servant to them when they grow old, bury them after death, and worship them afterwards [39].

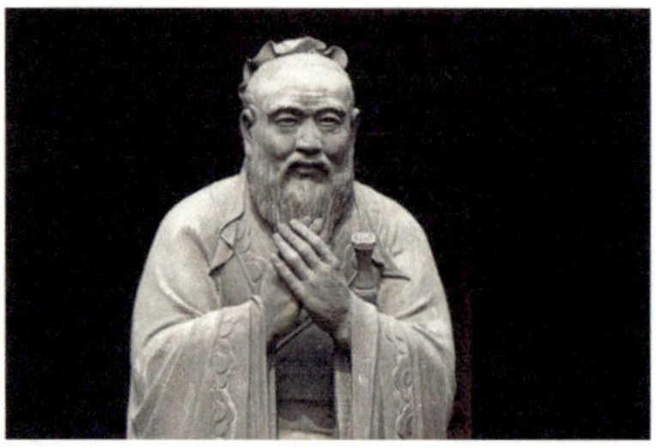

Figure 10. K◉ng Fūz◉.

The Confucian tradition assumes that one is born with a complete body and should end the same way as a form of filial piety. The body, hair, and skin are gifts from the parents and should not be damaged. This view will dictate that organ donation and transplantation are unfilial and disrespectful of parents. Therefore, Confucian beliefs could be considered as obstacles to organ donation [40].

Modern Confucian scholars have a different explanation. They stress on the words of Confucius who said, "The man of Jen is one who, desires to sustain himself, should sustain others". They view that Jen and righteousness are more valued than preserving the integrity of the dead body and therefore approve donation for organ transplantation [41].

8.8. Shintoism

Shinto is the predominant faith in Japan (**Figure 11**). There is debate as to whether Shintoism can be classed as a religion. Shintoism is very much concerned with the idea of purity. Shinto believe that humans are born pure while that living make their bodies impure. The body after death is thus impure and hazardous, and interfering with dead body brings bad luck and might injure the relationship between the theitai (the bereaved person) and the dead person. In view of this belief, the concept of brain death does not go with the Shintoism view of death [42].

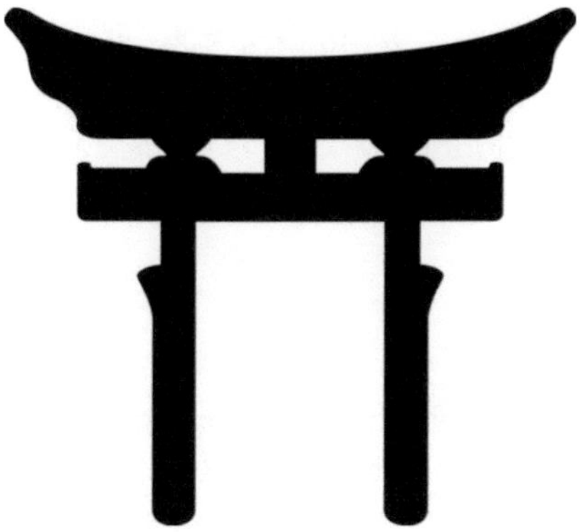

Figure 11. Tori, a traditional Japanese gate at the Shinto shrine, symbolically marks the transition from the profane to the sacred.

Until 1997, legislations in Japan used to forbid deceased donation. In 1997, the law has been changed to allow transplantation from deceased donors. However, deceased donation is still not often carried out in Japan and the percentage of Japanese who have an organ donor card is among the lowest in the world [43].

8.9. Taoism

Taoism embraces a variety of philosophical traditions and religious beliefs in Eastern Asia. Tao roughly translates as "path" (of life). This faith dates since more than 2000 years. The Taoist philosophy emphasizes naturalness, non-action (wu-wei), and peace. Wu-wei dictates not taking action against the path of nature. Organ donation may be viewed according to this tradition as an attempt to change the natural process. Modern Taoist scholars have indicated that the body itself is only a shelter to the soul and attempts to change the body cannot truly affect the nature of life and approved organ donation for transplantation. They also cite Laotze when he stated that "Let what is superfluous to fill what is insufficient" [44] (**Figure 12**).

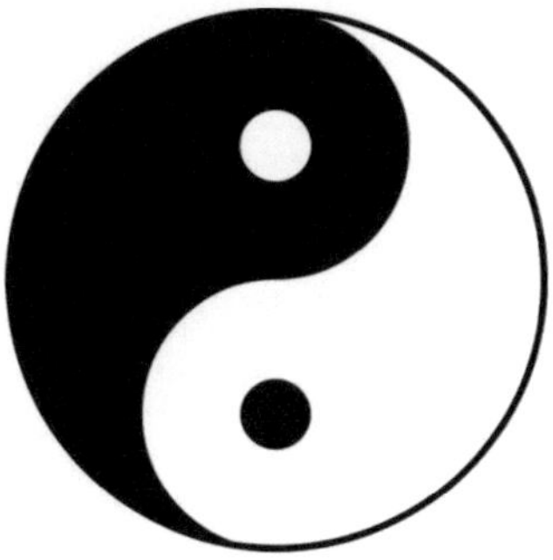

Figure 12. Ying Yang, a Taoism symbol representing a visual depiction of the intertwined duality of all things in nature.

8.10. Gypsies

Gypsies have different ethnic groups without a formalized religion. They share common beliefs and tend to oppose organ donation and transplantation. This may be related to their beliefs about the afterlife. Their traditional belief is that for 1 year after death the soul retraces its steps. Therefore, the body should remain intact so as the soul can maintain its physical shape.

8.11. Bahá'í Faith

There is no opposition in the Bahá'í Faith against organ donation. It is an issue that is left to the person's choice (Office of Public Information, Bahá'í International Community, November 10, 2005). The Bahá'í Faith assumes that organ donation is a noble act and insists on treating the donor's body respectfully and burying the remains within 1 hour of travel time (from the hospital to the funeral place) [45].

9. Conclusions

The interplay of faith, religion, and wider cultural attitudes and their relationship with views on organ donation is so complex. Engaging faith leaders and providing them accurate, clear, and detailed information about the concepts of brain death, organ donation, and transplantation is of great importance.

Acknowledgements

Most of contents of this chapter could be viewed as a form of common knowledge. However, the authors acknowledge that it, expands the information originally presented in the article presented by. Oliver M, Woywodt A, Ahmed A, Saif I. Organ donation, transplantation and religion. Nephrology Dialysis Transplantation. 2011;26(2):437–444. DOI: 10.1093/ndt/gfq628.

Author details

Hesham Abdeldayem[1*], Ahmed Farag El-Kased[2], Ahmed Elshaarawy[1],
Essam Salah Hammad[1], OmKolsoum Al-Haddad[1], Gihan Sobhi[1] and Naglaa Allam[1]

*Address all correspondence to: habdeldayem64@hotmail.com

1 National Liver Institute, Menoufia University, Al Minufya, Egypt

2 Faculty of Medicine, Menoufia University, Al Minufya, Egypt

References

[1] Feehally J. Ethnicity and renal replacement therapy. Blood Purif 2010; 29: 125–129.

[2] Rithalia A, McDaid C, Suekarran S, et al. Impact of presumed consent for organ donation on donation rates: a systematic review. BMJ 2009; 338: a3162.

[3] Bruzzone P. Religious aspects of organ transplantation. Transplant Proc 2008; 40: 1064–1067.

[4] Mueller PS, Case EJ, Hook CC. Responding to offers of altruistic living unrelated kidney donation by group associations: an ethical analysis. Transplant Rev (Orlando) 2008; 22: 200–205.

[5] Black J. Broaden your mind about death and bereavement in certain ethnic groups in Britain. Br Med J (Clin Res Ed) 1987; 295: 536–539.

[6] Daar AS. The body, the soul and organ donation beliefs of the major world religions. Nefrologia 1994; 14: 78–81.

[7] Truog RD. The ethics of organ donation by living donors. N Engl J Med 2005; 353: 444–446.

[8] Park L, Moon JI, Kim SI, et al. Exchange donor program in kidney transplantation. Transplantation 1999; 67: 336.

[9] Sprung CL, Maia P, Bulow HH, et al. The importance of religious affiliation and culture on end-of-life decisions in European intensive care units. Intensive Care Med 2007; 33: 1732–1739.

[10] van Gelder F, Manyalich M, Costa AN, et al. 2009 International Donation and Transplantation Activity IRODaT Preliminary Data. Cells Tissues Organs 2010; 13: 5–8.

[11] Owen R. Pope Benedict carries organ donor card as 'an act of love'. Times; 2008. Available at: http://www.timesonline.co.uk/tol/comment/faith/article4673438.ece.

[12] Pius XII: Address to a group of eye specialists, May 14, 1956. In the Monks of Johannes Paulus II. Evangelium Vitae; 1995. Available at: http://www.vatican.va/edocs/ENG0141/_INDEX.HTM.

[13] Bogdanovsky A. Press release regarding the head of the Greek Orthodox Church. Novosti Press; 2005.

[14] A Christian view of life and death: joint declaration by the German Conference of Catholic Bishops and the Council of the Protestant Church in Germany; 1990. Available at: http://www.dober.de/ethik-organspende/religionen.html#gem.

[15] Organ donation a Christian duty. Church of England; 2007. Available at: http://www.cofe.anglican.org/news/pr9607.html.

[16] Mason JO. Attitudes of the Church of Jesus Christ of Latter-day Saints Toward Certain Medical Problems. Salt Lake City: The Church of Jesus Christ of Latter-Day Saints; 1974.

[17] Rogers DM, Crookston KP. The approach to the patient who refuses blood transfusion. Transfusion 2006; 46: 1471–1477.

[18] Bramstedt KA. Transfusion contracts for Jehovah's Witnesses receiving organ transplants: ethical necessity or coercive pact? J Med Ethics 2006; 32: 193–195.

[19] Oliver M, Woywodt A, Ahmed A, Saif I. Organ donation, transplantation and religion. Nephrology Dialysis Transplantation. 2011;26(2):437–444. DOI: 10.1093/ndt/gfq628.

[20] Gatrad AR. Muslim customs surrounding death, bereavement, postmortem examinations, and organ transplants. BMJ 1994; 309: 521–523.

[21] Topbas M, Can G, Can MA, et al. Outmoded attitudes toward organ donation among Turkish health care professionals. Transplant Proc 2005; 37: 1998–2000.

[22] Alkhawari FS, Stimson GV, WarrensAN. Attitudes toward transplantation in U.K. Muslim Indo-Asians in west London. Am J Transplant 2005; 5: 1326–1331.

[23] Hassaballah AM. Definition of death, organ donation and interruption of treatment in Islam. Nephrol Dial Transplant 1996; 11: 964–965.

[24] Golmakani MM, Niknam MH, Hedayat KM. Transplantation ethics from the Islamic point of view. Med Sci Monit 2005; 11: 105–109.

[25] Rady MY, Verheijde JL. Islam and end-of-life organ donation. Asking the right questions. Saudi Med J 2009; 30: 882–886.

[26] Najafizadeh K, Ghorbani F, Hamidinia S, et al. Holy month of Ramadan and increase in organ donation willingness. Saudi J Kidney Dis Transpl 2010; 21: 443–446.

[27] Organ donation and Halacha (brochure): The Halachic Organ Donor Society. Available at: http://www.hods.org.

[28] CardsHaredim Issue Anti-Organ-Donor. Haaretz; 2008. Available at: http://www.haaretz.com/jewish/news/haredim-issue-anti-organ-donor-cards-1.251280.

[29] Jotkowitz A. Notes on the new Israeli organ donation law-2008. Transplant Proc 2008; 40: 3297–3298.

[30] MahlerK, BresnahanMJ. Ethical debate over organ donation in the context of brain death. Bioethics 2010; 24: 54–60.

[31] Ashkenazi T, Berman M, Ben Ami S, et al. A bridge between hearts: mutual organ donation by Arabs and Jews in Israel. Transplantation 2004; 77: 151–155.

[32] Teo B. Organs for transplantation: the Singapore experience. Hastings Centre Report 1991; 21: 10–13.

[33] Sugunasiri SH. The Buddhist view concerning the dead body. Transplant Proc 1990; 22: 947–949.

[34] Keon D. Buddhism, brain death, and organ transplantation. JBE 2010; 17: 1–36.

[35] Hardacre H. Response of Buddhism and Shinto to the issue of brain death and organ transplant. Camb Q Healthc Ethics 1994; 3: 585–601.

[36] PrabhupādāACBS. Bhagavad-gītā as It Is: With the Original Sanskrit Text, Roman Transliteration, English Equivalents, Translation and Elaborate Purports. Los Angeles: Bhaktivedanta Book Trust; 1986.

[37] NHS Blood and Transplant: Hindu Dharma and Organ Donation. Available at: http://www.organdonation.nhs.uk/ukt/how_to_become_a_donor/religious_perspectives/leaflets/hindu_dharma_and_organ_donation.jsp.

[38] Exley C, Sim J, Reid N, et al. Attitudes and beliefs within the Sikh community regarding organ donation: a pilot study. Soc Sci Med 1996; 43: 23–28.

[39] Chung CK, Ng CW, Li JY, et al. Attitudes, knowledge, and actions with regard to organ donation among Hong Kong medical students. Hong Kong Med J 2008; 14: 278–285.

[40] Kim JR, Elliott D, Hyde C. The influence of sociocultural factors on organ donation and transplantation in Korea: findings from key informant interviews. J Transcult Nurs 2004; 15: 147–154.

[41] Lam WA, McCullough LB. Influence of religious and spiritual values on the willingness of Chinese-Americans to donate organs for transplantation. Clin Transplant 2000; 14: 449–456.

[42] Namihira E. Shinto concept concerning the dead human body [Japanese]. Transplant Proc 1990; 22: 940–941

[43] DataDeceased Donation 2010. Japan Organ Transplant Network; 2010. Available at: http://www.jotnw.or.jp/english/data.html.

[44] Tai MC. An Asian perspective on organ transplantation. Wien Med Wochenschr 2009; 159: 452–456.

[45] Randhawa G, Brocklehurst A, Pateman R, et al. Faith leaders united in their support for organ donation: findings from the UK Organ Donation Taskforce study. Transpl Int 2010; 23: 140–146.

Section 2

Basic Issues

Chapter 2

Embryonic Organ Transplantation: The New Era of Xenotransplantation

Ximo García-Domínguez, Cesar D. Vera-Donoso, Luís García-Valero, Jose S. Vicente and Francisco Marco-Jimenez

Additional information is available at the end of the chapter

http://dx.doi.org/10.5772/62400

Abstract

Here, we review the recent advances towards the use of organs from embryonic donors, antecedent investigations, and the latest work from our own laboratory exploring the utility for transplantation of embryonic kidney as an organ replacement therapy. In addition, we have recently reported, for the first time, that it is possible to create a long-term biobank of kidney precursors as an unlimited source of organs for xenotransplantation, facilitating inventory control and the distribution of organs.

Kidney transplantation from deceased or living human donors has been limited by donor availability as opposed to the increasing demand. Simultaneously, the risk of loss of graft by rejection or toxicity of immunosuppressive therapy exacerbates this organ shortage. In recent years, xenotransplantation of developing pancreas and kidney precursor cells has offered a novel solution for the unlimited supply of human donor organs. Specifically, transplantation of kidney precursors in adult hosts showed that intact embryonic kidneys underwent maturation, exhibiting functional properties, and averted humoral rejection post-transplantation from non-immunosuppressed hosts.

Organ primordia engraft, attract a host vasculature, and differentiate following transplantation to ectopic sites. Attempts have been made to exploit these characteristics to achieve clinically relevant endpoints for end-stage renal disease using animal models. We focused on two main points: (a) performing transplantation by a minimally invasive laparoscopic procedure and (b) creating a long-term biobank of kidney precursors, as an unlimited source of organs for transplantation, facilitating the inventory control and the distribution of organs. Because even if supply and demand could be balanced using xenotransplants or laboratory-grown organs from regenerative medicine, the future of these treatments would still be compromised by the ability to physically distribute the organs to patients in need and to produce these products in a way that allows adequate inventory control and quality assurance.

Keywords: chronic renal failure, cryopreservation, laparoscopy, organogenesis, organ primordia, vitrification, xenotransplantation

1. Introduction

The functional failure of an organ has several origins, from malignancies to degenerative diseases. These latter ailments are non-infectious disorders characterised by progressive disability. Nowadays, more and more patients are suffering from degenerative processes that end in specific irreversible organ failure. Loss of function becomes irreversible once injury exceeds the inherent regenerative potential or redundancy of the affected organ system; in many instances, therapeutic options are limited to supportive measures and prevention of further damage [1]. Although substantial progress has been made in the minimisation of irreversible tissue loss in the acute phase of many disease processes, the restoration of lost tissue and organ function after critical damage has occurred has been less successful. In these cases, transplantation represents the ideal method of restoring full physiological organ function [2]. However, transplantation from deceased or living human donors has been limited by donor availability, as opposed to the increasing demand, by the risks of allograft loss rejection and immunosuppressive therapy toxicity [2,3]. These factors mean that many patients have to wait for long periods of time, entailing increased morbidity and mortality for tens of thousands of people each year [4], and a lot of patients die before receiving the desired organ. As proof, it is interesting to recall that, in April 2014 in the United States, approximately 122,000 patients were waiting for an organ transplant, but, a year later, less than 30,000 of them had received it [5].

Currently, in the field of urology, the prevalence of chronic renal failure continues to outpace the development of effective treatment strategies. In the European Union, in late 2011, more than 42,000 patients were on waiting lists for kidney transplant [6]. During this year, 18,712 transplants were performed, of which 20.6% came from living donors. This means that patients with advanced renal disease are habitually obliged to resort to renal replacement therapies, such as haemodialysis or peritoneal dialysis. However, these techniques fail to meet the functional endocrine and reabsorption demands of normal kidney function [2], also affecting the quality of patient's life [7]. In the United States, approximately 100,000 individuals are waiting for a kidney transplant and more than 400,000 individuals are suffering some kind of end-stage kidney disease requiring haemodialysis [8,9]. Nevertheless, the issue is even more severe than in the United States, being a universal problem affecting approximately 5–7% of the world population [10]. Two decades ago in Spain, a leading country in the field of transplants, approximately 4400 patients were on the waiting list for kidney transplantation [11]. Today, approximately 129 (incidence) and 1039 (prevalence) patients per million habitants still require renal replacement therapies [12]. The therapeutic alternatives to transplant (haemodialysis or peritoneal dialysis) represent a cost of €1518 million to the country's public services. Whereas this is a problem in Spain, the issue is much more serious in other countries, such as the United Kingdom, where organ donation rates are lower and the costs of renal replacement therapies amounted to £1.2 billion [13,14]. Therefore, seeking alternative solutions to this grave problem is indispensable.

2. Transplantation of embryonic organs as a novel solution to organ shortage

Even before obtaining an allogeneic organ, despite advances in renal transplant immunology, 20% of recipients will experience an episode of acute rejection within 5 years of transplantation, and approximately 40% of recipients will die or lose graft function within 10 years after transplantation [9]. Thus, the risk of graft rejection is still an obstacle in the field of kidney transplantation. Similarly, the use of xenotransplants has been considered for years as a possible solution to the organ shortage, but the risks of xenograft loss rejection and zoonosis have limited the clinical application of this kind of treatment [15,16]. The use of individual cells or groups of cells to repair damaged tissue (cellular therapies) offers an alternative for renal tissue replacement. However, the recapitulation of complex functions, such as glomerular filtration and reabsorption and secretion of solutes that are dependent on a three-dimensionally integrated kidney structure, is beyond the scope of most cellular replacement therapies [17].

The field of renal transplantation is exploring new frontiers. Recently, following this line, and together with the production of specific pathogen-free animals [18], xenotransplantation of developing kidney precursors has provided a novel solution for these troubles [17,19]. Unlike embryonic stem (ES) cells or induced pluripotent stem cells, developing metanephric kidney

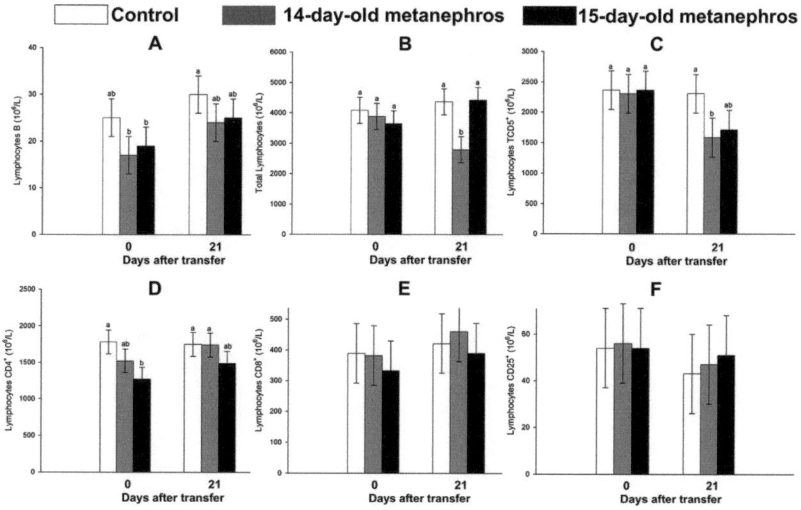

Figure 1. Effect of foetus metanephroi transplanted into 14- and 15-day-old rabbit on peripheral blood. (A) Total lymphocytes, (B) B lymphocytes (C), and T lymphocytes CD5⁺ (×10⁶/l), (D) CD4⁺ (×10⁶/l), (E) CD8⁺ (×10⁶/l), and (F) CD25⁺ cells (×10⁶/l) after 21 days in non-immunocompromised recipients. a,b significant differences ($P<0.05$).

cells are already committed to a genetic program of renal development and "knowing" its destination cell type and how it should be assembled [3], obviating the need to pre-program cell fate. Otherwise, transplantation of kidney precursors in adult hosts showed that intact embryonic kidneys underwent maturation, exhibiting functional properties and avoiding rejection from non-immunosuppressed hosts [17]. This happens because, in a developing kidney, antigen-presenting cells, which mediate direct host recognition of strange antigen, are absent because they would not have yet developed in the donor and migrated into the metanephroi [20,21]. Furthermore, metanephroi express fewer MHC class I and II antigens, which mediate host recognition, than the adult kidney [22,23] (**Figure 1**). In addition, the immunological response mediated by T helper lymphocytes is skewed when responding to a foetal organ compared to an adult organ [24].

Moreover, it is important to recall that metanephroi trigger the formation of a vascular system directly from the host [25,26], attenuating rejection and encouraging their transplantation across the species barrier [19,26–28]. Additionally, renal primordials do not require immediate vascular anastomosis upon transplantation, as is the case in a vascularised organ [29]. Finally, into the bargain, the use of animal cells avoids ethical barriers to human ES cell use [3]. Therefore, the results achieved with embryonic organs (**Figure 2**) have returned the use of xenotransplantation as a possible solution to the shortage of vital organs, such as the kidney, to the front line of research [30].

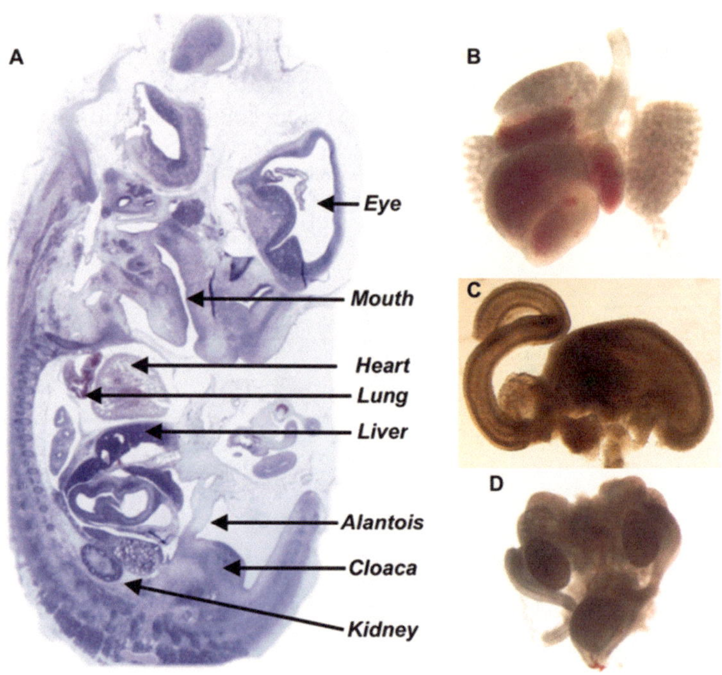

Figure 2. Histology of 15-day-old rabbit foetus and recovery organs. (A) Foetus. (B) Lung and heart. (C) Stomach and intestines. (D) Gonads and cloaca.

3. Experiences in embryonic organ transplantation

A major advantage inherent in the use of embryonic kidney or pancreas (**Figure 3**) for transplantation relative to more pluripotent undifferentiated cells is that the former differentiate spontaneously along defined organ-committed lines, albeit with a different outcome relative to what would occur if the primordia remained undisturbed within the embryo [31].

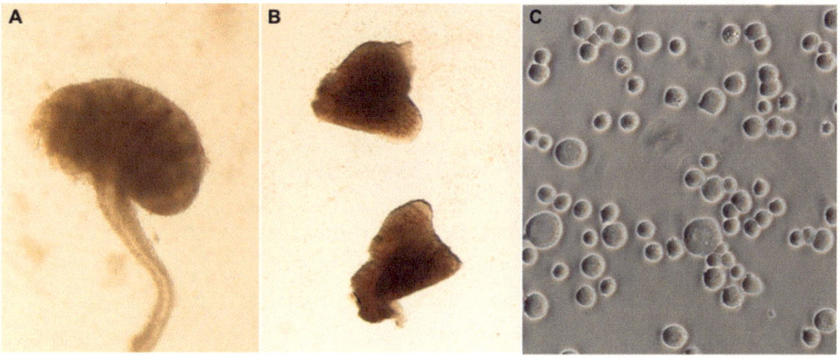

Figure 3. Detail of rabbit 15-day-old metanephros (A) and pancreas (B) and stem cells (C).

At present, experiences in this area revolve around the endocrine pancreas and kidney, the latter organ being the theme that will be the focus of this work. However, it is interesting to mention the major advances that have been achieved with embryonic pancreas to emphasise the potential of embryonic organ transplantation as a possible solution to solve many of today's diseases. Thus, it was reported that, when embryonic pancreas was transplanted through the species barrier (xenotransplantation), a selective development of endocrine tissue took place [32–38]. These developing β cells enter lymphatic vessels and engraft in mesenteric lymph nodes, secreting insulin in response to elevated blood glucose. Consequently, glucose intolerance can be corrected in formerly diabetic rats [32–35,37] and ameliorated in rhesus macaques [36,38] based on porcine insulin secreted in a glucose-dependent manner by β cells originating from transplants [31]. Furthermore, if embryonic pancreas were obtained in a specific time window of the embryonic development, these primordia were able to engraft in diabetic rats [32–35,37] and rhesus macaques [36,38] without immunosuppression treatment. However, although the results obtained in this field are promising, it is still too soon to predict the future of this line. This is because the experiences show that, depending on which xenogeneic barrier is crossed, the results will be different [31]: rat-to-mouse transplantation results in the formation of the new organ and requires host immunosuppression, whereas pig-to-rat or pig-to-rhesus macaque transplantation results in lymphatic dissemination of β cells and no immunosuppression is required. Therefore, further studies are required to clarify the matter and its therapeutic potential.

In the case of renal primordia, since Woolf et al. [39] reported a study of embryonic kidney tissue transplantation in 1990, several groups have investigated embryonic kidney transplantation, with surprising results [19,27,39–47] (**Figure 4**).

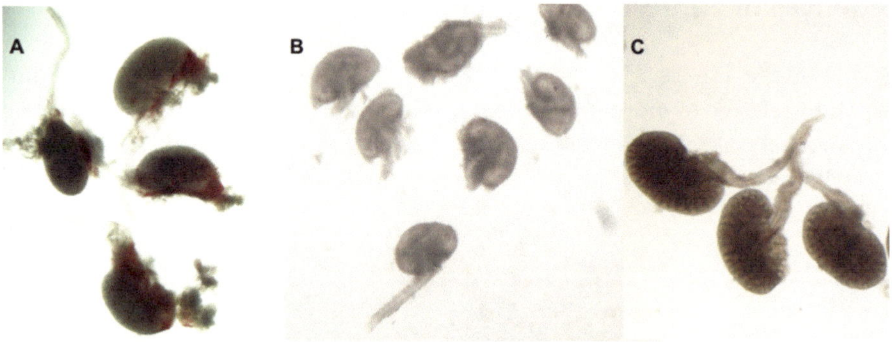

Figure 4. Image of metanephroi in different species. (A) Details of porcine 28-day-old metanephroi. (B) Details of rabbit 15-day-old metanephris. (C) Details of mouse 13.5-day-old metanephroi.

Woolf et al. [39] reported that mouse metanephroi continued to grow if transplanted into the renal cortex of a host mouse [39]. In this study, developed metanephroi showing vascularised glomeruli, mature proximal tubules, and extensions of metanephric tubules into the renal medulla were observed. This is a sufficiently encouraging result, which boosted research in this line. Later, Rogers et al. [27] reported in rats the first long-term survival (>10 days) after subcapsular transplantation of metanephroi into fully differentiated kidneys of animals in which nephron formation is no longer taking place as well as the first intraomental transplantation of metanephroi. Glomerular filtration in developed metanephroi transplanted was demonstrated both subcapsularily [39] and in the omentum [27]. Rogers et al. [40] demonstrated that pig metanephroi transplanted into pigs underwent growth and differentiation of nephrons over a 2-week period without the need for co-stimulatory blockade of hosts. Furthermore, pig metanephroi after 2 weeks of transplantation had enlarged, become vascularised, and formed mature tubules and glomeruli in host mice with the use of immunosuppressants. In the same year, Dekel et al. [19] transplanted metanephroi of both human and pig origins into mice, which differentiated into functional nephrons and their renal functionality, as evidenced by the dilute urine they produced. One year later, it was reported that the survival of rats with all native renal mass removed can be increased by prior metanephroi transplantation and ureteroureterostomy [41]. A couple of years later, Takeda et al. [42] confirmed experimentally that the predominant origin of endothelial cells after transplantation of embryonic pig metanephroi into rats is the host, whereas mesangial cells originate mainly from the donor. Recently, in 2012, the Hosoya et al. [43] group reported that transplantation of metanephroi produces plasma renin activity and contributes to raising arterial blood pressure in a rat model of acute hypotension and suppresses the progression of vascular calcification in rats with adenine-induced renal failure by significantly reducing vascular calcium and phosphorus content [44]. Thus, developed metanephroi in new renal tissue not only provide an excretion function but also an endocrine function, synthesising renal hormones such as renin and erythropoietin [43,45] Interestingly, it is known that xenotransplanted embryonic kidney also provides a niche for endogenous mesenchymal stem cell differentiation into erythropoietin-producing tissue [46]. Furthermore, using metanephroi from transgenic ER-E2F1 suicide-inducible mice, the xenotissue component could be eliminated, leaving autologous EPO-producing tissue. These findings may alleviate adverse effects due to long-lasting immunosuppression and help mitigate ethical concerns [46]. One of the most important obstacles in this field of renal primordia transplantation is that, due to the growth and functionality of the nascent kidney, it ultimately developed hydronephrosis and did not grow in size because it lacked a urine excretion channel [47]. However, through the method described by Yokote et al. [47], it is possible to avoid this end. If metanephroi were transplanted beside bladders (developed from cloacas), the tubular lumina dilatation and interstitial fibrosis were reduced in comparison to single metanephroi transplant. In addition, if cloacal-developed bladder was connected to the host ureters, it avoided hydronephrosis and permitted the cloacas to differentiate well, producing and excreting urine through the recipient ureter and allowing the metanephroi to continue their growth (**Figure 5**).

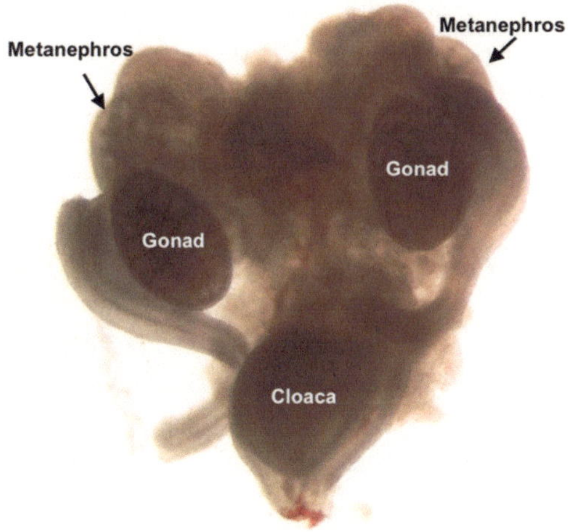

Figure 5. Detail of cloaca structure. (A) Cloaca-gonads-metanephroi.

4. Metanephroi transplant surgery and graft site

Initial studies have been performed using the renal subcapsular space and omentum, neither being an immunologically privileged site [48]. However, because the vasculature of the transplant is of host origin and the embryonic organ per se is less immunogenic [24], intense immunomodulation should not be required. Nonetheless, the influence of the insertion site of the kidney is not indifferent. Matsumoto et al. [45] reported that, when metanephroi were transplanted into the paraaortic area, where the developing kidney is exposed to hydrostatic pressure from the aorta, and in the omentum, where there is no hydrostatic pressure, renin production was greater in the metanephroi transplanted to the paraaortic area, although there were no site-specific differences in erythropoietin production. This result therefore suggests that renin production in our systems requires induction by vascular tension stimulus, whereas erythropoietin production can be achieved by transplanting tissue into the omentum, where it is easily accessed by endoscopy.

Nevertheless, although to date metanephroi have been transplanted into different sites, such as the anterior eye chamber [49], intrarenally [27,39,49–51], intra-abdominally [52], or intraomentally [27,53], all these experiments were performed through open surgery. To our best knowledge, our recent study [54] was the only experiment to tackle embryonic kidney transplantation through laparoscopic surgery.

5. Laparoscopic surgery for metanephroi transplantation

Taking into account all the information reported by some of the authors just mentioned, we have learnt that omentum is used mainly because it is not confined by a tight capsule, facilitating the growth of transplanted metanephroi [27,53] and the transplantation technique [45]. Until now, laparotomy was the sole method used to transfer metanephroi into recipients. In 2014, we developed a new minimally invasive laparoscopic procedure to transfer metanephroi into the retroperitoneal fat [54]. In addition, this new study was first conducted in rabbit as animal model, where our experience shows that size does play a crucial role. Choosing a healthy large animal more than 3–3.5 kg provides an experimental subject with a good capacity for the laparoscopic approach (**Figure 6**).

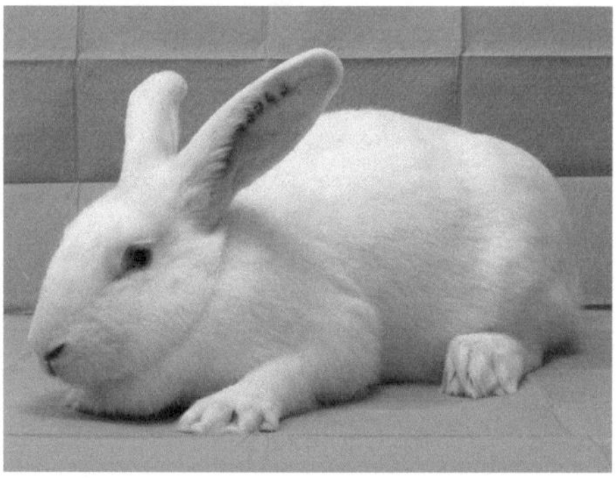

Figure 6. New Zealand rabbit.

The rabbit (*Oryctolagus cuniculus*) is the third mammal most used as experimental animal in Europe after the mouse (59%) and the rat (17%) [56]. Moreover, the rabbit is phylogenetically closer to primates than rodents are [57], and disease aetiologies exhibited by humans are more similar to those in rabbits than in mice [58]. This animal is very docile and non-aggressive and hence easy to handle and observe. Widely bred and very economical compared to the expense of larger animals, rabbits also have short life cycles (gestation, lactation, and puberty). Taking these reasons into account, we consider that the rabbit is an excellent animal model for the first steps in this field. Nevertheless, we do not lose sight of the fact that further development of the art, in higher species more similar anatomically and physiologically to the human species in an attempt to finally reach clinical use, is crucial.

The effectiveness of the minimally invasive laparoscopic procedure was recently reviewed [6,54]. Briefly, recipient animals were sedated by intramuscular injection of xylazine (5 mg/kg) and morphine chloride (3 mg/kg). As surgical preparation, anaesthesia was performed by intravenous injection of ketamine hydrochloride (35 mg/kg) into the marginal ear vein (**Figure 7**).

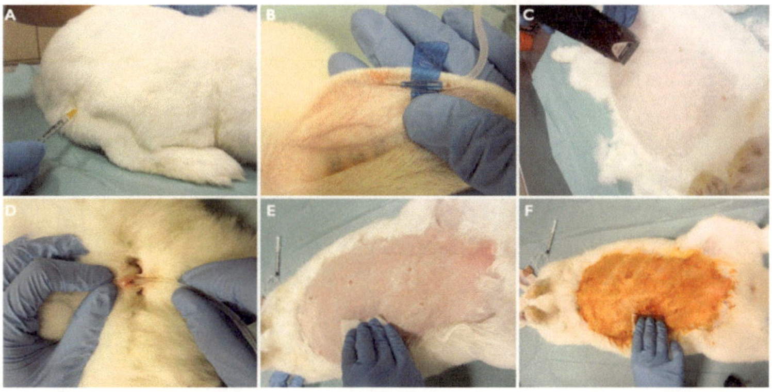

Figure 7. Receptor preparation. (A) Sedation. (B) Anaesthesia by intravenous injection into the marginal ear vein. (C) Skin. (D) Evacuating the bladder using a urinary catheter. (E) Cleaning surgical area. (F) Disinfection of the surgical area.

First, animals were placed in the stretcher in a vertical position (head down at 45° angle). Only one endoscope trocar was inserted into the abdominal cavity (**Figure 8**).

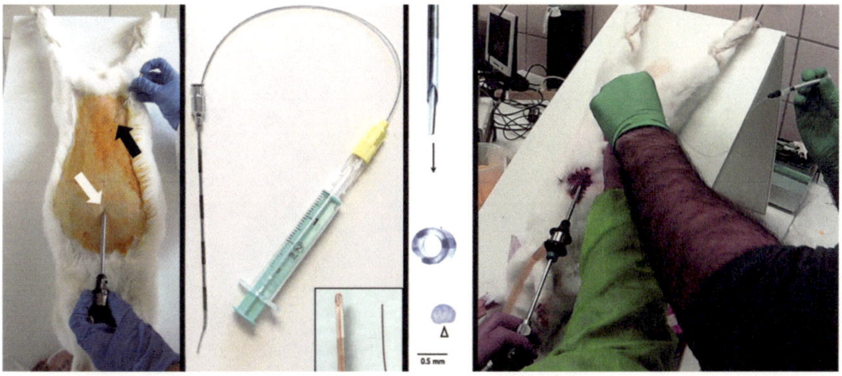

Figure 8. Laparoscopy procedure for metanephros transfers. (A) Allocation of the animal on the surgical table, trocar endoscope insertion position (white arrow) and epidural needle (black arrow). (B) Epidural needle (Perifix® 17 Ga × 4 in. (100 mm) and epidural catheter (17G, Vygon Corporate). (C) Epidural catheter, needle, and metanephros (white arrow). (D) Introduction of the catheter through the needle with the metanephros.

Then, a 17G epidural needle was inserted into the inguinal region (**Figure 9**). After identifying a vessel in the retroperitoneal fat, a hole was performed adjacent to the vessel (**Figure 9**). Then, kidney precursor was aspirated into an epidural catheter and the catheter was introduced through the epidural needle and inserted into the performed hole (**Figure 9**). Four kidney precursors were transplanted in each host without immunosuppression (one metanephros per hole). After surgery, analgesia was administered every 12 h for 3 days [6,54].

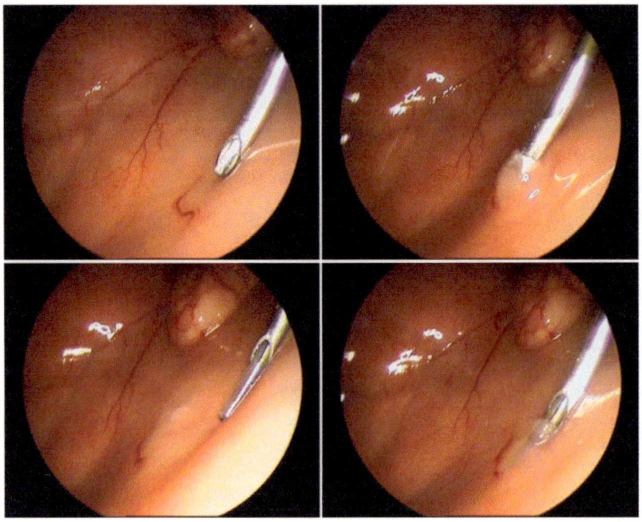

Figure 9. Laparoscopy procedure for metanephroi transfers. (A) Epidural needle. (B) Performing a hole into the retroperitoneal fat where the metanephros will be transferred. (C) Introduction of the catheter through the needle with the metanephros. (D) Insertion of the catheter with the metanephros into the hole and transfer.

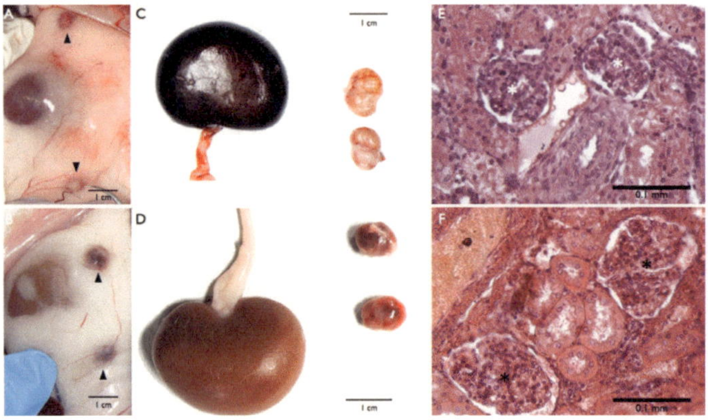

Figure 10. Successful development of new kidneys after allotransplantation of metanephroi. (A) Macroscopic view of kidney precursor 3 weeks after transplantation. Note massive growth and the blood vessels of a new kidney. Black arrowheads indicate the new kidneys. White asterisk indicates the host kidney. (B) Macroscopic view of a vitrified kidney precursor 3 weeks after transplantation. Black arrowhead indicates the new kidney. White asterisk indicates the host kidney. (C) Micrographs [haematoxylin and eosin (H&E)] showing glomeruli of the control kidney originating from a 5-week-old rabbit (coeval with the metanephroi age). (D) Micrograph (H&E) showing glomeruli of new kidney after fresh kidney precursor allotransplantation. (E) Micrograph (H&E) showing glomeruli of new kidney after allotransplantation of vitrified kidney precursor. Scale bar, 0.1 mm (C–E).

Following this protocol, we show that, 3 weeks after transplantation, 10 of 20 (50%) of 15-day-old and 12 of 26 (46.1%) of 16-day-old metanephroi grew and differentiated, presenting normally developed glomeruli, proximal and distal tubules, and collecting ducts [6,54,55] (**Figure 10**).

Thus, we describe, for the first time in the literature, laparoscopic allogeneic transplantation of metanephroi as a non-invasive and viable technique in receptors without immunosuppression [6,54]. In addition, our development of an appropriate research protocol reviewed by our institutional research ethics committee involving surgical procedures on white New Zealand rabbits has allowed us to carry out the project with good quality, control, and safety for both the researchers and the animals.

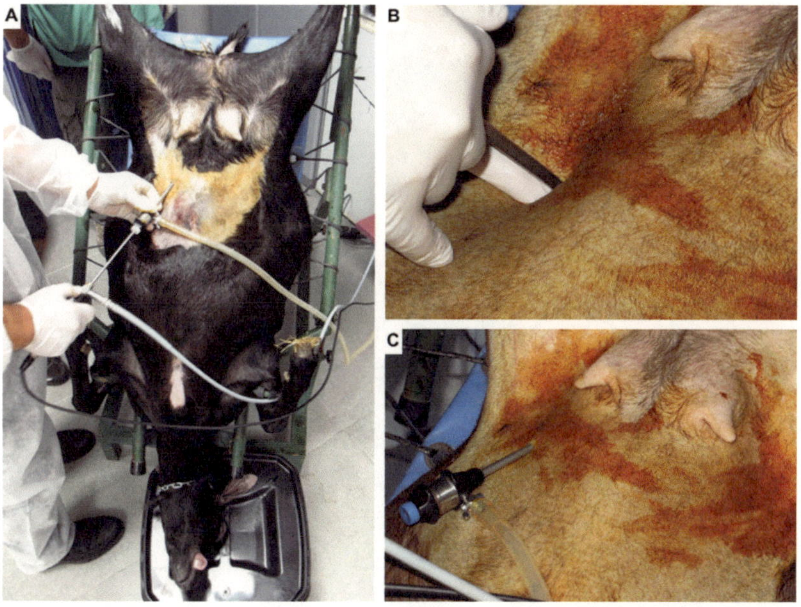

Figure 11. Laparoscopy procedure for metanephroi transfers. (A) Allocation of the animal on the stretcher. (B and C) Insertion of the trocar endoscope.

At the moment, successful embryo kidney transplantation tolerance has only been demonstrated previously in mice and rat. One attractive approach would be to apply this technology to large animals, whose nephron structure and size closely approximate human nephrons [3]. Larger animals, such as pigs, goats, sheep, and non-human primates, are ideal models. To the best of our knowledge, it has never been demonstrated in a large animal model. In this chapter, we develop a preliminary study in goat to provide a better test of the procedure feasibility for clinical application. As in the studies reported here in rabbit, we made use of our laparoscopy procedure adapted to this model. Briefly, recipient animals were sedated by intramuscular injection of xylazine (0.05 mg/kg) and butorphanol (0.1 mg/kg). As surgical preparation, anaesthesia was performed by intravenous injection of ketamine hydrochloride (0.5 mg/kg). First, animals were placed on an operating table in a vertical position (head down at 45° angle).

In Trendelenburg's position, rumen, stomach, and intestines do not cover the groin fat tissue into which metanephroi were transplanted. Only one endoscope trocar was inserted into the abdominal cavity (**Figure 11**).

Then, a 14G biopsy needle (Tru-Cut, 14G, 152 mm) was inserted into the inguinal region (**Figure 12**). After identifying a vessel in the retroperitoneal fat, a hole was performed adjacent to the vessel (**Figure 12**). Then, kidney precursor was aspirated in an adapted orogastric feeding catheter and the catheter was introduced through the biopsy needle and inserted into the aperture (**Figure 12**). Kidney precursors were transplanted in each host without immunosuppression (one metanephros per hole). After surgery, analgesia was administered every 12 h for 3 days [6,54].

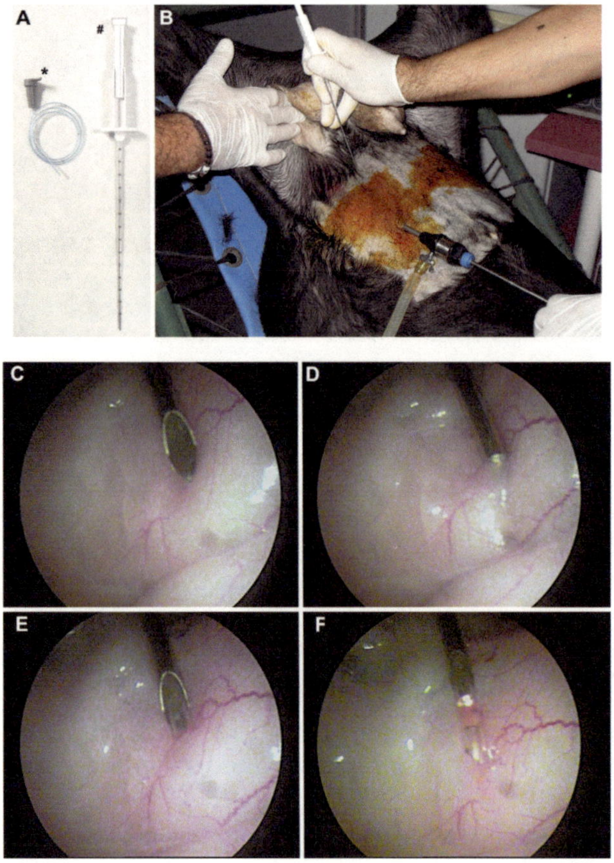

Figure 12. Laparoscopy procedure for metanephroi transfers. (A) Biopsy needle (Tru-Cut®, 14G, 152 mm) and orogastric feeding catheter. (B and C) Insertion of the biopsy needle. (D) Perform a hole into the fat where the metanephros will be transferred. (E) Introduction of the catheter through the needle with the metanephros. (D) Insertion of the catheter with the metanephros into the hole. (E) Metanephros transfer.

Following this protocol, we show that 6 weeks after transplantation of 15-day-old rabbit, metanephroi grew (**Figure 13**).

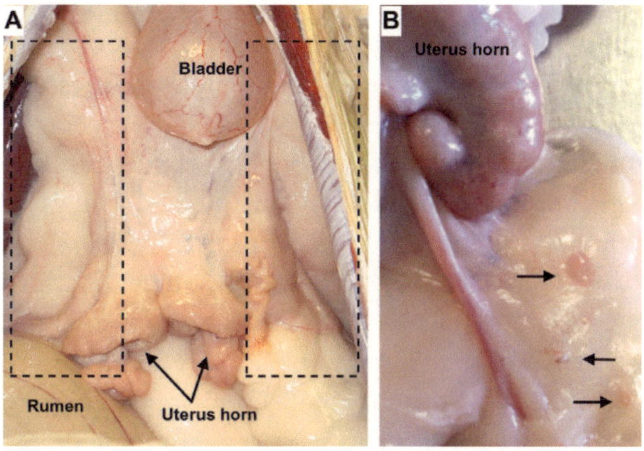

Figure 13. Successful development of new kidneys after xenotransplantation of rabbit metanephroi to goat. (A) Transplant area. (B) Growth.

6. Cryoconservation of embryonic kidney

Even if in a most favourable future situation the organ supply and demand could be balanced using xenotransplants or laboratory-grown organs from regenerative medicine, without proper cryopreservation procedures, the future of these treatments would still be compromised by the ability to physically distribute the organs to patients in need and produce these products in a way that allows adequate inventory control and quality assurance [59]. To this end, organ cryopreservation will be indispensable. Cryobiology is the study of the effects of low temperatures on living organisms. The aim of this discipline is to shift the pendulum from cell death to immortality at low temperatures. To achieve this, it is necessary to eliminate the two main causes of cell death associated with cryopreservation, ice crystal formation and lethal concentration of solutes, while maintaining the functional capacity of intracellular organelles [60–62] (**Figure 14**).

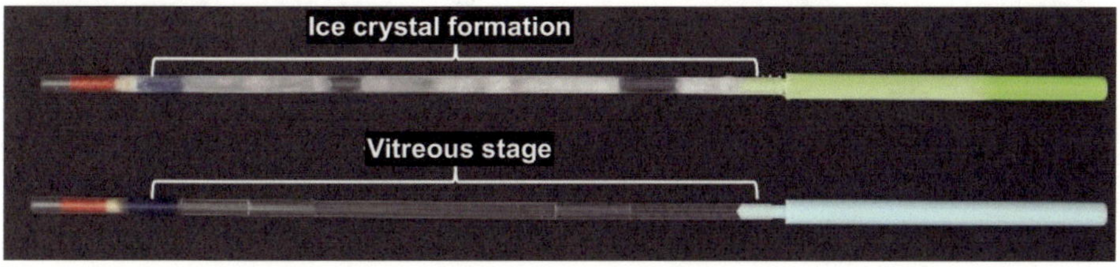

Figure 14. Successful development of new kidneys after xenotransplantation of rabbit metanephroi.

To date, small ovaries, blood vessels, heart valves, corneas, and similar structures are the only macroscopic structures having the capacity to recover, at least in part, after vitrification [63]. Fahy et al. [63] reported a case history of one rabbit kidney that survived vitrification and supported the life of a recipient animal for an indefinite period of time. Based on this knowledge, we recently described a method to cryopreserve metanephroi whole organs and generate kidneys after transplantation into a syngeneic non-immunosuppressed host [59]. Previously, to our best knowledge, only Bottomley et al. [64] evaluated the cryopreservation of metanephroi immediately after thawing, but only under in vitro conditions. Briefly, vitrification was performed following the minimum essential volume method using Cryotop® as device and VM3 as vitrification solution (**Figure 15**). Kidney precursors were first exposed for 3 min to equilibration solution containing 1.7% (w/v) ethylene glycol (EG), 1.3% (w/v) formamide, 2.2% (w/v) dimethyl sulfoxide (DMSO), 0.7% (w/v) PVP K12 (polyvinylpyrrolidone of Mr 5000 Da), and 0.1% (w/v) SuperCool X-1000 and SuperCool Z-1000 (ice blockers) in base medium [BM: Dulbecco's PBS + 20% foetal bovine serum (FBS)]. Then, the kidney precursors were exposed for 1 min to solution containing 4.7% (w/v) EG, 3.6% (w/v) formamide, 6.2% (w/v) DMSO, 1.9% (w/v) PVP K12, and 0.3% (w/v) ice blockers in BM. Finally, the kidney precursors were transferred to vitrification solution consisting of 16.84% (w/v) EG, 12.86% (w/v) formamide, 22.3% (w/v) DMSO, 7% (w/v) PVP K12, and 1% (w/v) ice blockers in BM before being loaded onto Cryotop® devices and directly plunged into liquid nitrogen within 1 min.

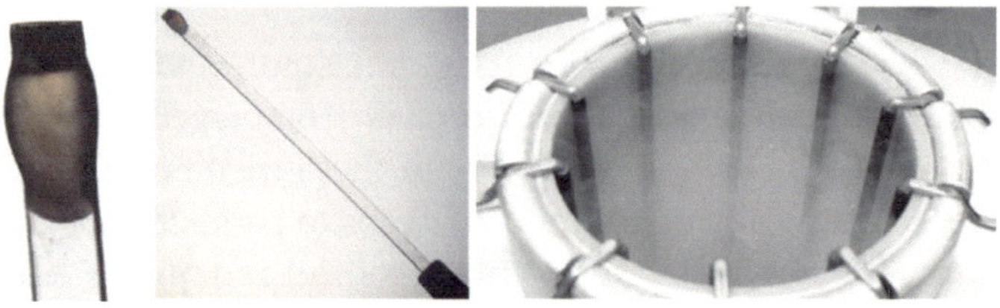

Figure 15. Details of 15-day-old metanephros loaded in a Cryotop® device. Details of metanephros loaded into film strip of Cryotop®.

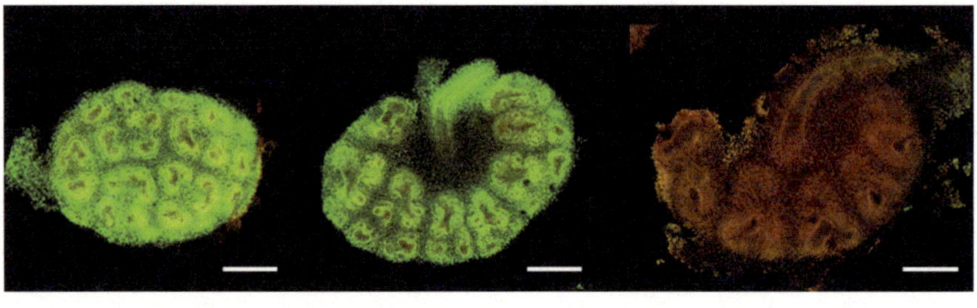

Figure 16. Kidney precursor viability analysis evaluated by a confocal microscope. Viability cells were evaluated by SYBR-14 (live) and propidium iodide (dead) fluorescence. (A) Fresh metanephros. (B) Live vitrified metanephros. (C) Dead vitrified metanephros. Scale bar, 1 mm.

For warming, kidney precursors were placed in a solution composed of 1.25 M sucrose in BM for 1 min and later transferred stepwise into decreasing sucrose solutions (0.6, 0.3, and 0.15 M sucrose in BM) for 30 s before and then washed twice in BM for 5 min. When the kidney

http://dx.doi.org/10.5772/62400

precursors were thawed and processed without further culture, a high percentage of kidney precursors was considered as viable (80%; **Figure 16**).

In our study, 14 metanephroi were transplanted after 3 months of vitrification (storage). Twenty-one days after transplant, the capacity for angiogenesis of the metanephros after laparoscopic transplantation was observed (**Figure 17**).

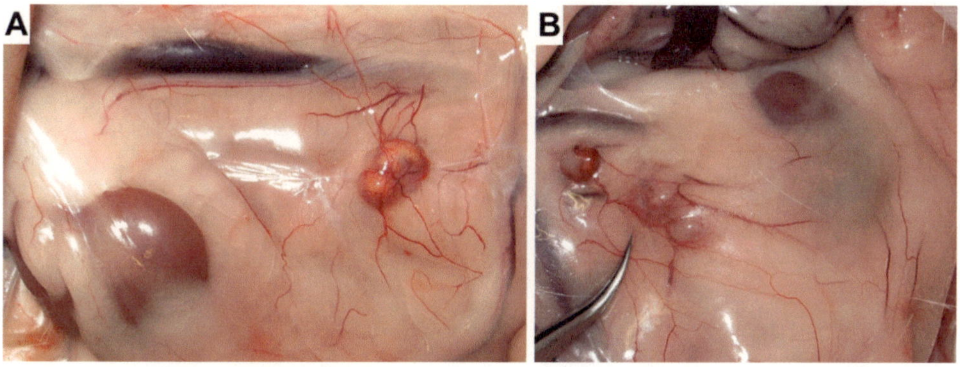

Figure 17. Generation of new kidneys using fresh (A) and vitrified (B) metanephroi after allotransplantation in rabbits. Note massive growth and blood vessels of the new kidney.

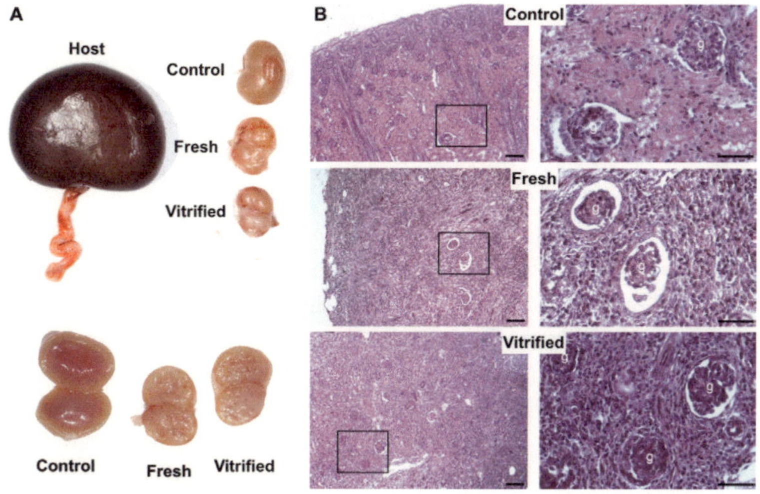

Figure 18. Generation of a kidney using vitrified kidney precursors after allotransplantation in rabbits. (A) Image showing the growth and shape of kidneys as well as the appearance of the renal cortex and renal medulla. Control kidney originating from a 5-week-old rabbit. (B) Histological analysis, by H&E staining, of the vitrified and fresh kidney precursors under in vivo culture for 3 weeks after transplantation. Control kidney originating from a 5-week-old rabbit. g, glomeruli. Scale bar, 0.1 mm.

In all of the recipients, new kidneys were recovered and examined. In total, 7 (50.0%) vitrified metanephroi were successfully grown. Similar rates were reached from fresh kidney precursors (43.7%; **Figure 18**). In all of them, new kidneys developed mature glomeruli whose histomorphometry analysis showed that vitrification has no significant effect on glomerular perimeter compared to the corresponding values in the control (**Figure 18**).

Finally, we examined whether kidneys had normal endocrine functionality. We analysed the expression profile of the renin and erythropoietin transcript by quantitative real-time PCR (RT-PCR). The expression of renin and erythropoietin was similar in vitrified new kidneys, consistent with previous reports (**Figure 19**).

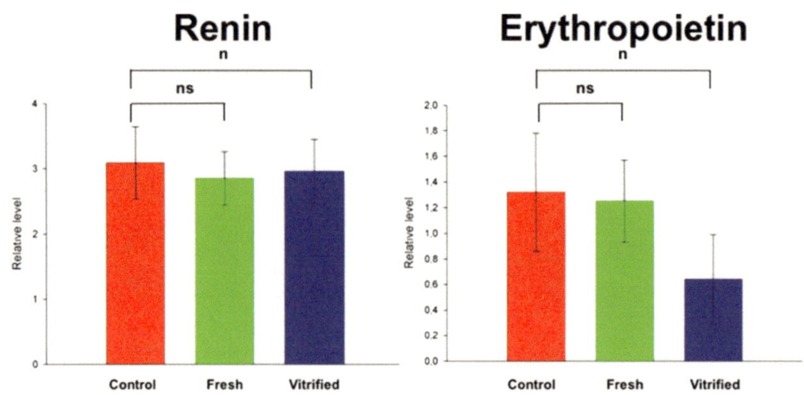

Figure 19. RT-PCR analysis of renin and erythropoietin transcript expression in kidneys from vitrified and fresh metanephroi and control kidney. Gapdh was used as reference gene. n=6; mean±SD. Student's t test: P value not significant (ns).

7. Conclusion

Our study essentially makes two innovative contributions in the field of transplantation of embryonic organs. First, we provide the first evidence of a successful long-term storage of an entire vital organ, enabling the generation of new kidneys after transplantation into a syngeneic non-immunosuppressed host. Our results therefore make a substantial contribution to the development of a long-term biobank of kidney precursors as an unlimited source of kidneys, facilitating sanitary and inventory control and the distribution of organs. Second, we show that a translational future application to transplant patients is possible using a very simple and minimally invasive laparoscopic procedure. Our present findings should also encourage the future development of bioengineering technologies to reconstitute primordial organs as an alternative approach to regenerative medicine.

Acknowledgements

This study was supported by a grant from ALCER-TURIA.

http://dx.doi.org/10.5772/62400

Author details

Ximo García-Domínguez[1], Cesar D. Vera-Donoso[2], Luís García-Valero[1], Jose S. Vicente[1] and Francisco Marco-Jimenez[1*]

*Address all correspondence to: fmarco@dca.upv.es

1 Institue for Animal Science and Technology, Politechnichal University of Valencia, Valencia, Spain

2 Urology, Hospital Universitari i Politècnic La Fe, Valencia, Spain

References

[1] Ott HC, Mathisen DJ. Bioartificial tissues and organs: are we ready to translate?. Lancet. 2011; 378: 1977–1978.

[2] Salvatori M, Peloso A, Katari R, Orlando G. Regeneration and bioengineering of the kidney: current status and future challenges. Curr Urol Rep. 2014; 15: 379.

[3] D'Agati VD. Growing new kidneys from embryonic cell suspensions: fantasy or reality? J Am Soc Nephrol. 2002; 11: 1763–1766.

[4] Badylak SF, Taylor D, Uygun K. Whole-organ tissue engineering: decellularization and recellularization of three-dimensional matrix scaffolds. Annu Rev Biomed Eng. 2011; 13: 27–53.

[5] Aznar Lucea J, Tudela Cuenca J, Sánchez García JL. Artificial organs production. Cuad Bioet. 2015; 26: 149–169.

[6] Vera-Donoso CD, García-Dominguez X, Jiménez-Trigos E, García-Valero L, Vicente JS, Marco-Jiménez F. Laparoscopic transplantation of metanephroi: a first step to kidney xenotransplantation. Actas Urol Esp. 2015; 39: 527–534.

[7] Jofré R. Factores que afectan a la calidad de vida en pacientes en prediálisis, diálisis y trasplante renal. Nefrologia. 1999; 19: 84–90.

[8] Organ Procurement and Transplantation Network. National waiting list passes 100 thousand [Internet]. 2008. Available from: https://optn.transplant.hrsa.gov/news/national-waiting-list-passes-100-thousand [Accessed: 2015-11-05].

[9] Song JJ, Guyette JP, Gilpin SE, Gonzalez G, Vacanti JP, Ott HC. Regeneration and experimental orthotopic transplantation of a bioengineered kidney. Nat Med. 2013; 19: 646–651.

[10] Xinaris C, Yokoo T. Reforming the kidney starting from a single-cell suspension. Nephron Exp Nephrol. 2014; 126: 107.

[11] Miranda B, Felipe C González-Posada JM, Ferández M, Naya MT. Evolución de las características de los donantes en España, y riñones desechados para trasplante. Nefrologia. 1998; 18: 196–205.

[12] Villa G, Rodríguez-Carmona A, Fernández-Ortiz L, Cuervo J, Rebollo P, Otero A, Arrieta J. Cost analysis of the Spanish renal replacement therapy programme. Nephrol Dial Transplant. 2011; 26: 3709–3714.

[13] Dilworth Mr, Clancy Mj, Marshall D, Ca Bravery, Pe Brenchley, Ashton N. Development and functional capacity of transplanted rat metanephroi. Nephrol Dial Transplant. 2008; 23: 871–879.

[14] Clancy Mj, Marshall D, Dilworth M, Bottomley M, Ashton N, Brenchley P. Immunosuppression is essential for successful allogeneic transplantation of the metanephroi. Transplantation. 2009; 88: 151–159.

[15] Cooper DK. A brief history of cross-species organ transplantation. Proc (Bayl Univ Med Cent). 2012; 25: 49–57.

[16] Costa MR, Fischer N, Gulich B, Tönjes RR. Comparison of porcine endogenous retroviruses infectious potential in supernatants of producer cells and in cocultures. Xenotransplantation. 2014; 21: 162–173.

[17] Hammerman MR. Transplantation of renal primordia: renal organogenesis. Pediatr Nephrol. 2007; 22: 1991–1998.

[18] Yasutomi Y. Establishment of specific pathogen-free macaque colonies in Tsukuba Primate Research Center of Japan for AIDS research. Vaccine. 2010; 28: 75–77.

[19] Dekel B, Burakova T, Arditti FD, Reich-Zeliger S, Milstein O, Aviel-Ronen S, Rechavi G, Friedman N, Kaminski N, Passwell JH, Reisner Y. Human and porcine early kidney precursors as a new source for transplantation. Nat Med. 2003; 9: 53–60.

[20] Naito M. Macrophage heterogeneity in development and differentiation. Arch Histol Cytol. 1993; 56: 331–351.

[21] Foglia RP, La Quaglia M, Statter MB, Donahoe PK. Fetal allograft survival in immunocompetent recipients is age dependent and organ specific. Ann Surg. 1986; 204: 402–410.

[22] Dekel B, Burakova T, Ben-Hur H, Marcus H, Oren R, Laufer J, Yair R. Engraftment of human kidney tissue in rat radiation chimera: II. Human fetal kidneys display reduced immunogenicity to adoptively transferred human peripheral blood mononuclear cells and exhibit rapid growth and development. Transplantation. 1997; 64: 1550–1558.

[23] Statter M, Fahrner KJ, Barksdale EM, Parks DE, Flavell RA, Donahoe PK. Correlation of fetal kidney and testis congenic graft survival with reduced major histocompatibility complex burden. Transplantation. 1989; 47: 651–660.

[24] Dekel B, Marcus H, Herzel BH, Bucher WO, Passwell J, Yair R. In vivo modulation of the allogeneic immune response by human fetal kidneys: The role of cytokines, chemokines, and cytolytic effector molecules. Transplantation. 2000; 69: 1470–1478.

[25] Rogers SA, Hammerman MR. Transplantation of rat metanephroi into mice. Am J Physiol. 2001; 280: 1865–1869.

[26] Hammerman MR. Renal organogenesis from transplanted metanephric primordia. J Am Soc Nephrol. 2004; 15: 1126–1132.

[27] Rogers SA, Lowell JA, Hammerman NA, Hammerman MR. Transplantation of developing metanephroi into adult rats. Kidney Int. 1998; 54: 27–37.

[28] Hammerman MR. Transplantation of embryonic kidneys. Clin Sci (Lond). 2002; 103: 599–612.

[29] Marshall D, Dilworth MR, Clancy M, Bravery CA, Ashton N. Increasing renal mass improves survival in anephric rats following metanephroi transplantation. Exp Physiol. 2007; 92: 263–271.

[30] De Francisco AL. Future directions in therapy for chronic kidney disease. Nefrologia. 2010; 30: 1–9.

[31] Hammerman MR. Classic and current opinion in embryonic organ transplantation. Curr Opin Organ Transplant. 2014; 19: 133–139.

[32] Rogers SA, Liapis H, Hammerman MR. Normalization of glucose post-transplantation of pig pancreatic anlagen into non-immunosuppressed diabetic rats depends on obtaining anlagen prior to embryonic day 35. Transplant Immunology. 2005; 14: 67–75.

[33] Rogers SA, Chen F, Talcott M, Hammerman MR. Islet cell engraftment and control of diabetes in rats following transplantation of pig pancreatic anlagen. Am J Physiol. 2004; 286: E502–E509.

[34] Rogers SA, Chen F, Talcott M, Liapis H, Hammerman MR. Glucose tolerance normalization following transplantation of pig pancreatic primordia into non-immunosuppressed diabetic ZDF rats. Transplant Immunol. 2006; 16: 176–184.

[35] Rogers SA, Hammerman MR. Normalization of glucose post-transplantation into diabetic rats of pig pancreatic primordia preserved in vitro. Organogenesis. 2008; 4: 48–51.

[36] Rogers SA, Chen F, Talcott MR, Faulkner C, Thomas JM, Thevis M, Hammerman MR. Long-term engraftment following transplantation of pig pancreatic primordia into non-immunosuppressed diabetic rhesus macaques. Xenotransplantation. 2007; 14: 591–602.

[37] Rogers SA, Mohanakumar T, Liapis H, Hammerman MR. Engraftment of cells from porcine islets of Langerhans and normalization of glucose tolerance following transplantation of pig pancreatic primordia in non-immune suppressed diabetic rats. Am J Pathol. 2010; 177: 854–864.

[38] Rogers SA, Tripathi P, Mohanakumar T, Liapis H, Chen F, Talcott MR, Faulkner C, Hammerman MR. Engraftment of cells from porcine islets of Langerhans following transplantation of pig pancreatic primordia in non-immune suppressed diabetic rhesus macaques. Organogenesis. 2011; 7: 154–162.

[39] Woolf AS, Palmer SJ, Snow ML, Fine LG. Creation of functioning chimeric mammalian kidney. Kidney Int. 1990; 38: 991–997.

[40] Rogers SA, Talcott M, Hammerman MR. Transplantation of pig metanephroi. ASAIO J. 2003; 49: 48–52.

[41] Rogers SA, Hammerman MR. Prolongation of life in anephric rats following de novo renal organogenesis. Organogenesis. 2004; 1: 22–25.

[42] Takeda S, Rogers SA, Hammerman MR. Differential origin for endothelial and mesangial cells after transplantation of pig fetal renal primordia into rats. Transpl Immunol. 2006; 15: 211–215.

[43] Yokote S, Yokoo T, Matsumoto K, Utsunomiya Y, Kawamura T, Hosoya T. The effect of metanephroi transplantation on blood pressure in anephric rats with induced acute hypotension. Nephrol Dial Transplant. 2012; 27: 3449–3455.

[44] Yokote S, Yokoo T, Matsumoto K, Ohkido I, Utsunomiya Y, Kawamura T, Hosoya T. Metanephroi transplantation inhibits the progression of vascular calcification in rats with adenine-induced renal failure. Nephron Exp Nephrol. 2012; 120: e32–e40.

[45] Matsumoto K, Yokoo T, Yokote S, Utsunomiya Y, Ohashi T, Hosoya T. Functional development of a transplanted embryonic kidney: effect of transplantation site. J Nephrol. 2012; 25: 50–55.

[46] Matsumoto K, Yokoo T, Matsunari H, Iwai S, Yokote S, Teratani T, Gheisari Y, Tsuji O, Okano H, Utsunomiya Y, Hosoya T, Okano HJ, Nagashima H, Kobayashi E. Xenotransplanted embryonic kidney provides a niche for endogenous mesenchymal stem cell differentiation into erythropoietin-producing tissue. Stem Cells. 2012; 30: 1228–1235.

[47] Yokote S, Matsunari H, Iwai S, Yamanaka S, Uchikura A, Fujimoto E, Matsumoto K, Nagashima H, Kobayashi E, Yokoo T. Urine excretion strategy for stem cell-generated embryonic kidneys. Proc Natl Acad Sci U S A. 2015; 112: 12980–12985.

[48] Streilen JW. Unravelling immune privilege. Science. 1995; 270: 1158–1159.

[49] Abrahamson DR. Glomerular development in intraocular and intrarenal graft of fetal kidney. Lab Invest. 1991; 64: 629–639.

[50] Robert B, St John PL, Hyink DP, Abrahamson DR. Evidence that embryonic kidney cells expressing flk-1 are intrinsic, vasculogenic angioblasts. Am J Physiol. 1996; 271: F744–F753.

[51] Koseki C, Herzlinger D, al-Awqati Q. Integration of embryonic nephrogenic cells carrying a reporter gene into functioning nephrons. Am J Physiol. 1991; 261: C550–C554.

[52] Barakat TL, Harrison RG. The capacity of fetal and neonatal renal tissues to regenerate and differentiate in a heterotropic allogenic subcutaneous tissue site in the rat. J Anat. 1971; 110: 393–407.

[53] Rogers SA, Liapis H, Hammerman MR. Transplantation of metanephroi across the major histocompatibility complex in rats. Am J Physiol Regul Integr Comp Physiol. 2001; 280: R132–R136.

[54] Garcia-Dominguez X, Vicente J.S., Vera-Donoso C., Jimenez-Trigos E., Marco-Jiménez F. First steps towards organ banks: Vitrification of renal primordia. CryoLetters 2016;37:47-52.

[55] Barak H, Boyle SC. Organ culture and immunostaining of mouse embryonic kidneys. Cold Spring Harb Protoc. 2011; doi: 10.1101/pbd.prot5558.

[56] Fischer B, Chavatte-Palmer P, Viebahn C, Navarrete Santos A, Duranthon V. Rabbit as a reproductive model for human health. Reproduction. 2012; 144: 1–10.

[57] Wang S, Tang X, Niu Y, Chen H, Li B, Li T, Zhang X, Hu Z, Zhou Q, Ji W. Generation and characterization of rabbit embryonic stem cells. Stem Cells. 2007; 25: 481–489.

[58] Honda A, Hirose M, Inoue K, Ogonuki N, Miki H, Shimozawa N, Hatori M, Shimizu N, Murata T, Hirose M, Katayama K, Wakisaka N, Miyoshi H, Yokoyama KK, Sankai T, Ogura A. Stable embryonic stem cell lines in rabbits: potential small animal models for human research. Reprod Biomed Online. 2008; 17: 706–715.

[59] Marco-Jiménez F, Garcia-Dominguez X, Jimenez-Trigos E, Vera-Donoso CD, Vicente JS. Vitrification of kidney precursors as a new source for organ transplantation. Cryobiology. 2015; 70: 278–282.

[60] Mazur P. Kinetics of water loss from cells at subzero temperatures and the likelihood of intracellular freezing. J Gen Physiol 1963;47:347–369.

[61] Kleinhans FW, Mazur P. Comparison of actual vs. synthesized ternary phase diagrams for solutes of cryobiological interest. Cryobiology 2007;54:212–222.

[62] Edgar DH, Gook DA. A critical appraisal of cryopreservation (slow cooling versus vitrification) of human oocytes and embryos. Hum Reprod Update. 2012;18:536–554.

[63] Fahy GM, Wowk B, Pagotan R, Chang A, Phan J, Thomson B, Phan L. Physical and biological aspects of renal vitrification. Organogenesis. 2009; 5: 167–175.

[64] Bottomley MJ, Baicu S, Boggs JM, Marshall DP, Clancy M, Brockbank KG, Bravery CA. Preservation of embryonic kidneys for transplantation. Transplant Proc. 2005; 37: 280–284.

Chapter 3

Tolerance in Organ Transplantation

Laetitia Boucault, Séverine Bézie, Jason Ossart and
Carole Guillonneau

Additional information is available at the end of the chapter

http://dx.doi.org/10.5772/62653

Abstract

Transplantation is often the best option to treat organ end stage failure. Transplanted patients need to take long-term immunosuppressive drugs to inhibit rejection and maintain their graft. But those therapies have numerous important side effects such as cancer induction and opportunistic infections. Thus, the development of novel therapies to induce specific rather than general immunosuppression and therefore, tipping the balance between effector and regulatory functions to inhibit transplant rejection is a major goal in the field. One major approach is the blockade of costimulatory signals to abort effector T-cell activation following TCR engagement and to promote regulatory T cells. Here we summarized the research to date that details immune mechanisms involved in tolerance in organ transplantation and strategies toward tolerance.

Keywords: Transplantation, Tolerance, Costimulation, Tregs, Immunointervention

1. Introduction

The primary role of the immune system is to protect against foreign antigens without reacting against self-antigens. In this objective, some mechanisms of immune tolerance have been set up. Immune tolerance is defined in general by a total absence of specific reaction against antigens, and particularly self-antigens and a break in immune tolerance can lead to autoimmune disorders. Understanding the mechanisms of immunological tolerance is crucial for the development of strategies to manipulate the immune system in the context of organ transplantation. Here, we provide a comprehensive summary of the immune mechanisms involved in transplant rejection and tolerance induction and the research to date leading to new strategies toward tolerance, as well as their translation to the clinics.

2. Tolerance in organ transplantation

In the context of transplantation, the graft is recognized as foreign antigens and immune responses are triggered. Immunosuppressive treatments can repress total immune responses, including responses against the graft, but these drugs are well known for inducing side effects such as cardiovascular diseases or increased opportunistic infections and malignancies, and lead to high morbidity and mortality, even when avoiding excessive immunosuppression [1]. In addition, current immunosuppressive regimens have marginal effects on long-term allograft survival with for example a half-life of 10 years for kidney transplantation. In fact, these drugs can even be deleterious in the establishment of tolerance. Some cases of tolerance spontaneously acquired by patients who stopped their immunosuppressive treatments because of side effects and noncompliance have been reported [2, 3]. Tolerance in transplantation is defined by the following criteria: the graft must be definitely accepted without any lesions of chronic rejection, and the recipient should not be on treatment at the moment of analysis and should be able to develop immune responses against any other foreign antigen (i.e. immunocompetent), and thus represents the center of immunologist efforts working in the field of transplantation. The most commonly transplanted solid organ is the kidney, but the field of solid organ transplantation also includes the heart, liver, pancreas, lung or intestine. Nowadays, transplantation still remains the best solution for organ failure, even in the face of graft rejection. There are three types of solid graft rejection:

- The quickest mechanism of rejection, said hyperacute rejection, takes place between minutes to hours after transplantation. It is mediated by the presence of pre-existent circulating antibodies against A, B molecules expressed by red blood cells [4, 5] and acquired antibodies against the human leukocyte antigen (HLA) [6, 7]. Those antibodies allow the immune system of the grafted patients to strongly recognize the molecules present at the surface of graft endothelium and lead to the destruction of this endothelium through complement cascade, neutrophils, and monocytes. Nowadays, hyperacute rejection is no longer a concern due to the establishment of pre-transplantation tests as cross-match test, where closest HLA compatibility between donor and recipient is ensured (concerning mainly HLA-A, B, and DR) and blood group typing.

- The months following transplantation, acute rejection can occur. Two mechanisms can be involved in this process. The cell-mediated rejection is induced by presentation of alloreactive molecules by APCs (Antigen Presenting Cells) to recipient's T lymphocytes, leading such activated lymphocytes to infiltrate and destroy the grafted organ [8]. The humoral mechanism acts through generation of alloantibodies directed mainly against MHC (major histocompatibility complex) class I by activated alloreactive B lymphocytes leading to antibody-dependent cellular cytotoxicity of endothelial cells (ADCC) [9]. Prevention of acute rejection is now ensured in more than 85% of cases by the current repertoire of immunosuppressive drugs available [10].

- Even though, the main problem in transplantation which remains unsolved is the long-term allograft dysfunction or chronic rejection. This phenomenon is slow and progressive but irreversible and cannot be controlled by immunosuppressive drugs. It is characterized by

http://dx.doi.org/10.5772/62653

an increase of the thickness of the intima's layer of graft vessels, leading to the ischemia of the tissue and finally to graft loss. Chronic rejection is mediated by the antigen-specific cellular and humoral immune responses against the graft. These immune responses lead to the recruitment of inflammatory mediators to the graft through the activation of the endothelium, and the secretion of free radicals and damage signals which activate muscle vessels proliferation.

Thus, T cells play an important role in graft rejection. In solid organ transplantation, naive T cells from the recipient are activated by recognition of blood group (ABO), donor major histocompatibility complex (MHC), minor histocompatibility complex (mHC, MICA, MICB, H-Y), or nonpolymorphic peptides (collagen, angiotensin II receptor) presented by professional APCs from the recipient or the donor or directly from endothelial cells of the graft (mostly MHC class I) [11]. Thus, T cells can be primed by three distinct pathways.

The direct allorecognition: when the transplanted organ is reperfused, intact MHC/peptide (MHCp) at the surface of APCs from the donor travel to the lymphoid organs of the recipients where they interact with $CD4^+$ and $CD8^+$ alloreactive naive T cells and active them [8, 12]. This pathway is generally associated with acute rejection because donor's APCs persist a few months following transplantation. In addition, intact MHCp at the surface of endothelial cells of the graft can activate and maintain allogeneic $CD8^+$ effector T-cell responses [13].

The indirect allorecognition: this pathway involves the presentation of allogeneic peptides derived from donor MHC molecules and presented by APCs of the recipient. Dominant peptides presented by this pathway are generally derived from hypervariable regions. This pathway involves capture, processing, and presentation of alloantigens and is predominantly used by $CD4^+$ T cells and most of the alloantigens are presented by MHC class II. However, cross-presentation on MHC class I can occur and $CD8^+$ T cells can also be activated [14–16]. The indirect allopresentation pathway is also necessary for B cells activation, since their activation depends on $CD4^+$ T cells help [17]. The indirect allorecognition is involved in both acute and chronic rejection since the alloantigens are present during all the life of the allograft [18–21].

The semi-direct allorecognition: Lechler's team reported that APCs from the recipient can capture entire intact MHC/peptide complexes expressed at the surface of the donor's APCs. Those complexes are internalized, processed, and presented directly to $CD8^+$ T cells or indirectly to $CD4^+$ T cells. This presentation pathway involves the phenomenon of trogocytosis, i.e. the exchange of membrane fragments between cells in contact [22–24]. Brown and al have reported *in vivo*, in a model of transplantation in mice, the presence of intact donor MHC-I and MHC-II on the surface of DCs, B cells, and macrophages [25].

2.1. The immune tolerance

To date, two elaborated and complementary mechanisms of immune tolerance have been described as central tolerance and peripheral tolerance (see **Figure 1**).

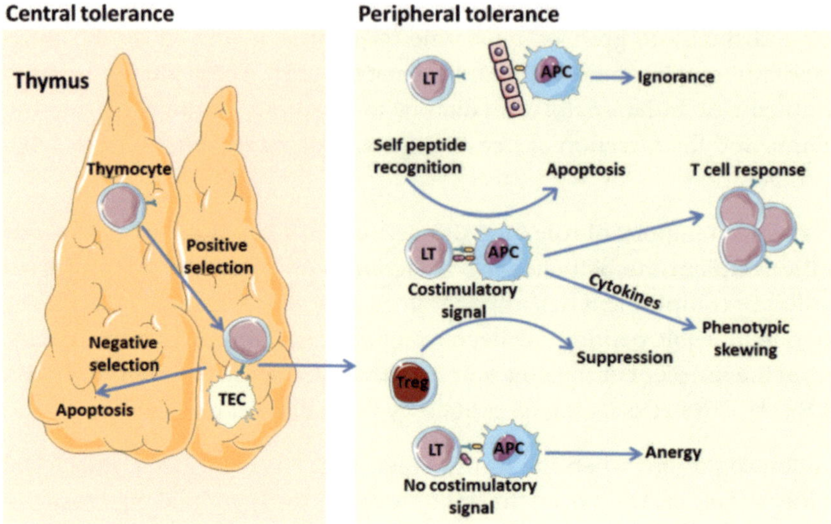

Figure 1. Central and peripheral tolerance. In the thymus, tight interactions between TCRs and self-antigens presented by thymic epithelial cells (TEC) induce thymocytes apoptosis. Four mechanisms induce peripheral tolerance: ignorance, apoptosis, phenotypic skewing and anergy. Appropriate combination of signals results in complete T-cell activation.

2.1.1. Central tolerance

In the context of immune tolerance, the T lymphocyte lineage is particularly important. T lymphocytes, B lymphocytes, and NK cells derive from a common hematopoietic precursor from foetal liver during embryogenesis of from adult bone marrow. The $CD3^-CD4^-CD8^-$ TCR^- thymocytes colonize the thymus and undergo different stages of maturation leading to TCR rearrangement. During their migration to the cortex, cells also acquire expression of CD3, CD4, and CD8 molecules and undergo a step of positive selection. All $CD4^+CD8^+$cells said double-positive (DP) thymocytes express a complete $\alpha\beta$TCR but only 20–25% of them are able to interact with the MHC [26, 27]. Cells that strongly interact with MHC class I become $CD8^+$ simple positive (SP) and the one which interact with MHC class II becomes $CD4^+$ SP [28–30]. This interaction provides a survival signal to thymocytes that can pursue their education by migrating into the thymic medulla. In this medulla, SP thymocytes undergo the second step of immune central tolerance called negative selection. After positive selection, the TCR repertoire is very large and uncontrolled; thymocytes are able to recognize a broad range of foreign antigens but also self-antigens. The maturation of thymocytes expressing a TCR against self-antigens can lead to autoimmune disease in the periphery. Negative selection consists in the inhibition of potentially autoreactive thymocytes by clonal deletion or by induction of anergy if receptor editing fail. This selection is mediated by medullary thymic epithelial cells (mTECs) that are the only antigens presenting cells (APCs) expressing a panel of ectopic tissue-specific antigens (TSA). The expression of those TSA is mainly under control of a transcription regulator named Auto-Immune REgulator (AIRE) [31]. Two mechanisms of TSA presentations can occur in the medulla. The first one is the direct presentation by mTEC that can be sufficient to induce negative selection of both CD4+ and CD8+ T cells [32, 33]. The second mechanism of presentation is mediated by thymic dendritic cells which are able to get TSAs from mTECs and to present them to thymocytes [34]. Thymocytes able to strongly recognize a TSA presented by mTECs or DCs receive a signal that leads to apoptosis [35]. After negative selection, approximately 5% of total thymocytes can finally go to the periphery.

2.1.2. Peripheral tolerance

Due to the absence of self-antigen presentation in the thymus [36], or the low affinity of T cells for self-antigens [37], autoreactive T cells escape sometimes from thymic negative selection. To complete the efficacy of central tolerance, the immune system developed many tools to neutralize these cells and avoid autoimmune diseases. These mechanisms are either passive, concerning antigen ignorance, T-cell anergy or apoptosis induction and phenotypic skewing, or active when mediated by regulatory cells [38].

Antigen ignorance allows autoreactive T cells to persist as functional circulating T cells while never primed by any antigen [39]. Indeed, antigens can be masked by anatomical barriers like lens proteins, spermatozoids, or nervous system protein protected by the meninges barrier. Besides, a low amount of antigens can be sufficient to activate cytotoxic T lymphocytes previously primed but not naive T lymphocytes [40].

On the contrary, a high amount of antigen can induce T-cell apoptosis. This mechanism called activation-induced cell death is induced by Fas signaling pathway [41]. Indeed, Fas expression deficiency results in autoimmunity [42]. Autoreactive T-cell peripheral deletion can also result from a lack of costimulatory signal or of growth factor. [43–45]. Likewise, the absence of costimulatory molecules induces a Fas-mediated apoptosis of autoreactive B cells [46], but anyway the autoreactive B cells escaping the clonal deletion are unlikely to meet the T cells specific to the same antigen they need to be completely primed [47, 48].

Autoreactive T cells can also be primed but functionally inactivated. This state of anergy is characterized by incapability to proliferate and to produce IL-2 following antigen stimulation [49, 50]. Antigens are required to maintain this inactive state [51], and large amounts of IL-2 or anti-OX40 antibodies can abrogate it [52]. Anergy results from either a lack of costimulatory signal by APCs, a low affinity of TCR for the antigen, or from CTLA4/B7 interaction. Indeed, interactions between CD28 expressed on T-cell surface and CD80-CD86 on antigen-presenting cells are essential for activation and proliferation of alloreactive T cells [53], allow generation of memory T cells and inhibit regulatory T (Tregs) suppressive activity [54, 55]. Without CD28/CD80-CD86 engagement, interactions between TCRs and alloantigens induce the anergy of T cells. CTLA-4 (CD152) has a large structural homology with CD28 and interacts with CD80-CD86 with better affinity than CD28 molecule and functions as a negative regulator of T-cell activation [56]. The expression of these two molecules regulates the balance between activation and inhibition of T cells and allows the control of an over-reaction of the immune system leading to inflammation or autoimmunity [57]. Similarly, the expression of Programmed Death-1 (PD-1) after antigenic stimulation and interaction with its ligand PDL-1 reduces IL-2 synthesis and induces T-cell anergy [58]. Another important co-stimulatory pathway is the CD40/CD40L co-stimulatory pathway. The CD40 molecule is a transmembrane protein that belongs to the TNF receptor family. It is expressed on vascular endothelial cells [59], activated DCs [60], monocytes/macrophages, platelets [61] and B lymphocytes [62]. The CD40L, also called CD154, exists in soluble form or at the cell membrane [63]. It is expressed on activated $CD4^+$ T cells, basophiles, eosinophils [64], DCs from the blood [65], endothelial cells, macrophages [66], and B lymphocytes [67]. The CD40-CD40L interaction is critical for T-cell–dependent effector functions [68]. Indeed, CD40/CD40L interaction acts with IL-12 to induce production of IFN-y by human T lymphocytes stimulated by anti-CD3/anti-CD28, as well as IL-2 production by Th1 and IL-4, IL-5 and IL-10 by Th2 lymphocytes [69]. Besides, interaction with CD40 activates the expression of adhesion molecules by T lymphocytes [70]. Many other co-stimulation pathways are well described such as RANK/RANKL or ICOS/ICOSL. These costimulatory pathways are crucial for T-cell activation inducing rejection, so inhibition of one or more of these pathways may inhibit rejection. Moreover, anergized T cells can inhibit DCs function [71], become IL-10 producing Tregs [72], and induce T-cell apoptosis [73]. Autoreactive B cells also undergo anergy induced by chronic stimulation of BCR(B cell receptor) by antigens [74].

Activated autoreactive T cells can persist in a nonpathogenic state. Indeed, Th2 cytokines expression is linked to lower autoimmunity [75, 76] and tolerance in transplantation [77–79], sometimes through Tregs induction [80]. By contrast, Th1 and Th17 are linked to allograft rejection [81]. Therefore, immunosuppressive treatments, like glucocorticoides or sirolimus, aim to inhibit Th1 responses and promote Th2 responses [82, 83].

Peripheral tolerance is also maintained by regulatory cells. Immune cells can acquire a regulatory function during development, such as "natural" Tregs in the thymus, or in periphery under the influence of the microenvironment, such as "induced" Tregs in the allograft or draining lymph nodes. Almost all type of cells have a regulatory counterpart, including T cells, B cells, myeloid cells (MDSCs, M2 macrophages), DCs. These regulatory cells limit effector cell responses to pathogens and self-antigens, acting by contact or by secretion of suppressive cytokines. In transplantation, regulatory cells are targets for therapeutic strategies to control innate immune responses triggered by ischemia/reperfusion of the graft, and adaptive responses triggered by the allograft.

3. Induction of tolerance

3.1. Animal models of tolerance

The immune system complexity is due to a large number of possible interactions and activation pathways. So, *in vitro* experiments provide primary results but they need to be confirmed by *in vivo* studies to overview all the potential effects on the organism. There are lots of rodent models of allograft transplantation and numerous strategies have been used successfully to induce tolerance in these models.

Kidney transplantation is often used between MHC mismatched rodents [84, 85]. General physical condition is observed during all the experiments. Serum creatinine levels and urine quality are measured after transplantation to evaluate kidney activity. Generally, this graft is realized in different steps. First, ablation of one recipient kidney and allograft of MCH mismatched kidney. The transplanted organ is not immediately efficient. So, ablation of the second recipient's kidney is realized few days after transplantation. At this time, the recipient has only one transplanted kidney. If the kidney is rejected, the rodent dies because of blood toxicity.

Cardiac allograft in rodent is also a good model [86–90]. In this case, it is a heterotopic graft. Recipients keep its heart and receive a MHC-mismatched heart in the abdomen. The heart is connected to recipient blood circulation. Heart allograft survival is evaluated by palpation through the abdominal wall and scoring of its beating. Just after transplantation, heart beats strongly. But, if there is activation of the recipient immune system against alloantigens, the heart tissue is stiffened and beating are less intense and frequent until their full arrest. The major advantage of this model is that the recipient survives even if rejection occurred, and thus mechanisms can be analyzed.

But, sometimes, results obtained in rodent models could not be reproduced in larger animal models, such as non-human primates (NHPs) or swine. Rodents are too different from human to serve as preclinical models. Indeed, rodents have 90% similarity with human genome while there are around 99% similarity between NHP and human. Thus, NHPs constitute a more relevant animal transplant model. But, using NHPs is considerably more expansive and restrictive than rodents. Indeed, NHPs need more time for reproduction and development and more place than rodents. Moreover, all protocols conducted on animals have to be approved by an ethical comity. NHPs are ethically largely more controlled than rodents. So, first experiments are generally conducted on rodent models to generate primary results and conclusion. Then, a model with immune system more reflective of the human immune system is essential for testing protocols before moving into clinical studies.

This was the case for anti-CD40L treatment. All results obtained in rodents have demonstrated a great potential for induction of transplant tolerance. However, similar experiments in primate and human have highlighted a major barrier. Indeed, CD40L is a molecule expressed on NHPs, and human platelets. So this treatment resulted in thrombosis in NHPs and could not be used in the clinic [91, 92]. New anti-CD40L antibodies are being engineered as alternatives given the potential of this strategy in multiple diseases [93–95].

An alternative possibility that has been developed in the last decade is the engineering of mouse with humanized immune system in which various types of human cells are engrafted and functional [96, 97]. These mice harbor a complete null mutation of the IL-2 receptor gamma chain, NOD/SCID IL-2r γ^{null} (NSG), or Rag $2^{-/-}\gamma^{null}$ and are characterized by an impaired development and function of murine T, B and NK cells. These mice can efficiently support the development of a functional human hemato-lymphopoiesis. There are different protocols, more and more efficient, to induce humanization in highly deficient mice, such as injection of $CD34^{+}$ cells or PBMCs. Mice humanized with PBMCs represent the fastest model of graft versus host disease (GVHD), due to direct injection of adult PBMCs. Indeed, these models allow the analysis of human immunology *in vivo* [98, 99]. The mice are monitored for weight loss and tissue damages.

Another important model is skin transplantation [100–102]. It is possible to graft tailskin on the recipient lateral flank in rodent models. After removal of the bandage, grafts are observed to analyse their evolution. It's considered as rejected when skin dries and falls, indeed no viable skin remains. This strategy is even more relevant in humanized mice model [103]. In this case, mice are grafted with human skin obtained from abdominal surgery from patients. In this kind of model, skins are left to engraft at least 15 days before rejection is triggered by injection of allogeneic PBMCs.

3.2. Co-stimulation blockade

The aim of transplantation research is to exploit mechanisms of self-tolerance to generate specific tolerance after transplantation. One of the most promising approaches is to inhibit co-stimulatory pathways to abort activation of T cells following TCR engagement. T cells are an essential component of the immune response against allogenic cells inducing allograft rejection. Interaction between TCR and MHC/antigen induces the first signal of stimulation. But this alloantigen recognition only is not sufficient for complete T cell activation. Co-stimulatory signals generated by the interaction between antigen and T cells and cytokine stimulation are also necessary for complete immune system activation [104]. There are 4 different co-stimulation molecules families: immunoglobulins superfamily, TNF receptors, integrin family, and T-cell immunoglobulin and mucin-containing domain (TIM) family.

Blockade of costimulatory pathways has been considered as a good strategy for the prevention of allograft rejection in transplantation by aborting activation following TCR engagement [52, 105]. These strategies have been studied in mice, rat, and NHPs and induces allograft tolerance [106, 107]. Blockade of both CD28/B7 and CD40/CD40L co-stimulatory pathways induces long-term allograft survival. In the '90s, the first CTLA-4Ig soluble molecule was generated [108]. This molecule corresponds to the fusion between CTLA-4 extracellular domain and a modified IgG1 constant fragment domain [109]. CTLA-4Ig interaction with CD80-CD86 inhibits T-cell activation and prevents rejection of cardiac and renal allografts in rodent models [87, 108, 110] and prolongs survival of human islets xenograft in mice [111]. But CTLA-4Ig is not sufficient to induce tolerance because all allograft were finally rejected. Besides, when this treatment is combined with donor-specific transfusion (DST), allograft tolerance is obtained in heart allograft rodent models [105, 112]. DST corresponds to injection of donor splenocytes during transplantation and induces a state of chimerism. CD28 blockade show interesting results in rodent models, but this strategy is not efficient enough in NHP models [113]. Furthermore, it has been described that CTLA-4 is important for Tregs functions [114] and also for induction of tolerance to allograft [115, 116]. Thus, it would be more benefic to target CD28 molecule on T cell than CD80/CD86. Different groups have demonstrated that specific targeting of CD28 prevented rejection and generated Tregs [115, 117, 118]. FR104 has been developed in our laboratory as a costimulatory inhibitor that target CD28 without altering CD80/CD86 [119]. There are important differences between murine and human CD28 in terms of expression and interactions [120]. Thus, FR104 has been studied in NOD/SCID mice and NHP models. FR104 is safe *in vitro* and *in vivo* on human cells and does not play agonistic function on T cells [99]. This point is really important because another anti-CD28 molecule (TGN1412) studied in a phase 1 clinical trial induced important cytokine storm that caused life threatening effects [121].

CD40-CD40L blockade has also been studied for induction of transplantation tolerance. There are different strategies to block this pathway (monoclonal antibodies, CD40Ig). Treatment with monoclonal antibody anti-CD40L induces skin, renal, and cardiac allograft survival in mice [86, 122] and in NHP models [123, 124] but only with long-term repeated injections [123]. Some groups have shown that these monoclonal antibodies deplete activated T cells through cytotoxicity [125] and apoptosis [126], and induce Tregs [102]. These blockades of the CD40-CD40L pathway induce prolongation of allograft survival but without real allograft tolerance. Effect of anti-CD40L treatment has been improved by association with DST in islet graft in mice [127]. Different studies have demonstrated the importance of treatment associated with DST, such as anti-CD4, anti-thymocytes, or anti-CD40L [128–130]. Another strategy uses CD40Ig molecule as treatment in allograft models. Our team has demonstrated that treatment with CD40Ig molecule or gene transfer induces allograft acceptance in cardiac allograft rat models [131] mediated by $CD8^{+}CD45RC^{low}$ Tregs [132]. Several approaches use combined protocols. Indeed, anti-CD40L and CTLA-4Ig treatment synergies in heart and skin allograft in rodents [86, 101] and in renal allograft in NHPs [113].

ICOS-ICOSL pathway is another costimulatory pathway. ICOS presents around 40% similarity with CD28 and CTLA-4. ICOSL is constitutively expressed by B lymphocytes and monocytes and induced after T-cell activation [133]. Mice knocked out for ICOS have shown weak humoral responses [134–136]. ICOS-ICOSL blockade alone does not really induce significant effect on graft outcomes [137]. Therefore, our team have demonstrated that blockade of both ICOS-ICOSL and CD40-CD40L induce long-term heart allograft survival in rat model and decreases chronic rejection lesions [138]. During acute rejection, RANK and RANKL molecules are increased. Moreover, RANKL blockade induce long-term heart allograft survival in both rats and mice [139], and blockade effect is stronger when associated with CD40 pathway. PD1 is expressed by activated T lymphocytes, B and NK cells and macrophages, while PDL1 and PDL2 are expressed by activated APCs. PD-L1Ig alone does not improve allograft survival but synergizes with cyclosporine A, rapamycin, and anti-CD40L [140]. This pathway seems to play a role in the generation of some Tregs [141, 142].

3.3. Regulatory cells, crucial players in tolerance

In the context of organ transplantation, the findings of the last decades have put lights on regulatory cells as key players in the induction and maintenance of tolerance in organ transplantation. Although it has become evident that several distinct subsets of regulatory cells have the capacity to finely and tightly regulate the anti-donor immune responses in organ transplantation, one subset has attracted most of the research, the $CD4^{+}CD25^{high}CD127^{low}$Tregs, thanks to the identification of a crucial mastergene necessary for their development, identity, and function, the Foxp3 (Forkhead box P3) transcription factor [143–146].

3.3.1. Regulatory T cells (Tregs)

Tregs suppression of immune responses has been unravelled in the '70s [147]. Several subsets of Tregs have been evidenced including $CD4^{+}CD25^{high}CD127^{low}$ Tregs, but also $CD8^{+}$ Tregs, among them the $CD8^{+}CD45RC^{low}$ and $CD8^{+}CD28^{-}$ Tregs are the most known, $CD4^{-}CD8^{-}$ Tregs, NKT cells and γδ T cells. Tregs can further be subdivided in characteristics (phenotype, repertoire...) and potential in organ transplantation depending of their emergence from the thymus (nTregs) or from the periphery (iTregs). While nTregs developed as a distinct lineage in the thymus, iTregs can be generated from naive cells in the periphery and can be *in vitro* or *in vivo* induced in transplantation under some conditions such as donor-specific blood transfusion, blockade of the CD40/CD40L pathway, or donor MHC-derived peptides [148–150].

Since the identification of the CD25 and Foxp3 markers, several other markers have been proposed to better define Tregs, such as for $CD4^{+}$ Tregs glucocorticoid-induced tumor necrosis factor receptor family-related protein (GITR), CTLA-4, CD62L, CD103 (alpha beta integrin), LAG-3 and CD127 (alpha chain of the IL-7 receptor) [151–155]. For $CD8^{+}$ Tregs, the identification of relevant markers has been more difficult and several markers have been proposed such as CD122, CD28, CD45RC, CD103, and PD-1 [156–160]. A major discovery for Tregs biology was the identification of the Foxp3 and its role in $CD4^{+}$ Tregs development, identity and function [161, 162]. Mutations of the Foxp3 gene lead to a lymphoproliferative pathology in mice and an immune dysregulation polyendocrinopathy enteropathy X linked (IPEX) syndrome in human [163]. To date, this gene remains the best marker to identify $CD4^{+}$ Tregs, although in human it has been demonstrated that it can be transitory upregulated in T lymphocytes upon activation without providing regulatory capacity [164]. The Helios and neuropilin-1 (Nrp-1) markers have also been proposed to distinguish nTregs from iTregs, and also more recently as an important marker for $CD8^{+}$ Tregs identity and function [165–167]. Indeed, the Cantor group demonstrated that Helios was a key transcription factor that stabilizes $CD8^{+}$ Tregs in the context of an inflammatory response and that Helios-deficient Tregs developed an unstable phenotype (reduced Foxp3 and increased effector cytokines expression) during inflammatory responses. Antigen specificity has also been proposed to play an important role to distinguish Tregs origins [168]. Tregs originating from the thymus were selected for their specificity toward self-antigens, and thus are susceptible to be continuously stimulated by the self-antigens in periphery, potentially explaining their high expression of activation markers such as CD25, while iTregs generated by environmental conditions (inflammation, tolerance. . .) have a higher affinity toward exogenous antigens and thus are less stable once the antigens have been eliminated. In the context of organ transplantation, the antigens remain and we have demonstrated that $CD8^{+}CD45RC^{low}$ iTregs were maintained and stable for a long time [132, 150].

Tregs use different mechanisms to suppress anti-donor immune responses; they can mediate their activity through cell contact, cytokines secretion, or metabolic disturbance. Suppression through cell contact is mediated by the CTLA-4 and LAG-3 molecules expressed by Tregs. Interaction of CTLA-4 with B7 modulates CD80-86 expression by APCs and tryptophan catabolism in DCs, thus inhibiting T-cell activation [169]. Tregs can also induce effector cells apoptosis by cytolysis mediated by cell contact and secretion of cytotoxic molecules such as granzyme B and perforin [170]. Suppression through metabolic disturbance consists in the modification of the biochemical and cytokine environment, leading to target cell death. Adenosine triphosphate (ATP), cyclic-adenosine-monophosphate (cAMP), or IL-2 deprivation has been shown has strong inhibitor of cell proliferation [171, 172]. Finally, immunosuppressive cytokines play a major role in Treg-mediated suppression. IL-10, TGF-β, IL-34, IL-35, FGL-2, and IFNγ are all involved in $CD4^+$ and/or $CD8^+$ Tregs function [89, 159, 173, 174]. We have demonstrated that IFNγ production by $CD8^+CD45RC^{low}$ Tregs in a model of cardiac allograft tolerance in rat resulted in indoleamine 2,3-dioxygenase (IDO) expression by DCs and endothelial cells of the graft [159]. We have shown that $CD8^+CD45RC^{low}$ iTregs also produced high levels of FGL-2 [89] and IL-34 in rat and we have demonstrated that IL-34 is a cytokine that is specifically expressed by human $Foxp3^+$ $CD4^+$ and $CD8^+$ Tregs [173].

3.3.2. Other subsets of regulatory cells

Clinical and experimental observations have highlighted the role and potential of non–T cells with regulatory properties, defined as regulatory B cells (Bregs), tolerogenic dendritic cells (Tol-DCs), or regulatory macrophages (Mregs) or myeloid-derived suppressor cells (MDSCs) (nonexhaustive list) [89, 175–179].

The role of Bregs has been particularly investigated in allograft models of tolerance by our laboratory and in tolerant transplanted patients. In these patients, high levels of B lymphocytes and B markers have been observed, while these patients were tolerant and displayed an absence of donor-specific antibodies (DSAs) [3, 180, 181]. The phenotypic profile of Bregs remains unclear, in contrast to Tregs, although a few markers have been identified including CD1d, CD21, CD24, and IgM and it has been demonstrated that they mostly display an immature phenotype [182, 183]. A common feature of Bregs is their ability to secrete IL-10 and IL-35, two cytokines playing a major role in their activity and initially demonstrated in autoimmune diseases [184]. Other mechanisms of action resulting in Bregs activation and suppression involve their BCR engagement, cooperation with T lymphocytes, signaling via CD40/CD40L, TLR activation, IFNγ from tolerogenic DCs, or granzyme B secretion [185–189]. The engagement of their function results in inhibition of effector $CD4^+$ T-cell proliferation, Th1 differentiation, APCs function, and monocytes activation. In addition, Bregs have been shown as able to induce Tregs and NKT cells [177, 190]. In the context of transplantation, the role of Bregs has been proven in a model of cardiac allograft tolerance in mice treated with anti-CD45RB [191]. In our laboratory, we have demonstrated that IgM^+IgG^- B cells with a regulatory activity accumulated in the cardiac allograft of tolerant rat recipients and can adoptively transfer allograft tolerance to newly grafted recipients [183, 189]. We have shown that those Bregs had a partial defect in CD40 signaling and overexpressed granzyme B. In a similar model of cardiac allograft, we have demonstrated that administration of an adenovirus encoding fibroleukin-2 (FGL-2), a cytokine associated with Treg function, can induce tolerance to the allograft, thought generation of Bregs capable of infectious tolerance [89]. Finally, we have also demonstrated in a model of $CD8^+$ Treg-mediated CD40Ig-induced allograft tolerance, depletion of CD8$^+$ Tregs resulted in maintenance of long-term survival induction through generation of Bregs and RegMCs [176].

Although DCs are mostly known to be immunogenic; they also have the capacity to be tolerogenic. They play a major role in central and peripheral tolerance since they are involved in clonal deletion of autoreactive T lymphocytes in the thymus and correlate with an increased risk of autoimmune diseases and decreased presence of CD4$^+$ Tregs when depleted in periphery [192]. They are defined by their expression of tolerogenic molecules, such as IL-10, indoleamine 2,3-dioxygenase (IDO), TGF-β or heme-oxygenase 1 (HO-1), their low expression of immunostimulatory molecules, such as MHC molecules or CD80 and CD86, and in general their ability to generate Tregs and to inhibit effector T-cell responses. Their tolerogenic properties have been linked with their maturation, exposure to immunosuppressive, or anti-inflammatory treatments and their environment [193]. In the last year, a number of protocols have been developed to generate Tol-DCs as therapeutic tools to induce a specific tolerance to antigens in autoimmune diseases and transplantation, and our laboratory is involved in the first clinical trial in kidney transplanted patients using Tol-DCs in the context of a European "ONE STUDY" funding involving several centers [194, 195].

Initially, the focus was on the potential of immature conventional DCs (cDCs) expressing low levels of MHC and costimulatory molecules and their potential to induce transplant tolerance to a cardiac graft in mice [196, 197]. Our laboratory has demonstrated that autologous DC combination with suboptimal dose of immunosuppressive drugs induces long-term allograft survival in rat [198]. We have shown that they require TMEM176B, an intracellular protein identified in tolerant recipients, to cross-present donor antigens and induce Tregs and prolong allograft survival [199]. We have also shown that the molecule HO-1 can inhibit DC maturation, while preserving their production of IL-10, and thus leading to inhibition of pro-inflammatory and allogeneic immune responses [200].

Although their tolerogenic properties in transplantation are less well defined, the role of plasmacytoid DCs (pDCs) has been demonstrated for the regulation and the maintenance of bone marrow and organ transplantation [201]. As for cDCs, they can be immunogenic or tolerogenic according to their receptor engagement and maturation status. We have demonstrated their preferential interaction with CD8$^+$ Tregs in a model of cardiac allotransplantation in rat treated with CD40Ig resulting in the superior suppressive potential of CD8$^+$CD45RC^{low} Tregs [159, 202]. A group has shown their involvement in a model of cardiac allograft tolerance in mice treated with DST and anti-CD40L. In this model, pDCs induced tolerance through generation of alloantigen-specific CD4$^+$CD25$^+$Foxp3$^+$ Tregs [203] and depletion of pDCs inhibited Treg development and tolerance induction. In human, pDCs stimulated through certain of their TLR (toll like receptor) or costimulatory molecules efficiently induced CD4$^+$ and CD8$^+$ Tregs inhibiting *in vitro* allogeneic T-cell stimulation [204–206]. Liver-transplanted patients tolerating their allograft displayed significantly more pDCs and CD4$^+$ Tregs [207].

Finally, Tregs can generate tolerogenic DCs, by modifying molecules expression such as inducing tolerogenic molecules expression like IDO, ILT3 or ILT4, changing their function [208]. We have demonstrated in several models of allograft tolerance that DCs were essential for establishment and maintenance of allograft tolerance [202, 209–211].

In transplantation, although macrophages activation is often associated with allograft destruction and rejection in the early phases, the existence of an alternative population of Mregs contributing to tissue reparation, activated by Th2-type cytokine such as IL-4 and IL-13 and inhibiting pro-inflammatory cytokines secreted by macrophages [212]. Mregs can be induced by Treg interactions, Tregs depletions, and can even induce in turn Tregs via IL-10 secretion for example [213, 214]. The reduction of macrophages in mice receiving hematopoietic stem cells aggravated the GVHD, whereas expansion of macrophages with CSF-1 resulted in the opposite effect [215]. Mregs isolated from peripheral blood are characterized by their morphology, specific markers, although unstable, and their capacity to inhibit T-cell proliferation *in vitro* [216]. A clinical pilot study is administering donor-derived Mregs to kidney-transplanted patients, allowing graft survival under minimal immunosuppression one year following administration without clinical signs of graft rejection [217]. We and others have shown the potential of M-CSF and IL-34, two cytokines involved in monocytes survival and differentiation to induce Mregs *in vitro* and *in vivo* in human, mice, and rat transplantation models, and that those Mregs induced in turn Tregs capable of tolerance induction [173, 218].

MDSCs are a heterogeneous population of immature hematopoietic progenitor cells presenting numerous suppressive functions, including alloantigen tolerance induction in cardiac and islet allograft model in mice and kidney allograft in rat [219, 220].

3.4. Tipping the balance between effector and regulatory functions

Allograft outcome depends on the balance between effectors, which attack alloantigenic tissues, and regulators, which are essential for regulation/inhibition of alloresponses and induction of tolerance [221]. Induction of tolerance might be induced by the diminution of alloreactive T cells to allow Tregs to suppress the immune system activation. A large number of protocols have been studied with more or less efficacy.

Several approaches have been based on the expression amount of CD45 molecule on T cells allowing to distinguish effector and Tregs [222]. Strategies using monoclonal antibodies have been tested in animal models, notably in mice models of transplantation targeting CD45RB, as $CD4^{+}CD45RC^{high}$ T cells from untreated mice have been shown as capable of inducing colitis, diabetes, and thyroiditis [223]. In all cases where $CD4^{+}CD45RB^{high}$ T cells have been shown to cause autoimmunity, their counterpart $CD4^{+}CD45RB^{low}$ T cells have been shown to prevent the induction of the disease. Anti-CD45RB antibody (MB23G2) caused transitory decrease of circulating lymphocytes expressing CD45RB and induced allograft survival with normal kidney allograft function [85]. This antibody induces also upregulation of CTLA-4 on lymphocytes [224]. This treatment has been studied in kidney, pancreatic islets, and heart allograft models. Lazarovits et al. have studied two different CD45RB mAb (MB23G2 and MB4B4). They have shown that the nondepleting MB4B4 is therapeutically ineffective while MB23G2 depletes $CD45RB^{high}$ lymphocytes and induces renal and islets allograft tolerance in mice model [85, 225].

Tipping the balance to favor regulatory functions is an interesting alternative to effector cells depletion. In our laboratory, we have developed and demonstrated the efficacy of different therapeutic strategies to modify the balance in favor of regulatory functions, such as CD40Ig, anti-CD28 (FR104), HO-1, FGL-2, or IL-34, for example [55, 89, 131, 173, 226]. Our team studied CD40Ig treatment in a cardiac allograft rat model. We have demonstrated that this treatment induces long-term survival by generation of $CD8^{+}CD45RC^{low}$[131]. CD45RC has been shown in rats, mice, and humans to be a marker of both $CD4^{+}$ and $CD8^{+}$ Tregs [98, 102–106]. Moreover, this cell population is able to transfer infectious tolerance to naive transplanted rats[159]. Anti-CD28 is a good candidate to prevent rejection in the clinic [115, 231]. Zhang and al have shown that anti-CD28 inhibits lymphocytes activation and increases the proportion of cells expressing Foxp3 in the allograft. Our team and others have proved that treatment with anti-CD28 acts through the increase of the proportion of Tregs [117, 118, 178]. Actually, FR104 is the most known molecule targeting CD28. This humanized molecule has no agonist activity on human T cells *in vitro* and it does not induce cytokine storm in NOD/SCID mice reconstituted with human PBMCs. Moreover, Poirier and al have demonstrated the potential of FR104 in GVHD humanized mice model. They have also administrated FR104 to NHPs. Their results indicated a good tolerance in NHP and excluded cytokines release [99]. Several nondepleting antibodies, such as anti-CD4 and anti-CD8 mAb, are efficient to induce tolerance [232] and have permitted the first proof of the possibility of infectious tolerance [233]. Moreover, different strategies should be combined to improve their effects. Indeed, anti-CD45RB mAb and anti-CD40L mAb synergized and improved long-term allograft survival in islets and skin allografts [234].

All these examples confirm the importance of the balance between effector and regulatory cells for graft outcome.

4. From the bench to the clinic

Regulatory cells are essential for tolerance in transplantation. Many animal models have highlighted the potential of such tools for preventing allograft rejection and GVHD development. Their human counterparts are a promising issue for following immune status and inducing tolerance in transplanted patients.

4.1. New biomarkers for a real-time adapted treatment

A biomarker is "a characteristic that is objectively measured and evaluated as an indicator of normal biological processes, pathogenic processes, or pharmacologic responses to a therapeutic intervention" [235]. Nowadays, the reliability of the prognosis to predict allograft survival/ rejection is low. For pancreas and liver transplantation, the measurement of lipase/amylase and liver enzymes respectively is recommended as routine post transplantation monitoring. The monitoring of cardiac enzymes is not recommended because of the poor sensitivity of these markers in the diagnosis of acute rejection, thus patients have to suffer endomyocardial biopsies 15 times during the first year after transplantation [236]. Echocardiography, diastolic function analysis, and quantitative measurement of changes of the transverse relaxation time T2 in the myocardium by magnetic resonance imaging are considered to improve cardiac allograft rejection prediction [237]. For renal allograft, the prognosis is generally based on creatinemia evolution and glomerular filtration. This prediction can be improved by calculating the kidney transplant failure score (KTFS) considering not only the creatinemia at 3 and 12 months post graft, but also the proteinuria at 12 months, the number of previous transplantations, the age and sex of the donor, the creatinemia of the donor at the harvesting time, and the incidence of an acute graft rejection in first year post transplantation [238].

Noncompliant patients spontaneously developing an operational tolerance to their graft are useful to identify new biomarkers and adapt in real time the care of patients. By comparing phenotypes of cells and cytokines from tolerant patients with healthy volunteers and patients rejecting their graft, we should be able to identify markers correlating with the immune status toward the graft. However, studies are limited to blood and urine analysis because of the ethical question of performing a biopsy of a tolerated graft. Kidney-grafted spontaneous operational tolerant patients are defined as having ceased all immunosuppressive drugs for more than one year, with no increase in serum creatinine during the last 12 months (CRT < 10%). Using microarray analysis, Brouard, Newell, and Sagoo compared genes differentially expressed in tolerant recipients with patients exhibiting chronic rejection [181, 239, 240]. Tolerant patients showed a reduction of activation markers of proinflammatory T cells, a down-regulation of pro-inflammatory cytokines [239], a GATA3 upregulation suggesting a Th2 deviation [241], and an increase in $CD4^{+}CD45RA^{-}Foxp3^{hi}$ memory Tregs versus patients with chronic rejection [3, 242, 243]. Interestingly, the three distinct studies and cohorts converge also with an increase of B cells in blood and CD20 transcript in urine in tolerant patients [180, 181, 240]. However, the phenotype of B cells named Bregs they described diverges [180, 181, 240, 244]. In liver-grafted spontaneous operational tolerant patients, higher numbers of $CD4^{+}CD25^{+}CD127^{-}$ T cells, $V\delta1^{+}$ T cells, and NK cells were detected [245, 246].

The heterogeneity of treatments, in terms of dose and type of immunosuppressors administered to patients during chronic rejection episodes, and the heterogeneity of the parameters selected to monitor regulatory cells activity in the recent trials, prevents comparison of the results. To define general tolerance signatures, consortiums as The ONE Study and EU COST Action "BM1305: action to focus and accelerate cell-based tolerance-inducing therapies," standardized immune monitoring of patients included in clinical trial [247]. Six panels of 7–9 markers designed are now standardized within 8 international laboratories to monitor T cells, B cells, and DCs [247].

Newly described cytokines associated with regulatory cells should be considered as prognostic markers. Recently, IL-34 has been closely associated with Tregs and M2 macrophages [173]. FGL2, produced by Tregs and generating Bregs, could also reflecting immune status of the graft [248]. Furthermore, nucleic acid analysis suggests new biomarkers for allograft rejection, such as donor-derived cell-free DNA (ddcfDNA) [249], OX40 [250], OX40L [250], PD-1 [250], Foxp3 [250] mRNA levels in urinary cells, and A20 [251], HO-1 [251], granzyme B [251], perforin [251], and Tim-3 mRNA [252] in both urinary cells and PBLs.

4.2. From patients observation to action

Many immunosuppressive drugs were developed these last decades. By targeting many cell types at different levels/pathways, their association largely contains the immune responses against the allograft. Briefly, glucocorticoids and calcineurin inhibitors (ciclosporin, tacrolimus) inhibit cytokine transcription in T lymphocytes and macrophages; mTOR inhibitors (rapamycin, everolimus [253]) inhibit expression of costimulatory molecules on APCs and T lymphocytes proliferation; cytostatics (cyclosphosphamide, methotrexate, azathioprine) and purines inhibitors (mycophenolate mofetil) inhibit T and B cell divisions; antibodies targeting thymocytes (ATG, thymoglobulin), CD3 or CD52 (Campath-1H) deplete T lymphocytes, CD25 (basiliximab, daclizumab) inhibit T lymphocytes activation, and CD20 (rituximab) and CD52 deplete B lymphocytes; sphingosine 1 phosphate inhibitor FTY720 (Fingolimod) retain lymphocytes in lymphoid organs and decrease their circulation in blood; efalizumab inhibits LFA-1 functions. However, drawbacks and side effects they induce are still unresolved.

The identification of new immunoregulatory mediators and the recent findings regarding regulatory cells over-represented in tolerant patients whereas lacking in graft-rejecting ones suggest new therapeutic strategies to control the immune balance. Several cytokines and antibodies have shown promising results in animal models. It has recently been shown that the cytokine IL-34 is able to induce Tregs through conversion of regulatory macrophages [173]. Similarly, FGL2 can induce Bregs [248]. In addition, antibodies blocking costimulatory pathway like CD28 antagonist (FR104) or antibodies targeting TCR-associated signaling (CD45RC [254]) or DR3 [255] marker seem efficient to decrease T-cell function whereas promoting Tregs [55, 99, 256]. The promotion of regulatory cells is likely to induce lower drawback than classical broad-spectrum drugs.

Immunoregulatory cell therapy may be able to support peripheral tolerance and aims to induce a donor-specific unresponsiveness. This personalized method consists in harvesting blood cells from a patient, isolating and expanding *ex vivo* regulatory cells before re-infusing them to the patient in order to control allogeneic response against the graft in solid organ transplantation, or to control allogeneic response against the recipient infused with hematopoietic stem cells (HSCT) to avoid a GVHD reactions.

The first clinical trial was realized in 2009 by Trzonkowski et al, using 10^5 Tregs/kg expanded $CD4^+CD25^+CD127^-$ Tregs to reduce chronic GVHD symptoms [257]. In 2011, Brunstein began a phase I clinical trial and to date showed that until 3×10^6 expanded Tregs would be safe and efficient to reduce the incidence of grade II–IV aGVHD [258]. The same year, Di anni showed that freshly purified $CD4^+CD25^+$ Tregs counteracts the GVHD potential of a high number of donor Tcons in HLA-haploidentical HSCT [259]. In 2014, Martelli confirmed in a phase II clinical trial that co-infusion of freshly purified $CD4^+CD25^+$ Tregs significantly reduces GVHD incidence without affecting GVL (graft versus leukemia) effect [260]. In 2014, Bacchetta infused 10^5 donor T lymphocytes pretreated with IL-10/kg into recipient of HSCT and showed the protective effect of TR1 cells against GVHD [261]. Whereas these first clinical studies focused on Tregs in HSCT, several alternative regulatory cell types have been identified as potential sources for immunotherapies in solid organ transplantation. The EU-funded international ONE study consortium considers several immunoregulatory cell-based therapies for clinical management of solid organ transplant recipients and shares a common clinical protocol design. The ONE Study project titled "A Unified Approach to Evaluating Cellular Immunotherapy in Solid Organ Transplantation" aims to compare the feasibility and the potential of cell therapy by using MDSCs, Mregs, DC-10, Tol-DCs [262], rapa-DCs, monocytes conditioned with mesenchymal stem cells [263], Tr1 [264], and $CD4^+$ Tregs [265]. $CD8^+$ Tregs are now approaching clinical tests [266–268] and Bregs are also considered as a tool for cell therapy [269].

Success of cell therapy to control allogeneic immune responses against the donor depends on regulatory properties of cells and on the number of regulatory cells infused into the recipient. Based on animal models and preclinical models of humanized mice, about 7 to 11×10^8 Tregs/kg would be necessary to control allogeneic response [270]. However, we have to consider the *in vivo* proliferation of Tregs after infusion [271]. Thus, the maximal infusible dose approved by The ONE Study for safety is 10^7 Tregs/kg [265]. Nowadays, Tregs from patients can be 100 to 1000 fold short-term expanded *ex vivo* while keeping their suppressive properties [272–274].

Importantly, clinical protocols also consider specificity of therapeutic cells against the graft donor. Indeed, antigen-specific Tregs have been shown more efficient in inhibiting anti-donor immune response [275]. The frequency of direct alloreactive Tregs has been estimated to 1–10% of total Tregs [276]. Injecting more donor-specific cells would amount to inject fewer cells, and to reduce nonspecific unwanted drawbacks. For Tang and Bluestone, the effect induced by 5×10^9 polyclonal $CD4^+$ Tregs would be equivalent to the effect induced by 1.5×10^8 to 1×10^9 allogeneic Tregs [277]. That is why processes have been developed to expand Tregs specifically with APCs or antigen derived from the HLA donor. Indeed, $CD4^+$ Tregs expanded with donor DCs or B cells, or by indirect presentation of donor cell lysate antigen onto recipient APCs [276], showed a higher suppressive activity compared to polyclonally expanded Tregs [275, 278–280]. Similar protocols were used to generate donor-specific $CD8^+$ Tregs [266]. Whereas TCR repertoire of donor APCs-expanded Tregs is still diverse, Tregs relatively efficiently reduce alloreactive T cell response without compromising general immunity according to mice models [266, 279]. Based on their capacity of infectious tolerance, Ag-specific Tregs can exert dominant tolerance to alloantigen *in vivo* by inducing regulatory properties in alloreactive T cells [281]. The identification of a unique shared peptide is of crucial interest today. Tregs with a unique antigen specificity can also be isolated and then expanded for cell therapy [282], or selected during the expansion by indirect presentation of one peptide [150, 267, 283]. Genetic engineering used to confer a TCR specificity to lymphocytes to redirect T cells in cancer immunotherapy [284, 285] offers new possibilities to obtain Tregs with an artificial specificity toward the graft donor Ag.

As cells will be re-infuse into the patient, all reagents used to culture cells have to be validated for "clinical grade," and after expansion, cells are analyzed for purity and stability. Tregs are phenotypically characterized for expression of helios [167], DNA methylation status of the TSDR (Treg specific demethylated region) [286], while Foxp3 expression is no more sufficient [287], and tested in *in vitro* suppression assay.

Cell therapy strategy would allow reducing the use of conventional immunosuppression in organ transplant recipients; nevertheless, clinical trials are rarely totally free of drugs for patients' safety. This could affect regulatory cells survival and functions. Indeed, tacrolimus, mycophenolate mofetil (MMF), and methylprednisolone do not affect phenotype, function, or stability of Tregs, but reduce their proliferative capacity, whereas rapamycin did not [288–290]. Moreover, rapamycin is sometimes used to maintain regulatory properties of Tregs during expansion culture and also to convert conventional $CD4^+$ T cells into Tregs *ex vivo* [291].

By targeting upstream IL-2 synthesis, cyclosporine A compromises the homeostatic behaviour of CD4$^+$ Tregs in peripheral immune compartments [292]. On the contrary, FTY720 synergizes with rapamycin for the conversion of CD4$^+$ Tregs [293]. Thus, the choice of drugs combined with cell therapy has to be considered.

5. Conclusion

Research in transplantation has made considerable progresses improving transplantation outcomes, but important obstacles remain. Induction of tolerance is considered as the key to reduce the impact of toxic side effects of general immunosuppressive drugs. Better definition of immune tolerance mechanisms in human should lead to a better understanding of the potential effects of targeting strategies.

Author details

Laetitia Boucault, Séverine Bézie, Jason Ossart and Carole Guillonneau*

*Address all correspondence to: carole.guillonneau@univ-nantes.fr

INSERM UMR1064, Center for Research in Transplantation and Immunology-ITUN, Nantes University Hospital, Medicine University, University of Nantes, France

References

[1] Marcén R. Immunosuppressive drugs in kidney transplantation: impact on patient survival, and incidence of cardiovascular disease, malignancy and infection. Drugs 2009;69(16):2227–43.

[2] Ashton-Chess J, Giral M, Brouard S, Soulillou J-P. Spontaneous operational tolerance after immunosuppressive drug withdrawal in clinical renal allotransplantation. Transplantation 2007;84(10):1215–9.

[3] Sagoo P, Perucha E, Sawitzki B, Tomiuk S, Stephens DA, Miqueu P, et al. Development of a cross-platform biomarker signature to detect renal transplant tolerance in humans. J Clin Invest. 2010;120(6):1848–61.

[4] Porter KA. Morphological aspects of renal homograft rejection. Br Med Bull. 1965;21:171–5.

[5] Kissmeyer-Nielsen F, Olsen S, Petersen VP, Fjeldborg O. Hyperacute rejection of kidney allografts, associated with pre-existing humoral antibodies against donor cells. Lancet 1966;2(7465):662–5.

[6] Halloran PF, Wadgymar A, Ritchie S, Falk J, Solez K, Srinivasa NS. The significance of the anti-class I antibody response. I. Clinical and pathologic features of anti-class I-mediated rejection. Transplantation 1990;49(1):85–91.

[7] Halloran PF, Schlaut J, Solez K, Srinivasa NS. The significance of the anti-class I response. II. Clinical and pathologic features of renal transplants with anti-class I-like antibody. Transplantation 1992;53(3):550–5.

[8] Lechler RI, Batchelor JR. Restoration of immunogenicity to passenger cell-depleted kidney allografts by the addition of donor strain dendritic cells. J Exp Med. 1982;155(1): 31–41.

[9] Hippen BE, DeMattos A, Cook WJ, Kew CE, Gaston RS. Association of CD20+ infiltrates with poorer clinical outcomes in acute cellular rejection of renal allografts. Am J Transplant Off J Am Soc Transplant Am Soc Transpl Surg. 2005;5(9):2248–52.

[10] Nankivell BJ, Kuypers DRJ. Diagnosis and prevention of chronic kidney allograft loss. Lancet Lond Engl. 2011;378(9800):1428–37.

[11] Zhang Q, Reed EF. Non-MHC antigenic targets of the humoral immune response in transplantation. Curr Opin Immunol. 2010;22(5):682–8.

[12] Larsen CP, Morris PJ, Austyn JM. Migration of dendritic leukocytes from cardiac allografts into host spleens. A novel pathway for initiation of rejection. J Exp Med. 1990;171(1):307–14.

[13] Kreisel D, Krupnick AS, Balsara KR, Riha M, Gelman AE, Popma SH, et al. Mouse vascular endothelium activates CD8+ T lymphocytes in a B7-dependent fashion. J Immunol Baltim Md 1950. 2002;169(11):6154–61.

[14] Celli S, Albert ML, Bousso P. Visualizing the innate and adaptive immune responses underlying allograft rejection by two-photon microscopy. Nat Med. 2011;17(6):744–9.

[15] He C, Heeger PS. CD8 T cells can reject major histocompatibility complex class I-deficient skin allografts. Am J Transplant Off J Am Soc Transplant Am Soc Transpl Surg. 2004;4(5):698–704.

[16] Joffre OP, Segura E, Savina A, Amigorena S. Cross-presentation by dendritic cells. Nat Rev Immunol. 2012;12(8):557–69.

[17] Steele DJ, Laufer TM, Smiley ST, Ando Y, Grusby MJ, Glimcher LH, et al. Two levels of help for B cell alloantibody production. J Exp Med. 1996;183(2):699–703.

[18] Auchincloss H, Lee R, Shea S, Markowitz JS, Grusby MJ, Glimcher LH. The role of "indirect" recognition in initiating rejection of skin grafts from major histocompatibility complex class II-deficient mice. Proc Natl Acad Sci U S A 1993;90(8):3373–7.

[19] Morón G, Dadaglio G, Leclerc C. New tools for antigen delivery to the MHC class I pathway. Trends Immunol. 2004;25(2):92–7.

[20] Fluck N, Witzke O, Morris PJ, Wood KJ. Indirect allorecognition is involved in both acute and chronic allograft rejection. Transplant Proc. 1999;31(1–2):842–3.

[21] Dalchau R, Fangmann J, Fabre JW. Allorecognition of isolated, denatured chains of class I and class II major histocompatibility complex molecules. Evidence for an important role for indirect allorecognition in transplantation. Eur J Immunol. 1992;22(3):669–77.

[22] Issa F, Schiopu A, Wood KJ. Role of T cells in graft rejection and transplantation tolerance. Expert Rev Clin Immunol. 2010;6(1):155–69.

[23] Herrera OB, Golshayan D, Tibbott R, Salcido Ochoa F, James MJ, Marelli-Berg FM, et al. A novel pathway of alloantigen presentation by dendritic cells. J Immunol Baltim Md 1950. 2004;173(8):4828–37.

[24] Jiang S, Herrera O, Lechler RI. New spectrum of allorecognition pathways: implications for graft rejection and transplantation tolerance. Curr Opin Immunol. 2004;16(5):550–7.

[25] Brown K, Sacks SH, Wong W. Coexpression of donor peptide/recipient MHC complex and intact donor MHC: evidence for a link between the direct and indirect pathways. Am J Transplant Off J Am Soc Transplant Am Soc Transpl Surg. 2011;11(4):826–31.

[26] Huesmann M, Scott B, Kisielow P, von Boehmer H. Kinetics and efficacy of positive selection in the thymus of normal and T cell receptor transgenic mice. Cell 1991;66(3):533–40.

[27] Merkenschlager M, Graf D, Lovatt M, Bommhardt U, Zamoyska R, Fisher AG. How many thymocytes audition for selection? J Exp Med. 1997;186(7):1149–58.

[28] Cosgrove D, Chan SH, Waltzinger C, Benoist C, Mathis D. The thymic compartment responsible for positive selection of CD4+ T cells. Int Immunol. 1992;4(6):707–10.

[29] Laufer TM, DeKoning J, Markowitz JS, Lo D, Glimcher LH. Unopposed positive selection and autoreactivity in mice expressing class II MHC only on thymic cortex. Nature 1996;383(6595):81–5.

[30] Capone M, Romagnoli P, Beermann F, MacDonald HR, van Meerwijk JP. Dissociation of thymic positive and negative selection in transgenic mice expressing major histocompatibility complex class I molecules exclusively on thymic cortical epithelial cells. Blood 2001;97(5):1336–42.

[31] Anderson MS, Venanzi ES, Klein L, Chen Z, Berzins SP, Turley SJ, et al. Projection of an immunological self shadow within the thymus by the aire protein. Science 2002;298(5597):1395–401.

[32] Gallegos AM, Bevan MJ. Central tolerance to tissue-specific antigens mediated by direct and indirect antigen presentation. J Exp Med. 2004;200(8):1039–49.

[33] Hinterberger M, Aichinger M, Prazeres da Costa O, Voehringer D, Hoffmann R, Klein L. Autonomous role of medullary thymic epithelial cells in central CD4(+) T cell tolerance. Nat Immunol. 2010;11(6):512–9.

[34] Koble C, Kyewski B. The thymic medulla: a unique microenvironment for intercellular self-antigen transfer. J Exp Med. 2009;206(7):1505–13.

[35] Liu GY, Fairchild PJ, Smith RM, Prowle JR, Kioussis D, Wraith DC. Low avidity recognition of self-antigen by T cells permits escape from central tolerance. Immunity 1995;3(4):407–15.

[36] Klein L, Klugmann M, Nave KA, Tuohy VK, Kyewski B. Shaping of the autoreactive T-cell repertoire by a splice variant of self protein expressed in thymic epithelial cells. Nat Med. 2000;6(1):56–61.

[37] Bouneaud C, Kourilsky P, Bousso P. Impact of negative selection on the T cell repertoire reactive to a self-peptide: a large fraction of T cell clones escapes clonal deletion. Immunity 2000;13(6):829–40.

[38] Walker LSK, Abbas AK. The enemy within: keeping self-reactive T cells at bay in the periphery. Nat Rev Immunol. 2002;2(1):11–9.

[39] Ohashi PS, Oehen S, Buerki K, Pircher H, Ohashi CT, Odermatt B, et al. Ablation of "tolerance" and induction of diabetes by virus infection in viral antigen transgenic mice. Cell 1991;65(2):305–17.

[40] Kurts C, Miller JF, Subramaniam RM, Carbone FR, Heath WR. Major histocompatibility complex class I-restricted cross-presentation is biased towards high dose antigens and those released during cellular destruction. J Exp Med. 1998;188(2):409–14.

[41] Dhein J, Walczak H, Bäumler C, Debatin KM, Krammer PH. Autocrine T-cell suicide mediated by APO-1/(Fas/CD95). Nature 1995;373(6513):438–41.

[42] Rieux-Laucat F, Le Deist F, Hivroz C, Roberts IA, Debatin KM, Fischer A, et al. Mutations in Fas associated with human lymphoproliferative syndrome and autoimmunity. Science 1995;268(5215):1347–9.

[43] Ferber I, Schönrich G, Schenkel J, Mellor AL, Hämmerling GJ, Arnold B. Levels of peripheral T cell tolerance induced by different doses of tolerogen. Science 1994;263(5147):674–6.

[44] Förster I, Hirose R, Arbeit JM, Clausen BE, Hanahan D. Limited capacity for tolerization of CD4+ T cells specific for a pancreatic beta cell neo-antigen. Immunity 1995;2(6):573–85.

[45] Alexander-Miller MA, Leggatt GR, Sarin A, Berzofsky JA. Role of antigen, CD8, and cytotoxic T lymphocyte (CTL) avidity in high dose antigen induction of apoptosis of effector CTL. J Exp Med. 1996;184(2):485–92.

[46] Rathmell JC, Townsend SE, Xu JC, Flavell RA, Goodnow CC. Expansion or elimination of B cells in vivo: dual roles for CD40- and Fas (CD95)-ligands modulated by the B cell antigen receptor. Cell 1996;87(2):319–29.

[47] Russell DM, Dembić Z, Morahan G, Miller JF, Bürki K, Nemazee D. Peripheral deletion of self-reactive B cells. Nature 1991;354(6351):308–11.

[48] Cyster JG, Hartley SB, Goodnow CC. Competition for follicular niches excludes self-reactive cells from the recirculating B-cell repertoire. Nature 1994;371(6496):389–95.

[49] Jenkins MK, Schwartz RH. Antigen presentation by chemically modified splenocytes induces antigen-specific T cell unresponsiveness in vitro and in vivo. J Exp Med. 1987;165(2):302–19.

[50] Schwartz RH. A cell culture model for T lymphocyte clonal anergy. Science 1990;248(4961):1349–56.

[51] Schwartz RH. T cell anergy. Annu Rev Immunol. 2003;21:305–34.

[52] Schwartz RH. T cell anergy. Annu Rev Immunol. 2003;21:305–34.

[53] Greenfield EA, Nguyen KA, Kuchroo VK. CD28/B7 costimulation: a review. Crit Rev Immunol. 1998;18(5):389–418.

[54] Zheng Y, Manzotti CN, Liu M, Burke F, Mead KI, Sansom DM. CD86 and CD80 differentially modulate the suppressive function of human regulatory T cells. J Immunol Baltim Md 1950. 2004;172(5):2778–84.

[55] Poirier N, Azimzadeh AM, Zhang T, Dilek N, Mary C, Nguyen B, et al. Inducing CTLA-4-dependent immune regulation by selective CD28 blockade promotes regulatory T cells in organ transplantation. Sci Transl Med. 2010;2(17):17ra10.

[56] Walunas TL, Lenschow DJ, Bakker CY, Linsley PS, Freeman GJ, Green JM, et al. CTLA-4 can function as a negative regulator of T cell activation. Immunity 1994;1(5):405–13.

[57] Wood KJ, Goto R. Mechanisms of rejection: current perspectives. Transplantation 2012;93(1):1–10.

[58] Chikuma S, Terawaki S, Hayashi T, Nabeshima R, Yoshida T, Shibayama S, et al. PD-1-mediated suppression of IL-2 production induces CD8+ T cell anergy in vivo. J Immunol Baltim Md 1950. 2009;182(11):6682–9.

[59] Hollenbaugh D, Mischel-Petty N, Edwards CP, Simon JC, Denfeld RW, Kiener PA, et al. Expression of functional CD40 by vascular endothelial cells. J Exp Med. 1995;182(1): 33–40.

[60] McLellan AD, Sorg RV, Williams LA, Hart DN. Human dendritic cells activate T lymphocytes via a CD40: CD40 ligand-dependent pathway. Eur J Immunol. 1996;26(6): 1204–10.

[61] Inwald DP, McDowall A, Peters MJ, Callard RE, Klein NJ. CD40 is constitutively expressed on platelets and provides a novel mechanism for platelet activation. Circ Res. 2003;92(9):1041–8.

[62] Kehry MR. CD40-mediated signaling in B cells. Balancing cell survival, growth, and death. J Immunol Baltim Md 1950. 1996;156(7):2345–8.

[63] Ludewig B, Henn V, Schröder JM, Graf D, Kroczek RA. Induction, regulation, and function of soluble TRAP (CD40 ligand) during interaction of primary CD4+ CD45RA + T cells with dendritic cells. Eur J Immunol. 1996;26(12):3137–43.

[64] Gauchat JF, Henchoz S, Fattah D, Mazzei G, Aubry JP, Jomotte T, et al. CD40 ligand is functionally expressed on human eosinophils. Eur J Immunol. 1995;25(3):863–5.

[65] Pinchuk LM, Klaus SJ, Magaletti DM, Pinchuk GV, Norsen JP, Clark EA. Functional CD40 ligand expressed by human blood dendritic cells is up-regulated by CD40 ligation. J Immunol Baltim Md 1950. 1996;157(10):4363–70.

[66] Mach F, Schönbeck U, Sukhova GK, Bourcier T, Bonnefoy JY, Pober JS, et al. Functional CD40 ligand is expressed on human vascular endothelial cells, smooth muscle cells, and macrophages: implications for CD40-CD40 ligand signaling in atherosclerosis. Proc Natl Acad Sci U S A. 1997;94(5):1931–6.

[67] Grammer AC, Bergman MC, Miura Y, Fujita K, Davis LS, Lipsky PE. The CD40 ligand expressed by human B cells costimulates B cell responses. J Immunol Baltim Md 1950. 1995;154(10):4996–5010.

[68] Grewal IS, Flavell RA. The role of CD40 ligand in costimulation and T-cell activation. Immunol Rev. 1996;153:85–106.

[69] Peng X, Kasran A, Warmerdam PA, de Boer M, Ceuppens JL. Accessory signaling by CD40 for T cell activation: induction of Th1 and Th2 cytokines and synergy with interleukin-12 for interferon-gamma production. Eur J Immunol. 1996;26(7):1621–7.

[70] Barrett TB, Shu G, Clark EA. CD40 signaling activates CD11a/CD18 (LFA-1)-mediated adhesion in B cells. J Immunol Baltim Md 1950. 1991;146(6):1722–9.

[71] Vendetti S, Chai JG, Dyson J, Simpson E, Lombardi G, Lechler R. Anergic T cells inhibit the antigen-presenting function of dendritic cells. J Immunol Baltim Md 1950. 2000;165(3):1175–81.

[72] Buer J, Lanoue A, Franzke A, Garcia C, von Boehmer H, Sarukhan A. Interleukin 10 secretion and impaired effector function of major histocompatibility complex class II-restricted T cells anergized in vivo. J Exp Med. 1998;187(2):177–83.

[73] Chai JG, Bartok I, Scott D, Dyson J, Lechler R. T:T antigen presentation by activated murine CD8+ T cells induces anergy and apoptosis. J Immunol Baltim Md 1950. 1998;160(8):3655–65.

[74] Gauld SB, Benschop RJ, Merrell KT, Cambier JC. Maintenance of B cell anergy requires constant antigen receptor occupancy and signaling. Nat Immunol. 2005;6(11):1160–7.

[75] Bradley LM, Asensio VC, Schioetz LK, Harbertson J, Krahl T, Patstone G, et al. Islet-specific Th1, but not Th2, cells secrete multiple chemokines and promote rapid induction of autoimmune diabetes. J Immunol Baltim Md 1950. 1999;162(5):2511–20.

[76] Young DA, Lowe LD, Booth SS, Whitters MJ, Nicholson L, Kuchroo VK, et al. IL-4, IL-10, IL-13, and TGF-beta from an altered peptide ligand-specific Th2 cell clone down-regulate adoptive transfer of experimental autoimmune encephalomyelitis. J Immunol Baltim Md 1950. 2000;164(7):3563–72.

[77] Karczewski J, Karczewski M, Glyda M, Wiktorowicz K. Role of TH1/TH2 cytokines in kidney allograft rejection. Transplant Proc. 2008;40(10):3390–2.

[78] Yin H, Li X-Y, Jin X-B, Zhang B-B, Gong Q, Yang H, et al. IL-33 prolongs murine cardiac allograft survival through induction of TH2-type immune deviation. Transplantation 2010;89(10):1189–97.

[79] Amarnath S, Chen H, Foley JE, Costanzo CM, Sennesh JD, Solomon MA, et al. Host-based Th2 cell therapy for prolongation of cardiac allograft viability. PLoS One 2011;6(4):e18885.

[80] Zhang D, Sanchez-Fueyo A, Kawamoto K, Alexopoulos SP, Zhang W, Zheng XX. Th1 to Th2 immune deviation facilitates, but does not cause, islet allograft tolerance in mice. Cytokine 2010;51(3):311–9.

[81] Xie A, Wang S, Zhang K, Wang G, Ye P, Li J, et al. Treatment with interleukin-12/23p40 antibody attenuates acute cardiac allograft rejection. Transplantation 2011;91(1):27–34.

[82] Franchimont D. Overview of the actions of glucocorticoids on the immune response: a good model to characterize new pathways of immunosuppression for new treatment strategies. Ann N Y Acad Sci. 2004;1024:124–37.

[83] Libetta C, Sepe V, Zucchi M, Portalupi V, Meloni F, Rampino T, et al. The effect of sirolimus- or cyclosporine-based immunosuppression effects on T-cell subsets in vivo. Kidney Int. 2007;72(1):114–20.

[84] Sayegh MH, Akalin E, Hancock WW, Russell ME, Carpenter CB, Linsley PS, et al. CD28-B7 blockade after alloantigenic challenge in vivo inhibits Th1 cytokines but spares Th2. J Exp Med. 1995;181(5):1869–74.

[85] Lazarovits AI, Poppema S, Zhang Z, Khandaker M, Le Feuvre CE, Singhal SK, et al. Prevention and reversal of renal allograft rejection by antibody against CD45RB. Nature 1996;380(6576):717–20.

[86] Hancock WW, Sayegh MH, Zheng XG, Peach R, Linsley PS, Turka LA. Costimulatory function and expression of CD40 ligand, CD80, and CD86 in vascularized murine cardiac allograft rejection. Proc Natl Acad Sci U S A. 1996;93(24):13967–72.

[87] Baliga P, Chavin KD, Qin L, Woodward J, Lin J, Linsley PS, et al. CTLA4Ig prolongs allograft survival while suppressing cell-mediated immunity. Transplantation 1994;58(10):1082–90.

[88] Chen L, Wang T, Zhou P, Ma L, Yin D, Shen J, et al. TLR engagement prevents transplantation tolerance. Am J Transplant Off J Am Soc Transplant Am Soc Transpl Surg. 2006;6(10):2282–91.

[89] Bézie S, Picarda E, Tesson L, Renaudin K, Durand J, Ménoret S, et al. Fibrinogen-like protein 2/fibroleukin induces long-term allograft survival in a rat model through regulatory B cells. PloS One 2015;10(3):e0119686.

[90] Lin H, Bolling SF, Linsley PS, Wei RQ, Gordon D, Thompson CB, et al. Long-term acceptance of major histocompatibility complex mismatched cardiac allografts induced by CTLA4Ig plus donor-specific transfusion. J Exp Med. 1993;178(5):1801–6.

[91] Kawai T, Andrews D, Colvin RB, Sachs DH, Cosimi AB. Thromboembolic complications after treatment with monoclonal antibody against CD40 ligand. Nat Med. 2000;6(2):114.

[92] Boumpas DT, Furie R, Manzi S, Illei GG, Wallace DJ, Balow JE, et al. A short course of BG9588 (anti-CD40 ligand antibody) improves serologic activity and decreases hematuria in patients with proliferative lupus glomerulonephritis. Arthritis Rheum. 2003;48(3):719–27.

[93] Shock A, Burkly L, Wakefield I, Peters C, Garber E, Ferrant J, et al. CDP7657, an anti-CD40L antibody lacking an Fc domain, inhibits CD40L-dependent immune responses without thrombotic complications: an in vivo study. Arthritis Res Ther. 2015;17:234.

[94] Tocoian A, Buchan P, Kirby H, Soranson J, Zamacona M, Walley R, et al. First-in-human trial of the safety, pharmacokinetics and immunogenicity of a PEGylated anti-CD40L antibody fragment (CDP7657) in healthy individuals and patients with systemic lupus erythematosus. Lupus 2015;24(10):1045–56.

[95] Xie JH, Yamniuk AP, Borowski V, Kuhn R, Susulic V, Rex-Rabe S, et al. Engineering of a novel anti-CD40L domain antibody for treatment of autoimmune diseases. J Immunol Baltim Md 1950. 2014;192(9):4083–92.

[96] Shultz LD, Ishikawa F, Greiner DL. Humanized mice in translational biomedical research. Nat Rev Immunol. 2007;7(2):118–30.

[97] Legrand N, Cupedo T, van Lent AU, Ebeli MJ, Weijer K, Hanke T, et al. Transient accumulation of human mature thymocytes and regulatory T cells with CD28 superagonist in "human immune system" Rag2(-/-)gammac(-/-) mice. Blood 2006;108(1):238–45.

[98] Ji M, Jin X, Phillips P, Yi S. A humanized mouse model to study human immune response in xenotransplantation. Hepatobiliary Pancreat Dis Int HBPD INT. 2012;11(5): 494–8.

[99] Poirier N, Mary C, Dilek N, Hervouet J, Minault D, Blancho G, et al. Preclinical efficacy and immunological safety of FR104, an antagonist anti-CD28 monovalent Fab' antibody. Am J Transplant Off J Am Soc Transplant Am Soc Transpl Surg. 2012;12(10):2630–40.

[100] Kingsley CI, Karim M, Bushell AR, Wood KJ. CD25+CD4+ regulatory T cells prevent graft rejection: CTLA-4- and IL-10-dependent immunoregulation of alloresponses. J Immunol Baltim Md 1950. 2002;168(3):1080–6.

[101] Larsen CP, Elwood ET, Alexander DZ, Ritchie SC, Hendrix R, Tucker-Burden C, et al. Long-term acceptance of skin and cardiac allografts after blocking CD40 and CD28 pathways. Nature 1996;381(6581):434–8.

[102] Honey K, Cobbold SP, Waldmann H. CD40 ligand blockade induces CD4+ T cell tolerance and linked suppression. J Immunol Baltim Md 1950. 1999;163(9):4805–10.

[103] Feng G, Nadig SN, Bäckdahl L, Beck S, Francis RS, Schiopu A, et al. Functional regulatory T cells produced by inhibiting cyclic nucleotide phosphodiesterase type 3 prevent allograft rejection. Sci Transl Med. 2011;3(83):83ra40.

[104] Lafferty KJ, Woolnough J. The origin and mechanism of the allograft reaction. Immunol Rev. 1977;35:231–62.

[105] Turka LA, Linsley PS, Lin H, Brady W, Leiden JM, Wei RQ, et al. T-cell activation by the CD28 ligand B7 is required for cardiac allograft rejection in vivo. Proc Natl Acad Sci U S A. 1992;89(22):11102–5.

[106] Ford ML, Larsen CP. Translating costimulation blockade to the clinic: lessons learned from three pathways. Immunol Rev. 2009;229(1):294–306.

[107] Li XC, Strom TB, Turka LA, Wells AD. T cell death and transplantation tolerance. Immunity 2001;14(4):407–16.

[108] Linsley PS, Brady W, Urnes M, Grosmaire LS, Damle NK, Ledbetter JA. CTLA-4 is a second receptor for the B cell activation antigen B7. J Exp Med. 1991;174(3):561–9.

[109] Lenschow DJ, Walunas TL, Bluestone JA. CD28/B7 system of T cell costimulation. Annu Rev Immunol. 1996;14:233–58.

[110] Azuma H, Chandraker A, Nadeau K, Hancock WW, Carpenter CB, Tilney NL, et al. Blockade of T-cell costimulation prevents development of experimental chronic renal allograft rejection. Proc Natl Acad Sci U S A 1996;93(22):12439–44.

[111] Lenschow DJ, Zeng Y, Thistlethwaite JR, Montag A, Brady W, Gibson MG, et al. Long-term survival of xenogeneic pancreatic islet grafts induced by CTLA4lg. Science 1992;257(5071):789–92.

[112] Sayegh MH, Zheng XG, Magee C, Hancock WW, Turka LA. Donor antigen is necessary for the prevention of chronic rejection in CTLA4Ig-treated murine cardiac allograft recipients. Transplantation 1997;64(12):1646–50.

[113] Kirk AD, Harlan DM, Armstrong NN, Davis TA, Dong Y, Gray GS, et al. CTLA4-Ig and anti-CD40 ligand prevent renal allograft rejection in primates. Proc Natl Acad Sci U S A 1997;94(16):8789–94.

[114] Wing K, Onishi Y, Prieto-Martin P, Yamaguchi T, Miyara M, Fehervari Z, et al. CTLA-4 control over Foxp3+ regulatory T cell function. Science 2008;322(5899):271–5.

[115] Zhang T, Fresnay S, Welty E, Sangrampurkar N, Rybak E, Zhou H, et al. Selective CD28 blockade attenuates acute and chronic rejection of murine cardiac allografts in a CTLA-4-dependent manner. Am J Transplant Off J Am Soc Transplant Am Soc Transpl Surg. 2011;11(8):1599–609.

[116] Markees TG, Phillips NE, Gordon EJ, Noelle RJ, Shultz LD, Mordes JP, et al. Long-term survival of skin allografts induced by donor splenocytes and anti-CD154 antibody in thymectomized mice requires CD4(+) T cells, interferon-gamma, and CTLA4. J Clin Invest. 1998;101(11):2446–55.

[117] Guillonneau C, Séveno C, Dugast A-S, Li X-L, Renaudin K, Haspot F, et al. Anti-CD28 antibodies modify regulatory mechanisms and reinforce tolerance in CD40Ig-treated heart allograft recipients. J Immunol Baltim Md 1950. 2007;179(12):8164–71.

[118] Haspot F, Séveno C, Dugast A-S, Coulon F, Renaudin K, Usal C, et al. Anti-CD28 antibody-induced kidney allograft tolerance related to tryptophan degradation and TCR class II B7 regulatory cells. Am J Transplant Off J Am Soc Transplant Am Soc Transpl Surg. 2005;5(10):2339–48.

[119] Mary C, Coulon F, Poirier N, Dilek N, Martinet B, Blancho G, et al. Antagonist properties of monoclonal antibodies targeting human CD28. mAbs 2013;5(1):47–55.

[120] Yao S, Zhu Y, Zhu G, Augustine M, Zheng L, Goode DJ, et al. B7-H2 Is a Costimulatory ligand for CD28 in human. Immunity 2011;34(5):729–40.

[121] Suntharalingam G, Perry MR, Ward S, Brett SJ, Castello-Cortes A, Brunner MD, et al. Cytokine storm in a phase 1 trial of the anti-CD28 monoclonal antibody TGN1412. N Engl J Med. 2006;355(10):1018–28.

[122] Markees TG, Phillips NE, Noelle RJ, Shultz LD, Mordes JP, Greiner DL, et al. Prolonged survival of mouse skin allografts in recipients treated with donor splenocytes and antibody to CD40 ligand. Transplantation 1997;64(2):329–35.

[123] Kirk AD, Burkly LC, Batty DS, Baumgartner RE, Berning JD, Buchanan K, et al. Treatment with humanized monoclonal antibody against CD154 prevents acute renal allograft rejection in nonhuman primates. Nat Med. 1999;5(6):686–93.

[124] Elster EA, Xu H, Tadaki DK, Montgomery S, Burkly LC, Berning JD, et al. Treatment with the humanized CD154-specific monoclonal antibody, hu5C8, prevents acute

rejection of primary skin allografts in nonhuman primates. Transplantation 2001;72(9): 1473–8.

[125] Monk NJ, Hargreaves REG, Marsh JE, Farrar CA, Sacks SH, Millrain M, et al. Fc-dependent depletion of activated T cells occurs through CD40L-specific antibody rather than costimulation blockade. Nat Med. 2003;9(10):1275–80.

[126] Blair PJ, Riley JL, Harlan DM, Abe R, Tadaki DK, Hoffmann SC, et al. Cd40 ligand (Cd154) triggers a short-term Cd4+ T cell activation response that results in secretion of immunomodulatory cytokines and apoptosis. J Exp Med. 2000;191(4):651–60.

[127] Parker DC, Greiner DL, Phillips NE, Appel MC, Steele AW, Durie FH, et al. Survival of mouse pancreatic islet allografts in recipients treated with allogeneic small lymphocytes and antibody to CD40 ligand. Proc Natl Acad Sci U S A 1995;92(21):9560–4.

[128] Omoto K, Nishimura Y, Nomoto K, Kong YY, Umesue M, Murakami Y, et al. Anti-CD4 monoclonal antibody reduces the dose of cyclophosphamide required to induce tolerance to H-2 haplotype identical skin allografts in mice. Immunobiology 1996;195(1):16–32.

[129] Mayumi H, Good RA. The necessity of both allogeneic antigens and stem cells for cyclophosphamide-induced skin allograft tolerance in mice. Immunobiology 1989;178(4-5):287–304.

[130] Seung E, Mordes JP, Rossini AA, Greiner DL. Hematopoietic chimerism and central tolerance created by peripheral-tolerance induction without myeloablative conditioning. J Clin Invest. 2003;112(5):795–808.

[131] Guillot C, Guillonneau C, Mathieu P, Gerdes CA, Ménoret S, Braudeau C, et al. Prolonged blockade of CD40-CD40 ligand interactions by gene transfer of CD40Ig results in long-term heart allograft survival and donor-specific hyporesponsiveness, but does not prevent chronic rejection. J Immunol Baltim Md 1950. 2002;168(4):1600–9.

[132] Guillonneau C, Hill M, Hubert F-X, Chiffoleau E, Hervé C, Li X-L, et al. CD40Ig treatment results in allograft acceptance mediated by CD8CD45RC T cells, IFN-gamma, and indoleamine 2,3-dioxygenase. J Clin Invest. 2007;117(4):1096–106.

[133] Yoshinaga SK, Whoriskey JS, Khare SD, Sarmiento U, Guo J, Horan T, et al. T-cell co-stimulation through B7RP-1 and ICOS. Nature 1999;402(6763):827–32.

[134] Dong C, Juedes AE, Temann UA, Shresta S, Allison JP, Ruddle NH, et al. ICOS co-stimulatory receptor is essential for T-cell activation and function. Nature 2001;409(6816):97–101.

[135] Dong C, Temann UA, Flavell RA. Cutting edge: critical role of inducible costimulator in germinal center reactions. J Immunol Baltim Md 1950. 2001;166(6):3659–62.

[136] Tafuri A, Shahinian A, Bladt F, Yoshinaga SK, Jordana M, Wakeham A, et al. ICOS is essential for effective T-helper-cell responses. Nature 2001;409(6816):105–9.

[137] Salama AD, Yuan X, Nayer A, Chandraker A, Inobe M, Uede T, et al. Interaction between ICOS-B7RP1 and B7-CD28 costimulatory pathways in alloimmune responses in vivo. Am J Transplant Off J Am Soc Transplant Am Soc Transpl Surg. 2003;3(4):390–5.

[138] Guillonneau C, Aubry V, Renaudin K, Séveno C, Usal C, Tezuka K, et al. Inhibition of chronic rejection and development of tolerogenic T cells after ICOS-ICOSL and CD40-CD40L co-stimulation blockade. Transplantation 2005;80(4):546–54.

[139] Guillonneau C, Louvet C, Renaudin K, Heslan J-M, Heslan M, Tesson L, et al. The role of TNF-related activation-induced cytokine–receptor activating NF-κB interaction in acute allograft rejection and CD40L-independent chronic allograft rejection. J Immunol. 2004;172(3):1619–29.

[140] Ozkaynak E, Wang L, Goodearl A, McDonald K, Qin S, O'Keefe T, et al. Programmed death-1 targeting can promote allograft survival. J Immunol Baltim Md 1950. 2002;169(11):6546–53.

[141] Aramaki O, Shirasugi N, Takayama T, Shimazu M, Kitajima M, Ikeda Y, et al. Programmed death-1-programmed death-L1 interaction is essential for induction of regulatory cells by intratracheal delivery of alloantigen. Transplantation 2004;77(1):6–12.

[142] Wang L, Pino-Lagos K, de Vries VC, Guleria I, Sayegh MH, Noelle RJ. Programmed death 1 ligand signaling regulates the generation of adaptive Foxp3+CD4+ regulatory T cells. Proc Natl Acad Sci U S A 2008;105(27):9331–6.

[143] Sakaguchi S, Sakaguchi N, Asano M, Itoh M, Toda M. Immunologic self-tolerance maintained by activated T cells expressing IL-2 receptor alpha-chains (CD25). Breakdown of a single mechanism of self-tolerance causes various autoimmune diseases. J Immunol Baltim Md 1950. 1995;155(3):1151–64.

[144] Shevach EM. The resurrection of T cell-mediated suppression. J Immunol Baltim Md 1950. 2011;186(7):3805–7.

[145] Fontenot JD, Rasmussen JP, Williams LM, Dooley JL, Farr AG, Rudensky AY. Regulatory T cell lineage specification by the forkhead transcription factor foxp3. Immunity 2005;22(3):329–41.

[146] Hori S, Nomura T, Sakaguchi S. Control of regulatory T cell development by the transcription factor Foxp3. Science 2003;299(5609):1057–61.

[147] Gershon RK, Kondo K. Cell interactions in the induction of tolerance: the role of thymic lymphocytes. Immunology 1970;18(5):723–37.

[148] Paiva RS, Lino AC, Bergman M-L, Caramalho I, Sousa AE, Zelenay S, et al. Recent thymic emigrants are the preferential precursors of regulatory T cells differentiated in the periphery. Proc Natl Acad Sci U S A 2013;110(16):6494–9.

[149] Curotto de Lafaille MA, Lafaille JJ. Natural and adaptive foxp3+ regulatory T cells: more of the same or a division of labor? Immunity 2009;30(5):626–35.

[150] Picarda E, Bézie S, Venturi V, Echasserieau K, Mérieau E, Delhumeau A, et al. MHC-derived allopeptide activates TCR-biased CD8+ Tregs and suppresses organ rejection. J Clin Invest. 2014;124(6):2497–512.

[151] Shimizu J, Yamazaki S, Takahashi T, Ishida Y, Sakaguchi S. Stimulation of CD25(+)CD4(+) regulatory T cells through GITR breaks immunological self-tolerance. Nat Immunol. 2002;3(2):135–42.

[152] Takahashi T, Tagami T, Yamazaki S, Uede T, Shimizu J, Sakaguchi N, et al. Immunologic self-tolerance maintained by CD25(+)CD4(+) regulatory T cells constitutively expressing cytotoxic T lymphocyte-associated antigen 4. J Exp Med. 2000;192(2):303–10.

[153] Szanya V, Ermann J, Taylor C, Holness C, Fathman CG. The subpopulation of CD4+CD25+ splenocytes that delays adoptive transfer of diabetes expresses L-selectin and high levels of CCR7. J Immunol Baltim Md 1950. 2002;169(5):2461–5.

[154] Huang C-T, Workman CJ, Flies D, Pan X, Marson AL, Zhou G, et al. Role of LAG-3 in regulatory T cells. Immunity 2004;21(4):503–13.

[155] Liu W, Putnam AL, Xu-Yu Z, Szot GL, Lee MR, Zhu S, et al. CD127 expression inversely correlates with FoxP3 and suppressive function of human CD4+ T reg cells. J Exp Med. 2006;203(7):1701–11.

[156] Ligocki AJ, Niederkorn JY. Advances on Non-CD4 + Foxp3+ T regulatory cells: CD8+, type 1, and double negative t regulatory cells in organ transplantation. Transplantation 2015;99(8):1553–9.

[157] Ménoret S, Guillonneau C, Bezié S, Caron L, Anegon I, Li X-L. Phenotypic and functional characterization of CD8(+) T regulatory cells. Methods Mol Biol Clifton NJ. 2011;677:63–83.

[158] Niederkorn JY. Emerging concepts in CD8(+) T regulatory cells. Curr Opin Immunol. 2008;20(3):327–31.

[159] Guillonneau C, Hill M, Hubert F-X, Chiffoleau E, Hervé C, Li X-L, et al. CD40Ig treatment results in allograft acceptance mediated by CD8CD45RC T cells, IFN-gamma, and indoleamine 2,3-dioxygenase. J Clin Invest. 2007;117(4):1096–106.

[160] Guillonneau C, Picarda E, Anegon I. CD8+ regulatory T cells in solid organ transplantation. Curr Opin Organ Transplant. 2010;15(6):751–6.

[161] Fontenot JD, Gavin MA, Rudensky AY. Foxp3 programs the development and function of CD4+CD25+ regulatory T cells. Nat Immunol. 2003;4(4):330–6.

[162] Hori S, Takahashi T, Sakaguchi S. Control of autoimmunity by naturally arising regulatory CD4+ T cells. Adv Immunol. 2003;81:331–71.

[163] Bacchetta R, Passerini L, Gambineri E, Dai M, Allan SE, Perroni L, et al. Defective regulatory and effector T cell functions in patients with FOXP3 mutations. J Clin Invest. 2006;116(6):1713–22.

[164] Morgan ME, van Bilsen JHM, Bakker AM, Heemskerk B, Schilham MW, Hartgers FC, et al. Expression of FOXP3 mRNA is not confined to CD4+CD25+ T regulatory cells in humans. Hum Immunol. 2005;66(1):13–20.

[165] Thornton AM, Korty PE, Tran DQ, Wohlfert EA, Murray PE, Belkaid Y, et al. Expression of Helios, an Ikaros transcription factor family member, differentiates thymic-derived from peripherally induced Foxp3+ T regulatory cells. J Immunol Baltim Md 1950. 2010;184(7):3433–41.

[166] Yadav M, Louvet C, Davini D, Gardner JM, Martinez-Llordella M, Bailey-Bucktrout S, et al. Neuropilin-1 distinguishes natural and inducible regulatory T cells among regulatory T cell subsets in vivo. J Exp Med. 2012;209(10):1713–22, S1–19.

[167] Kim H-J, Barnitz RA, Kreslavsky T, Brown FD, Moffett H, Lemieux ME, et al. Stable inhibitory activity of regulatory T cells requires the transcription factor Helios. Science 2015;350(6258):334–9.

[168] Lee WT, Prasad A, Watson ARO. Anergy in CD4 memory T lymphocytes. II. Abrogation of TCR-induced formation of membrane signaling complexes. Cell Immunol. 2012;276(1-2):26–34.

[169] Mellor AL, Munn DH. IDO expression by dendritic cells: tolerance and tryptophan catabolism. Nat Rev Immunol. 2004;4(10):762–74.

[170] Grossman WJ, Verbsky JW, Tollefsen BL, Kemper C, Atkinson JP, Ley TJ. Differential expression of granzymes A and B in human cytotoxic lymphocyte subsets and T regulatory cells. Blood. 2004;104(9):2840–8.

[171] Deaglio S, Dwyer KM, Gao W, Friedman D, Usheva A, Erat A, et al. Adenosine generation catalyzed by CD39 and CD73 expressed on regulatory T cells mediates immune suppression. J Exp Med. 2007;204(6):1257–65.

[172] Pandiyan P, Zheng L, Ishihara S, Reed J, Lenardo MJ. CD4+CD25+Foxp3+ regulatory T cells induce cytokine deprivation-mediated apoptosis of effector CD4+ T cells. Nat Immunol. 2007;8(12):1353–62.

[173] Bézie S, Picarda E, Ossart J, Tesson L, Usal C, Renaudin K, et al. IL-34 is a Treg-specific cytokine and mediates transplant tolerance. J Clin Invest. 2015;125(10):3952–64.

[174] Chaturvedi V, Collison LW, Guy CS, Workman CJ, Vignali DAA. Cutting edge: human regulatory T cells require IL-35 to mediate suppression and infectious tolerance. J Immunol Baltim Md 1950. 2011;186(12):6661–6.

[175] Chesneau M, Michel L, Dugast E, Chenouard A, Baron D, Pallier A, et al. Tolerant kidney transplant patients produce b cells with regulatory properties. J Am Soc Nephrol JASN. 2015;26(10):2588–98.

[176] Bézie S, Picarda E, Ossart J, Martinet B, Anegon I, Guillonneau C. Compensatory regulatory networks between CD8 T, B, and myeloid cells in organ transplantation tolerance. J Immunol Baltim Md 1950. 2015;195(12):5805–15.

[177] Durand J, Chiffoleau E. B cells with regulatory properties in transplantation tolerance. World J Transplant. 2015;5(4):196–208.

[178] Dugast A-S, Haudebourg T, Coulon F, Heslan M, Haspot F, Poirier N, et al. Myeloid-derived suppressor cells accumulate in kidney allograft tolerance and specifically suppress effector T cell expansion. J Immunol Baltim Md 1950. 2008;180(12):7898–906.

[179] Dilek N, Poirier N, Usal C, Martinet B, Blancho G, Vanhove B. Control of transplant tolerance and intragraft regulatory T cell localization by myeloid-derived suppressor cells and CCL5. J Immunol Baltim Md 1950. 2012;188(9):4209–16.

[180] Pallier A, Hillion S, Danger R, Giral M, Racapé M, Degauque N, et al. Patients with drug-free long-term graft function display increased numbers of peripheral B cells with a memory and inhibitory phenotype. Kidney Int. 2010;78(5):503–13.

[181] Newell KA, Asare A, Kirk AD, Gisler TD, Bourcier K, Suthanthiran M, et al. Identification of a B cell signature associated with renal transplant tolerance in humans. J Clin Invest. 2010;120(6):1836–47.

[182] Mauri C, Blair PA. Regulatory B cells in autoimmunity: developments and controversies. Nat Rev Rheumatol. 2010;6(11):636–43.

[183] Le Texier L, Thebault P, Lavault A, Usal C, Merieau E, Quillard T, et al. Long-term allograft tolerance is characterized by the accumulation of B cells exhibiting an inhibited profile. Am J Transplant Off J Am Soc Transplant Am Soc Transpl Surg. 2011;11(3):429–38.

[184] Bouaziz J-D, Le Buanec H, Saussine A, Bensussan A, Bagot M. IL-10 producing regulatory B cells in mice and humans: state of the art. Curr Mol Med. 2012;12(5):519–27.

[185] Qian L, Qian C, Chen Y, Bai Y, Bao Y, Lu L, et al. Regulatory dendritic cells program B cells to differentiate into CD19hiFcγIIbhi regulatory B cells through IFN-β and CD40L. Blood. 2012;120(3):581–91.

[186] Fillatreau S, Gray D, Anderton SM. Not always the bad guys: B cells as regulators of autoimmune pathology. Nat Rev Immunol. 2008;8(5):391–7.

[187] Yanaba K, Bouaziz J-D, Matsushita T, Tsubata T, Tedder TF. The development and function of regulatory B cells expressing IL-10 (B10 cells) requires antigen receptor diversity and TLR signals. J Immunol Baltim Md 1950. 2009;182(12):7459–72.

[188] Blair PA, Noreña LY, Flores-Borja F, Rawlings DJ, Isenberg DA, Ehrenstein MR, et al. CD19(+)CD24(hi)CD38(hi) B cells exhibit regulatory capacity in healthy individuals but are functionally impaired in systemic Lupus Erythematosus patients. Immunity 2010;32(1):129–40.

[189] Durand J, Huchet V, Merieau E, Usal C, Chesneau M, Remy S, et al. Regulatory B Cells with a Partial Defect in CD40 Signaling and Overexpressing Granzyme B Transfer Allograft Tolerance in Rodents. J Immunol Baltim Md 1950. 2015;195(10):5035–44.

[190] Kim JI, Rothstein DM, Markmann JF. Role of B cells in tolerance induction. Curr Opin Organ Transplant. 2015;20(4):369–75.

[191] Deng S, Moore DJ, Huang X, Lian M-M, Mohiuddin M, Velededeoglu E, et al. Cutting edge: transplant tolerance induced by anti-CD45RB requires B lymphocytes. J Immunol Baltim Md 1950. 2007 May 15;178(10):6028–32.

[192] Darrasse-Jèze G, Deroubaix S, Mouquet H, Victora GD, Eisenreich T, Yao K, et al. Feedback control of regulatory T cell homeostasis by dendritic cells in vivo. J Exp Med. 2009;206(9):1853–62.

[193] Manicassamy S, Pulendran B. Dendritic cell control of tolerogenic responses. Immunol Rev. 2011;241(1):206–27.

[194] Maldonado RA, von Andrian UH. How tolerogenic dendritic cells induce regulatory T cells. Adv Immunol. 2010;108:111–65.

[195] Moreau A, Varey E, Bouchet-Delbos L, Cuturi M-C. Cell therapy using tolerogenic dendritic cells in transplantation. Transplant Res. 2012;1(1):13.

[196] Fu F, Li Y, Qian S, Lu L, Chambers F, Starzl TE, et al. Costimulatory molecule-deficient dendritic cell progenitors (MHC class II+, CD80dim, CD86-) prolong cardiac allograft survival in nonimmunosuppressed recipients. Transplantation 1996;62(5):659–65.

[197] Lutz MB, Suri RM, Niimi M, Ogilvie AL, Kukutsch NA, Rössner S, et al. Immature dendritic cells generated with low doses of GM-CSF in the absence of IL-4 are maturation resistant and prolong allograft survival in vivo. Eur J Immunol. 2000;30(7):1813–22.

[198] Hill M, Thebault P, Segovia M, Louvet C, Bériou G, Tilly G, et al. Cell therapy with autologous tolerogenic dendritic cells induces allograft tolerance through interferon-gamma and epstein-barr virus-induced gene 3. Am J Transplant Off J Am Soc Transplant Am Soc Transpl Surg. 2011;11(10):2036–45.

[199] Segovia M, Louvet C, Charnet P, Savina A, Tilly G, Gautreau L, et al. Autologous dendritic cells prolong allograft survival through Tmem176b-dependent antigen cross-presentation. Am J Transplant Off J Am Soc Transplant Am Soc Transpl Surg. 2014;14(5):1021–31.

[200] Chauveau C, Rémy S, Royer PJ, Hill M, Tanguy-Royer S, Hubert F-X, et al. Heme oxygenase-1 expression inhibits dendritic cell maturation and proinflammatory function but conserves IL-10 expression. Blood 2005;106(5):1694–702.

[201] Rogers NM, Isenberg JS, Thomson AW. Plasmacytoid dendritic cells: no longer an enigma and now key to transplant tolerance? Am J Transplant Off J Am Soc Transplant Am Soc Transpl Surg. 2013;13(5):1125–33.

[202] Li XL, Ménoret S, Bezie S, Caron L, Chabannes D, Hill M, et al. Mechanism and localization of CD8 regulatory T cells in a heart transplant model of tolerance. J Immunol Baltim Md 1950. 2010;185(2):823–33.

[203] Ochando JC, Homma C, Yang Y, Hidalgo A, Garin A, Tacke F, et al. Alloantigen-presenting plasmacytoid dendritic cells mediate tolerance to vascularized grafts. Nat Immunol. 2006;7(6):652–62.

[204] Moseman EA, Liang X, Dawson AJ, Panoskaltsis-Mortari A, Krieg AM, Liu Y-J, et al. Human plasmacytoid dendritic cells activated by CpG oligodeoxynucleotides induce the generation of CD4+CD25+ regulatory T cells. J Immunol Baltim Md 1950. 2004;173(7):4433–42.

[205] Boor PPC, Metselaar HJ, Jonge S de, Mancham S, van der Laan LJW, Kwekkeboom J. Human plasmacytoid dendritic cells induce $CD8^+$ LAG-3^+ Foxp3^+ CTLA-4^+ regulatory T cells that suppress allo-reactive memory T cells. Eur J Immunol. 2011;41(6):1663–74.

[206] Gilliet M, Liu Y-J. Generation of human CD8 T regulatory cells by CD40 ligand-activated plasmacytoid dendritic cells. J Exp Med. 2002;195(6):695–704.

[207] Tokita D, Mazariegos GV, Zahorchak AF, Chien N, Abe M, Raimondi G, et al. High PD-L1/CD86 ratio on plasmacytoid dendritic cells correlates with elevated T-regulatory cells in liver transplant tolerance. Transplantation 2008;85(3):369–77.

[208] Manavalan JS, Kim-Schulze S, Scotto L, Naiyer AJ, Vlad G, Colombo PC, et al. Alloantigen specific CD8+CD28- FOXP3+ T suppressor cells induce ILT3+ ILT4+ tolerogenic endothelial cells, inhibiting alloreactivity. Int Immunol. 2004;16(8):1055–68.

[209] Chiffoleau E, Bériou G, Dutartre P, Usal C, Soulillou J-P, Cuturi MC. Role for thymic and splenic regulatory CD4+ T cells induced by donor dendritic cells in allograft tolerance by LF15-0195 treatment. J Immunol Baltim Md 1950. 2002;168(10):5058–69.

[210] Degauque N, Lair D, Dupont A, Moreau A, Roussey G, Moizant F, et al. Dominant tolerance to kidney allografts induced by anti-donor MHC class II antibodies: cooperation between T and non-T CD103+ cells. J Immunol Baltim Md 1950. 2006;176(7):3915–22.

[211] Josien R, Heslan M, Brouard S, Soulillou JP, Cuturi MC. Critical requirement for graft passenger leukocytes in allograft tolerance induced by donor blood transfusion. Blood 1998;92(12):4539–44.

[212] Broichhausen C, Riquelme P, Geissler EK and Hutchinson JA. Regulatory macrophages as therapeutic targets and therapeutic agents in solid organ transplantation. Curr. Opin. Organ Transplant. 2012;17(4):332–342.

[213] Elhage R, Cheraï M, Levacher B, Darrasse-Jeze G, Baillou C, Zhao X, et al. C-terminal cleavage of human Foxp3 at a proprotein convertase motif abrogates its suppressive function. Scand J Immunol. 2015;81(4):229–39.

[214] Liu G, Duan K, Ma H, Niu Z, Peng J, Zhao Y. An instructive role of donor macrophages in mixed chimeras in the induction of recipient CD4(+)Foxp3(+) Treg cells. Immunol Cell Biol. 2011;89(8):827–35.

[215] Hashimoto D, Chow A, Greter M, Saenger Y, Kwan W-H, Leboeuf M, et al. Pretransplant CSF-1 therapy expands recipient macrophages and ameliorates GVHD after allogeneic hematopoietic cell transplantation. J Exp Med. 2011;208(5):1069–82.

[216] Wood KJ, Bushell A, Hester J. Regulatory immune cells in transplantation. Nat Rev Immunol. 2012;12(6):417–30.

[217] Darrasse-Jèze G, Darasse-Jèze G, Klatzmann D, Charlotte F, Salomon BL, Cohen JL. CD4+CD25+ regulatory/suppressor T cells prevent allogeneic fetus rejection in mice. Immunol Lett. 2006;102(1):106–9.

[218] Taieb J, Chaput N, Schartz N, Roux S, Novault S, Ménard C, et al. Chemoimmunotherapy of tumors: cyclophosphamide synergizes with exosome based vaccines. J Immunol Baltim Md 1950. 2006;176(5):2722–9.

[219] Dilek N, Vuillefroy de Silly R, Blancho G, Vanhove B. Myeloid-derived suppressor cells: mechanisms of action and recent advances in their role in transplant tolerance. Front Immunol. 2012;3:208.

[220] Dilek N, van Rompaey N, Le Moine A, Vanhove B. Myeloid-derived suppressor cells in transplantation. Curr Opin Organ Transplant. 2010;15(6):765–8.

[221] Jiang S, Lechler RI, He X-S, Huang J-F. Regulatory T cells and transplantation tolerance. Hum Immunol. 2006;67(10):765–76.

[222] Ordonez L, Bernard I, L'faqihi-Olive F-E, Tervaert JWC, Damoiseaux J, Saoudi A. CD45RC isoform expression identifies functionally distinct T cell subsets differentially distributed between healthy individuals and AAV patients. PloS One 2009;4(4):e5287.

[223] Kamanaka M, Huber S, Zenewicz LA, Gagliani N, Rathinam C, O'Connor W, et al. Memory/effector (CD45RB(lo)) CD4 T cells are controlled directly by IL-10 and cause IL-22-dependent intestinal pathology. J Exp Med. 2011;208(5):1027–40.

[224] Fecteau S, Basadonna GP, Freitas A, Ariyan C, Sayegh MH, Rothstein DM. CTLA-4 up-regulation plays a role in tolerance mediated by CD45. Nat Immunol. 2001;2(1):58–63.

[225] Auersvald LA, Rothstein DM, Oliveira SC, Khuong CQ, Basadonna GP. Anti-CD45RB treatment prolongs islet allograft survival in mice. Transplant Proc. 1997;29(1–2):771.

[226] Moreau A, Hill M, Thébault P, Deschamps JY, Chiffoleau E, Chauveau C, et al. Tolerogenic dendritic cells actively inhibit T cells through heme oxygenase-1 in rodents and in nonhuman primates. FASEB J. 2009;23(9):3070–7.

[227] Spickett GP, Brandon MR, Mason DW, Williams AF, Woollett GR. MRC OX-22, a monoclonal antibody that labels a new subset of T lymphocytes and reacts with the high molecular weight form of the leukocyte-common antigen. J Exp Med. 1983;158(3): 795–810.

[228] Xystrakis E, Bernard I, Dejean AS, Alsaati T, Druet P, Saoudi A. Alloreactive CD4 T lymphocytes responsible for acute and chronic graft-versus-host disease are contained within the CD45RChigh but not the CD45RClow subset. Eur J Immunol. 2004;34(2): 408–17.

[229] Xystrakis E, Dejean AS, Bernard I, Druet P, Liblau R, Gonzalez-Dunia D, et al. Identification of a novel natural regulatory CD8 T-cell subset and analysis of its mechanism of regulation. Blood 2004;104(10):3294–301.

[230] Powrie F, Mason D. OX-22high CD4+ T cells induce wasting disease with multiple organ pathology: prevention by the OX-22low subset. J Exp Med. 1990;172(6):1701–8.

[231] Laskowski IA, Pratschke J, Wilhelm MJ, Dong VM, Beato F, Taal M, et al. Anti-CD28 monoclonal antibody therapy prevents chronic rejection of renal allografts in rats. J Am Soc Nephrol JASN. 2002;13(2):519–27.

[232] Cobbold SP, Adams E, Marshall SE, Davies JD, Waldmann H. Mechanisms of peripheral tolerance and suppression induced by monoclonal antibodies to CD4 and CD8. Immunol Rev. 1996;149:5–33.

[233] Qin S, Cobbold SP, Pope H, Elliott J, Kioussis D, Davies J, et al. "Infectious" transplantation tolerance. Science 1993;259(5097):974–7.

[234] Rothstein DM, Livak MF, Kishimoto K, Ariyan C, Qian HY, Fecteau S, et al. Targeting signal 1 through CD45RB synergizes with CD40 ligand blockade and promotes long term engraftment and tolerance in stringent transplant models. J Immunol Baltim Md 1950. 2001;166(1):322–9.

[235] Biomarkers Definitions Working Group. Biomarkers and surrogate endpoints: preferred definitions and conceptual framework. Clin Pharmacol Ther. 2001;69(3):89–95.

[236] Costanzo MR, Dipchand A, Starling R, Anderson A, Chan M, Desai S, et al. The International Society of Heart and Lung Transplantation Guidelines for the care of heart transplant recipients. J Heart Lung Transplant Off Publ Int Soc Heart Transplant. 2010;29(8):914–56.

[237] Bonnemains L, Cherifi A, Girerd N, Odille F, Felblinger J. Design of the DRAGET Study: a multicentre controlled diagnostic study to assess the detection of acute rejection in patients with heart transplant by means of T2 quantification with MRI in comparison to myocardial biopsies. BMJ Open. 2015;5(10):e008963.

[238] Foucher Y, Daguin P, Akl A, Kessler M, Ladrière M, Legendre C, et al. A clinical scoring system highly predictive of long-term kidney graft survival. Kidney Int. 2010;78(12): 1288–94.

[239] Brouard S, Mansfield E, Braud C, Li L, Giral M, Hsieh S, et al. Identification of a peripheral blood transcriptional biomarker panel associated with operational renal allograft tolerance. Proc Natl Acad Sci U S A 2007;104(39):15448–53.

[240] Sagoo P, Perucha E, Sawitzki B, Tomiuk S, Stephens DA, Miqueu P, et al. Development of a cross-platform biomarker signature to detect renal transplant tolerance in humans. J Clin Invest. 2010;120(6):1848–61.

[241] Moraes-Vieira PMM, Takenaka MCS, Silva HM, Monteiro SM, Agena F, Lemos F, et al. GATA3 and a dominant regulatory gene expression profile discriminate operational tolerance in human transplantation. Clin Immunol Orlando Fla. 2012;142(2):117–26.

[242] Braza F, Dugast E, Panov I, Paul C, Vogt K, Pallier A, et al. Central role of CD45RA-Foxp3hi memory regulatory T cells in clinical kidney transplantation tolerance. J Am Soc Nephrol JASN. 2015;26(8):1795–805.

[243] Moraes-Vieira PMM, Silva HM, Takenaka MCS, Monteiro SM, Lemos F, Saitovitch D, et al. Differential monocyte STAT6 activation and CD4(+)CD25(+)Foxp3(+) T cells in kidney operational tolerance transplanted individuals. Hum Immunol. 2010;71(5):442–50.

[244] Martínez-Llordella M, Puig-Pey I, Orlando G, Ramoni M, Tisone G, Rimola A, et al. Multiparameter immune profiling of operational tolerance in liver transplantation. Am J Transplant Off J Am Soc Transplant Am Soc Transpl Surg. 2007;7(2):309–19.

[245] Braza F, Soulillou J-P, Brouard S. Gene expression signature in transplantation tolerance. Clin Chim Acta Int J Clin Chem. 2012;413(17–18):1414–8.

[246] Bohne F, Martínez-Llordella M, Lozano J-J, Miquel R, Benítez C, Londoño M-C, et al. Intra-graft expression of genes involved in iron homeostasis predicts the development of operational tolerance in human liver transplantation. J Clin Invest. 2012;122(1):368–82.

[247] Streitz M, Miloud T, Kapinsky M, Reed MR, Magari R, Geissler EK, et al. Standardization of whole blood immune phenotype monitoring for clinical trials: panels and methods from the ONE study. Transplant Res. 2013;2(1):17.

[248] Bézie S, Picarda E, Tesson L, Renaudin K, Durand J, Ménoret S, et al. Fibrinogen-like protein 2/fibroleukin induces long-term allograft survival in a rat model through regulatory B cells. PloS One 2015;10(3):e0119686.

[249] Gielis EM, Ledeganck KJ, De Winter BY, Del Favero J, Bosmans J-L, Claas FHJ, et al. Cell-Free DNA: An Upcoming Biomarker in Transplantation. Am J Transplant Off J Am Soc Transplant Am Soc Transpl Surg. 2015;15(10):2541–51.

[250] Afaneh C, Muthukumar T, Lubetzky M, Ding R, Snopkowski C, Sharma VK, et al. Urinary cell levels of mRNA for OX40, OX40L, PD-1, PD-L1, or PD-L2 and acute rejection of human renal allografts. Transplantation 2010;90(12):1381–7.

[251] Bodonyi-Kovacs G, Strom TB, Putheti P. A20--a biomarker of allograft outcome: a showcase in kidney transplantation. Adv Exp Med Biol. 2014;809:103–16.

[252] Manfro RC, Aquino-Dias EC, Joelsons G, Nogare AL, Carpio VN, Gonçalves LFS. Noninvasive Tim-3 messenger RNA evaluation in renal transplant recipients with graft dysfunction. Transplantation 2008;86(12):1869–74.

[253] Bertoni E, Larti A, Rosso G, Zanazzi M, Di Maria L, Salvadori M. Good outcomes with cyclosporine very low exposure with everolimus high exposure in renal transplant patients. J Nephrol. 2011;24(5):613–8.

[254] Guillonneau C, Hill M, Hubert F-X, Chiffoleau E, Hervé C, Li X-L, et al. CD40Ig treatment results in allograft acceptance mediated by CD8CD45RC T cells, IFN-gamma, and indoleamine 2,3-dioxygenase. J Clin Invest. 2007;117(4):1096–106.

[255] Kim B-S, Nishikii H, Baker J, Pierini A, Schneidawind D, Pan Y, et al. Treatment with agonistic DR3 antibody results in expansion of donor Tregs and reduced graft-versus-host disease. Blood 2015;126(4):546–57.

[256] Vincenti F, Larsen C, Durrbach A, Wekerle T, Nashan B, Blancho G, et al. Costimulation blockade with belatacept in renal transplantation. N Engl J Med. 2005;353(8):770–81.

[257] Trzonkowski P, Bieniaszewska M, Juścińska J, Dobyszuk A, Krzystyniak A, Marek N, et al. First-in-man clinical results of the treatment of patients with graft versus host disease with human ex vivo expanded CD4+CD25+CD127- T regulatory cells. Clin Immunol Orlando Fla. 2009;133(1):22–6.

[258] Brunstein CG, Miller JS, Cao Q, McKenna DH, Hippen KL, Curtsinger J, et al. Infusion of ex vivo expanded T regulatory cells in adults transplanted with umbilical cord blood: safety profile and detection kinetics. Blood 2011;117(3):1061–70.

[259] Di Ianni M, Falzetti F, Carotti A, Terenzi A, Castellino F, Bonifacio E, et al. Tregs prevent GVHD and promote immune reconstitution in HLA-haploidentical transplantation. Blood 2011;117(14):3921–8.

[260] Martelli MF, Di Ianni M, Ruggeri L, Falzetti F, Carotti A, Terenzi A, et al. HLA-haploidentical transplantation with regulatory and conventional T-cell adoptive immunotherapy prevents acute leukemia relapse. Blood 2014;124(4):638–44.

[261] Bacchetta R, Lucarelli B, Sartirana C, Gregori S, Lupo Stanghellini MT, Miqueu P, et al. Immunological outcome in haploidentical-HSC transplanted patients treated with IL-10-anergized donor T cells. Front Immunol. 2014;5:16.

[262] Moreau A, Varey E, Bouchet-Delbos L, Cuturi M-C. Cell therapy using tolerogenic dendritic cells in transplantation. Transplant Res. 2012;1(1):13.

[263] Tobin LM, Healy ME, English K, Mahon BP. Human mesenchymal stem cells suppress donor CD4(+) T cell proliferation and reduce pathology in a humanized mouse model of acute graft-versus-host disease. Clin Exp Immunol. 2013;172(2):333–48.

[264] Petrelli A, Tresoldi E, Mfarrej BG, Paganelli A, Spotti D, Caldara R, et al. Generation of donor-specific T regulatory type 1 cells from patients on dialysis for cell therapy after kidney transplantation. Transplantation 2015;99(8):1582–9.

[265] Geissler EK. The ONE Study compares cell therapy products in organ transplantation: introduction to a review series on suppressive monocyte-derived cells. Transplant Res. 2012;1(1):11.

[266] Zheng J, Liu Y, Liu Y, Liu M, Xiang Z, Lam K-T, et al. Human CD8+ regulatory T cells inhibit GVHD and preserve general immunity in humanized mice. Sci Transl Med. 2013;5(168):168ra9.

[267] Picarda É, Ossart J, Bézie S, Guillonneau C. [Key role of allopeptide-specific CD8(+) Tregs in transplantation]. Médecine Sci MS. 2015;31(1):22–4.

[268] Dai Z, Zhang S, Xie Q, Wu S, Su J, Li S, et al. Natural CD8+CD122+ T cells are more potent in suppression of allograft rejection than CD4+CD25+ regulatory T cells. Am J Transplant Off J Am Soc Transplant Am Soc Transpl Surg. 2014;14(1):39–48.

[269] Nouël A, Simon Q, Jamin C, Pers J-O, Hillion S. Regulatory B cells: an exciting target for future therapeutics in transplantation. Front Immunol. 2014;5:11.

[270] Tang Q, Lee K. Regulatory T-cell therapy for transplantation: how many cells do we need? Curr Opin Organ Transplant. 2012;17(4):349–54.

[271] Nguyen VH, Zeiser R, Dasilva DL, Chang DS, Beilhack A, Contag CH, et al. In vivo dynamics of regulatory T-cell trafficking and survival predict effective strategies to control graft-versus-host disease following allogeneic transplantation. Blood 2007;109(6):2649–56.

[272] Nadig SN, Wieckiewicz J, Wu DC, Warnecke G, Zhang W, Luo S, et al. In vivo prevention of transplant arteriosclerosis by ex vivo-expanded human regulatory T cells. Nat Med. 2010;16(7):809–13.

[273] Issa F, Hester J, Goto R, Nadig SN, Goodacre TE, Wood K. Ex vivo-expanded human regulatory T cells prevent the rejection of skin allografts in a humanized mouse model. Transplantation 2010;90(12):1321–7.

[274] Wu DC, Hester J, Nadig SN, Zhang W, Trzonkowski P, Gray D, et al. Ex vivo expanded human regulatory T cells can prolong survival of a human islet allograft in a humanized mouse model. Transplantation 2013;96(8):707–16.

[275] Sagoo P, Ali N, Garg G, Nestle FO, Lechler RI, Lombardi G. Human regulatory T cells with alloantigen specificity are more potent inhibitors of alloimmune skin graft damage than polyclonal regulatory T cells. Sci Transl Med. 2011;3(83):83ra42.

[276] Veerapathran A, Pidala J, Beato F, Yu X-Z, Anasetti C. Ex vivo expansion of human Tregs specific for alloantigens presented directly or indirectly. Blood 2011;118(20): 5671–80.

[277] Tang Q, Bluestone JA. Regulatory T-cell therapy in transplantation: moving to the clinic. Cold Spring Harb Perspect Med. 2013;3(11) a015552

[278] Cheraï M, Hamel Y, Baillou C, Touil S, Guillot-Delost M, Charlotte F, et al. Generation of human alloantigen-specific regulatory T-cells under good manufacturing practice-compliant conditions for cell therapy. Cell Transplant 2015;24(12):2527–40.

[279] Putnam AL, Safinia N, Medvec A, Laszkowska M, Wray M, Mintz MA, et al. Clinical grade manufacturing of human alloantigen-reactive regulatory T cells for use in transplantation. Am J Transplant Off J Am Soc Transplant Am Soc Transpl Surg. 2013;13(11):3010–20.

[280] Peters JH, Hilbrands LB, Koenen HJPM, Joosten I. Ex vivo generation of human alloantigen-specific regulatory T cells from CD4(pos)CD25(high) T cells for immunotherapy. PloS One 2008;3(5):e2233.

[281] Qin S, Cobbold SP, Pope H, Elliott J, Kioussis D, Davies J, et al. "Infectious" transplantation tolerance. Science 1993;259(5097):974–7.

[282] Noyan F, Lee Y-S, Zimmermann K, Hardtke-Wolenski M, Taubert R, Warnecke G, et al. Isolation of human antigen-specific regulatory T cells with high suppressive function. Eur J Immunol. 2014;44(9):2592–602.

[283] Veerapathran A, Pidala J, Beato F, Betts B, Kim J, Turner JG, et al. Human regulatory T cells against minor histocompatibility antigens: ex vivo expansion for prevention of graft-versus-host disease. Blood 2013;122(13):2251–61.

[284] Sangiolo D. Redirected T cells in cancer therapy. Expert Opin Biol Ther. 2015;15(12): 1667–70.

[285] Duong CPM, Yong CSM, Kershaw MH, Slaney CY, Darcy PK. Cancer immunotherapy utilizing gene-modified T cells: From the bench to the clinic. Mol Immunol. 2015;67(2 Pt A):46–57.

[286] Baron U, Floess S, Wieczorek G, Baumann K, Grützkau A, Dong J, et al. DNA demethylation in the human FOXP3 locus discriminates regulatory T cells from activated FOXP3(+) conventional T cells. Eur J Immunol. 2007;37(9):2378–89.

[287] Allan SE, Crome SQ, Crellin NK, Passerini L, Steiner TS, Bacchetta R, et al. Activation-induced FOXP3 in human T effector cells does not suppress proliferation or cytokine production. Int Immunol. 2007;19(4):345–54.

[288] Scottà C, Fanelli G, Hoong SJ, Romano M, Lamperti EN, Sukthankar M, et al. Impact of immunosuppressive drugs on the therapeutic efficacy of ex vivo expanded human regulatory T cells. Haematologica. 2016;101(1):91–100.

[289] Hester J, Schiopu A, Nadig SN, Wood KJ. Low-dose rapamycin treatment increases the ability of human regulatory T cells to inhibit transplant arteriosclerosis in vivo. Am J Transplant Off J Am Soc Transplant Am Soc Transpl Surg. 2012;12(8):2008–16.

[290] Scottà C, Esposito M, Fazekasova H, Fanelli G, Edozie FC, Ali N, et al. Differential effects of rapamycin and retinoic acid on expansion, stability and suppressive qualities of human CD4(+)CD25(+)FOXP3(+) T regulatory cell subpopulations. Haematologica 2013;98(8):1291–9.

[291] Hippen KL, Merkel SC, Schirm DK, Nelson C, Tennis NC, Riley JL, et al. Generation and large-scale expansion of human inducible regulatory T cells that suppress graft-versus-host disease. Am J Transplant Off J Am Soc Transplant Am Soc Transpl Surg. 2011;11(6):1148–57.

[292] Coenen JJA, Koenen HJPM, van Rijssen E, Kasran A, Boon L, Hilbrands LB, et al. Rapamycin, not cyclosporine, permits thymic generation and peripheral preservation of CD4+ CD25+ FoxP3+ T cells. Bone Marrow Transplant. 2007;39(9):537–45.

[293] Wu T, Zhang L, Xu K, Sun C, Lei T, Peng J, et al. Immunosuppressive drugs on inducing Ag-specific CD4(+)CD25(+)Foxp3(+) Treg cells during immune response in vivo. Transpl Immunol. 2012;27(1):30–8.

Chapter 4

Subnormothermic and Normothermic Ex Vivo Liver Perfusion as a Novel Preservation Technique

Nicolas Goldaracena, Andrew S. Barbas and Markus Selzner

Additional information is available at the end of the chapter

http://dx.doi.org/10.5772/63811

Abstract

Due to the worldwide organ shortage, interest in the use of marginal liver allografts has increased. More widespread use of marginal grafts is limited by graft injury from cold storage and the risk of poor outcomes after transplantation. Warm (subnormothermic and normothermic) ex vivo liver perfusion has emerged as a novel preservation strategy to recover marginal organs and potentially increase the organ pool. Over the last decade, advances in the field have taken warm ex vivo liver perfusion from the laboratory to clinical trials. While most investigation thus far has focused on the rescue of marginal grafts for expansion of the donor pool, warm perfusion (WP) preservation also has great potential to facilitate novel graft interventions prior to transplantation.

Keywords: ex vivo liver perfusion, warm perfusion, machine perfusion, ischemia-reperfusion injury, organ preservation, subnormothermic machine perfusion, normothermic machine perfusion

1. Introduction

Liver transplantation (LT) is the treatment of choice for patients with end-stage liver disease. Since its origin in the 1960s, outcomes after LT have improved dramatically. Advances in surgical technique, anesthetic management, critical care, and immunosuppression have led to consistently safe performance of LT in the modern era.

However, in the last few decades, the number of patients on liver transplant waiting lists (WL) worldwide has increased significantly, greatly exceeding the number of available liver grafts.

This discrepancy between supply and demand has resulted in increasing mortality on the liver transplant WL. The severe organ shortage has triggered interest in increasing the donor pool by expanding donor criteria. These extended criteria organs include grafts donated after cardiocirculatory death (DCD), grafts with higher degrees of steatosis, grafts from elderly donors, and grafts with prolonged cold storage time. Preclinical and clinical experience with extended criteria grafts demonstrates an increased susceptibility to preservation injury during cold static storage and higher rates of graft dysfunction after transplantation [1,2].

Historically, cold static storage has been the preferred method of preservation due to its simplicity, low cost, and acceptable transplant outcomes with good-quality organs. The fundamental principle underlying hypothermic organ preservation is the reduction of cellular metabolism and oxygen demand. This prolongs organ viability by slowing down progression of ischemic injury. While cellular metabolism is significantly reduced at 4°C, ongoing low-level metabolic processes continue and lead to the development of energy debt and depletion of adenosine triphosphate (ATP) stores. ATP depletion results in dysfunction of Na^+/K^+ cell membrane pumps, accumulation of toxic products derived from anaerobic metabolism, mitochondrial injury, and cell swelling. At the time of graft reperfusion, restoration of oxygen supply to dysfunctional mitochondria results in the generation of reactive oxygen species (ROS), leading to cellular damage and activation of pro-inflammatory pathways. Depending on the initial quality of the graft and the duration of cold ischemic injury, the effects of ischemia-reperfusion injury range from minor cellular dysfunction to primary nonfunction of the graft.

While standard criteria donor organs typically have the physiologic reserve to tolerate the injury associated with cold storage preservation, the diminished ability of marginal grafts to tolerate this process has triggered research to improve organ preservation. The shortcomings of cold static storage coupled with advances in organ perfusion technology have resulted in increased interest in warm ex vivo liver perfusion as an alternative to cold static storage. Warm perfusion (WP) preservation can potentially reduce injury from cold ischemia, facilitate a window of graft assessment during the preservation period, and serve as a platform for graft modification before LT.

2. Basic principles of warm liver perfusion

The primary objective of WP preservation is restoration of physiologic conditions and cellular function. The graft is supplied with nutrients and oxygen to restore and maintain cellular metabolism at physiologic or near-physiologic temperature. Simultaneously, toxic products from the cellular milieu are continuously eliminated. Under these conditions, ATP and glycogen reserves can be actively restored. If pro-inflammatory mediators are excluded from the perfusate (cytokines, leukocytes, platelets), reperfusion injury is minimized. The mechanisms underlying the observed benefit of WP have not yet been elucidated, but preclinical data suggest improved preservation of the graft endothelium may be contributory [3,4].

A second important characteristic of WP is the ability to perform an assessment of the graft during the preservation period. Since the organ is metabolically active, its performance can be evaluated by vascular flow parameters, injury markers, and functional indicators like bile production and lactate clearance. By assessing graft injury and metabolic function during organ perfusion, transplant physicians and surgeons can accept or decline liver grafts based on performance data, rather than purely clinical history and graft appearance. Perhaps most relevant for future research, the active metabolism during warm ex vivo perfusion also offers the opportunity to apply repair strategies to improve the quality of liver grafts.

3. Technical aspects of warm liver perfusion

Liver perfusion involves two separate inflow vessels (the hepatic artery and portal vein) with different pressures and flow requirements. While the hepatic artery requires high pressure (50–70 mmHg) and moderate flow (300–600 mL/min), the portal venous system has low pressure (3–5 mmHg) with higher flow (600–900 mL/min). Most groups have used continuous flow as opposed to a pulsatile flow in the hepatic artery. So far, there are no data available demonstrating superiority of either system. Clinical experience from left ventricular assist devices suggests that continuous flow devices are simpler to implement and more reliable, with comparable functional results, making it reasonable to assume similar outcomes for warm liver perfusion.

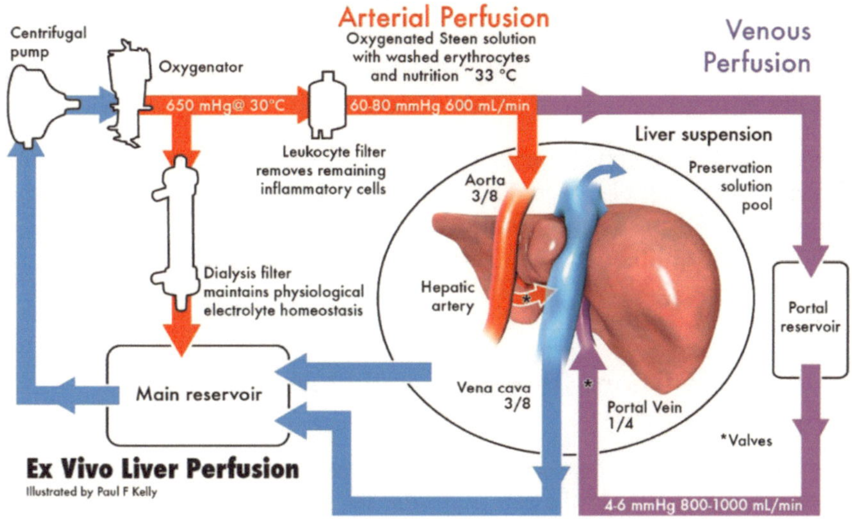

Figure 1. University of Toronto ex vivo liver perfusion system.

Regarding venous drainage, two different systems have been applied. In the simplest system, the venous blood drains directly into the organ basin, from where it is collected and recirculated. Alternatively, the venous blood can be drained through a closed tubing system either by dual vena cava outflow (infrahepatic and suprahepatic cannulas) or single vena cava outflow (**Figure 1**, Toronto perfusion scheme).

Ideally, warm organ perfusion should be initiated immediately after organ retrieval in order to avoid prolonged cold ischemic injury. Preclinical studies have demonstrated improved outcomes if cold storage is minimized prior to WP preservation for DCD grafts [1]. In clinical practice, however, in order to initiate warm perfusion immediately at the time of organ retrieval, a portable perfusion machine that can be transported to the donor hospital is required. Warm perfusion during organ ground transportation adds complexity to the preservation process and requires a safe and reliable system to maintain stability during this period. The cost of system failure is high, as this would lead to graft loss. An alternative strategy that has been employed to circumvent this issue is an initial period of cold storage, followed by transport and delayed start of WP at the transplant center. This strategy may require a modified perfusion solution to compensate for the inflammatory stimulus of the cold storage period.

4. Perfusate alternatives for warm ex vivo liver perfusion

Different perfusates have been explored in preclinical models. Due to its significant metabolism and large size, the liver requires a robust oxygen supply that cannot be provided without the addition of oxygen carriers. This is in contrast to normothermic lung perfusion, in which sufficient oxygen levels can be achieved by ventilation. While some preclinical studies have used whole blood from the donor animal for WP, most studies have used isolated RBCs as the primary oxygen carrier to avoid inflammatory mediators found in whole blood. Alternative cell-free oxygen carriers have been developed and incorporated in WP strategies with success in the preclinical setting [5].

The RBCs or alternative oxygen carriers are typically mixed with a colloid solution to replace the plasma component of whole blood. Examples of such colloid solutions include fresh frozen plasma, albumin-rich Steen solution, or starch-based solutions. Additional perfusate components typically include antibiotics, amino acids, glucose, anticoagulants, and antioxidants.

5. Temperature conditions for warm ex vivo liver perfusion

Two temperature settings have been explored for warm ex vivo liver perfusion. Normothermic perfusion is conducted at 37°C, while subnormothermic ex vivo liver perfusion (SNP) is carried out at lower temperatures (20–34°C). Both approaches have relative pros and cons, which will be highlighted below.

5.1. Subnormothermic ex vivo liver perfusion (SNP)

At the intermediate temperatures used in SNP, graft cellular activity and metabolism are greatly increased over cold storage, facilitating a window of observation of graft function prior to transplantation. The primary theoretical advantage of perfusion under subnormothermic conditions is that increased solubility of oxygen at lower temperatures (relative to 37°C) facilitates the use of perfusate solutions without the need for oxygen carriers.

5.1.1. Preclinical studies

Several groups have developed preclinical models in the pig, which is thought to most closely approximate human liver transplantation. Below, we highlight some of the most recent advances from these preclinical studies. In 2013, Minor and colleagues compared the effects of hypothermic perfusion (4°C), SNP (20°C), and controlled oxygenated rewarming, in which perfusion temperature was gradually increased from 4 to 20°C during perfusion [6]. Graft preservation consisted of an initial period of cold storage for 18 hours, followed by 90 minutes of machine perfusion preservation. Graft reperfusion was performed ex vivo with blood-containing perfusate for a period of 4 hours to simulate transplantation. Tissue ATP and energy charge were improved in the controlled rewarming and subnormothermic machine perfusion groups. Aspartate aminotransferase (AST) release and bile production were significantly improved in the controlled rewarming group relative to the other groups. These findings suggest there may be value in gradually increasing perfusion temperature to subnormothermic levels during preservation. In 2014, Knaak and colleagues at the University of Toronto reported a DCD study comparing cold storage versus SNP at 33°C [3]. After 45 minutes of in situ warm ischemia, livers underwent either cold storage for 10 versus 7 hours of cold storage followed by 3 hours of SNP. Grafts were then transplanted, and recipients followed for 7 days post transplant. SNP improved bile duct preservation and function with lower serum alkaline phosphatase (ALP) and bilirubin, lower LDH levels in bile, and the absence of biliary necrosis on histologic examination. Additionally, SNP had beneficial effects on graft endothelium. In 2015, Fontes and colleagues investigated SNP at 21°C using a novel hemoglobin-based oxygen carrier in a standard criteria donor model [5]. Grafts were preserved by SNP versus cold storage for 9 hours, followed by transplantation. Posttransplant survival at 5 days was significantly increased for SNP-preserved grafts (100 % SNP versus 33 % cold storage). SNP recipients demonstrated improved serum markers of cellular injury (AST), alanine aminotransferase (ALT) significantly increased bile production, and significantly decreased ischemia-reperfusion injury by histologic analysis. In recent report, Spetzler and colleagues at the University of Toronto performed a study with the objective of establishing the safety of SNP for standard criteria grafts [4]. In this study, heart-beating donor grafts were preserved by either 3 hours cold storage followed by 3 hours of SNP at 33°C versus 6 hours of cold storage, followed by transplantation. Following transplantation, serum levels of AST, ALP, and hyaluronic acid were lower in the SNP group. Immunohistochemistry demonstrated decreased apoptosis of sinusoidal cells in the SNP group.

5.1.2. Human studies

Thus far, SNP has not been studied in the clinical setting, although studies are likely forthcoming given the preclinical success described above. Human studies have been limited to examining the effects of SNP in discarded allografts. In 2014, Bruinsma and colleagues reported their experience with seven discarded grafts (five DCD, two DBD). SNP was carried out for

3 hours at 21°C using a bloodless perfusate [7]. Observations included increasing oxygen uptake, increased clearance of lactate, increased volume of bile production, and improved ATP content of the liver tissue during the course of perfusion, suggesting improvement in organ function. Histologic analysis demonstrated preservation of hepatocyte morphology and the sinusoidal endothelium.

5.2. Normothermic ex vivo liver perfusion (NMP)

Normothermic perfusion is performed at physiologic body temperature. The advantages of perfusion under normothermic conditions include rapid restoration of normal organ function, the ability to assess organ performance at full metabolic activity, and being a potential platform for organ repair/modification interventions (**Figure 2**).

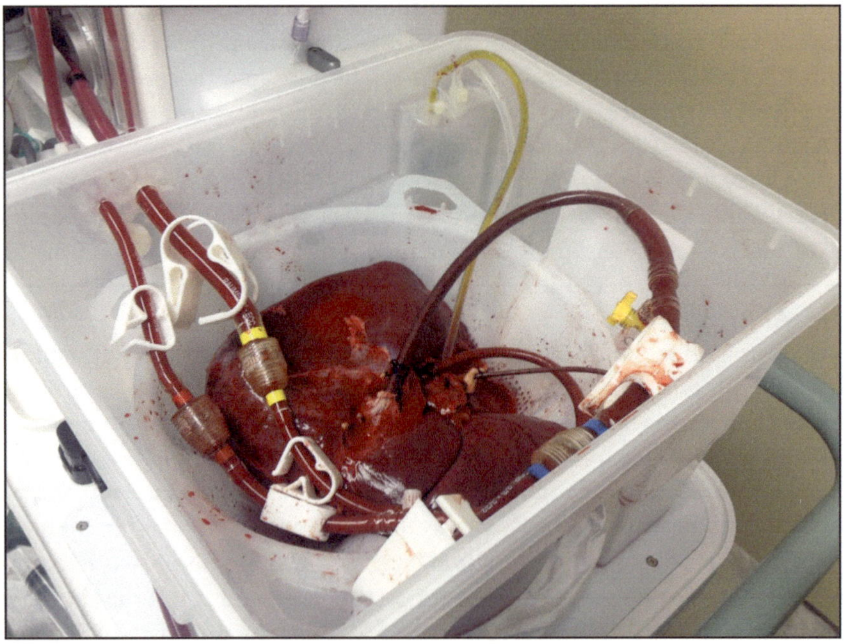

Figure 2. Liver graft connected to the Metra device being actively perfused.

5.2.1. Preclinical studies

Several preclinical studies have examined the effects and mechanisms of NMP, and encouraging results have prompted further investigation in clinical trials. The most clinically relevant preclinical experiments have been performed in porcine models, and below we highlight some of the most important studies in the preclinical setting.

Schon and colleagues reported one of the earliest studies describing the potential benefits of NMP in 2001 [8]. In this study, the effects of NMP were assessed in a DCD model with 1 hour of in situ warm ischemia. Grafts were preserved by cold storage for 4 hours versus NMP for

4 hours, followed by transplantation. In the cold storage group, all grafts exhibited primary nonfunction and recipient death. In contrast, the NMP grafts demonstrated normal graft function with 100 % recipient survival. Histologic examination demonstrated confluent necrosis in the cold storage group, while the NMP group demonstrated preservation of liver architecture. In 2005, Reddy and colleagues highlighted the detrimental effect of an initial period of cold storage prior to NMP in a DCD model [1]. In this study, grafts were retrieved after 1 hour of in situ warm ischemia and preserved either by 1 hour cold storage then 23 hours NMP or 24 hours of NMP. Markers of cellular injury (AST, ALT), sinusoidal dysfunction (hyaluronic acid), and Kupffer cell injury (β-galactosidase) were significantly higher in the grafts initially preserved with 1 hour of cold storage prior to NMP. These findings suggest that minimizing cold storage time as much as possible may improve preservation. In 2009, Brockmann and colleagues reported a study comparing NMP to cold storage in a DCD model (in situ warm ischemia of 40 versus 60 min) and also assessed the effect of extended preservation times (20 hours) [9]. At extended preservation times (20 hours), there was a significant improvement in recipient survival in the NMP group (86 % versus 27 % for grafts with no warm ischemia, 83 % versus 0 % for grafts with 40 minutes of warm ischemia). For longer warm ischemic times (60 minutes), there were no survivors in either group. An analysis of factors available during NMP that distinguished survivors from non-survivors demonstrated that bile output, base excess, AST, ALT, hyaluronic acid, portal venous pressure, and portal venous resistance were all significantly different between survivors and non-survivors. In 2013, Boehnert and colleagues at the University of Toronto reported results from a DCD study assessing the impact of NMP after an initial period of cold storage [10]. The goal of this study design was to more closely approximate the timeline of events in actual clinical practice. In the study, grafts were subjected to 1 hour of in situ warm ischemia, followed by either 4 hours of cold storage or 4 hours cold storage plus 8 hours NMP using an acellular colloid perfusate. After a period of ex vivo reperfusion to simulate transplantation, NMP-preserved grafts demonstrated lower ALT, higher oxygen extraction, more physiologic biliary composition, and less bile duct necrosis. CT angiography demonstrated superior hepatic artery perfusion in NMP grafts. In 2014, Liu and colleagues investigated the effect of NMP on bile duct preservation [11]. DCD grafts (1 hour in situ warm ischemia) were preserved by 10 hours of cold storage versus NMP. Grafts were reperfused ex vivo for an extended time period (24 hours). Histologic examination demonstrated the well-preserved parenchyma in NMP grafts, while cold-stored grafts demonstrated significant hepatocyte and biliary necrosis. In a novel analysis, the authors demonstrated increased Ki-67 staining in the biliary system of NMP grafts, consistent with biliary regeneration [11].

5.2.2. Human studies

Based on the encouraging results from several of the preclinical studies described above, normothermic ex vivo liver perfusion has entered the clinical setting. The results from a phase I trial using the transportable OrganOx Metra device (Oxford, UK) were recently reported by Ravikumar and colleagues in 2016 [12]. In this study, clinical outcomes of 20 liver transplants performed after graft preservation by NMP were compared with 40 matched controls transplanted after standard cold storage. Thirty-day graft survival was similar between groups

(100 % NMP versus 97 % cold storage), with significant improvements observed in posttransplant peak AST in the NMP group. Importantly, NMP was demonstrated to be safe, with no device-related failures in 20 consecutive cases. A second European study led by Dr. Peter Friend is currently underway comparing NMP to standard cold storage in randomized fashion. In North America, a prospective, non-randomized phase I clinical trial has been recently initiated at the University of Toronto and the University of Alberta, also using the OrganOx Metra device (**Figure 3**).

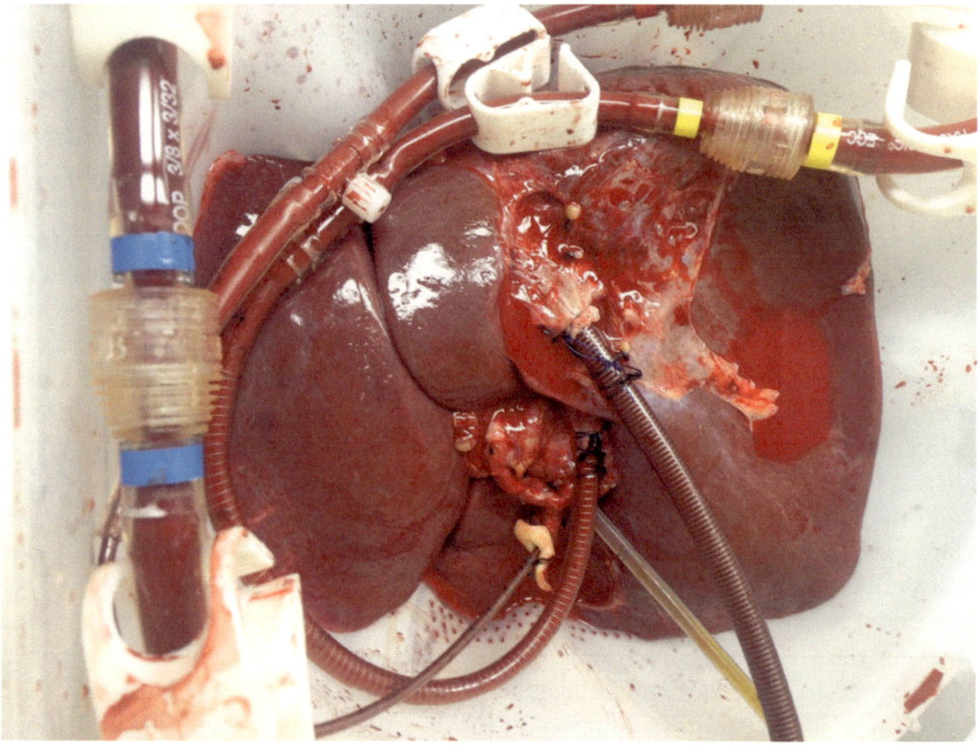

Figure 3. Normothermic perfusion of a DCD organ at the University of Toronto using the Metra device.

While clinical trials are necessary to establish the safety and efficacy of NMP, recent case studies describing the use of NMP to rescue extremely marginal grafts highlight what may become possible in the future. In 2016, Perera and colleagues in the UK reported the use of NMP to resuscitate a DCD graft with extended warm and cold ischemia time far outside of traditionally accepted parameters (109 minutes of in situ warm ischemia followed by 422 minutes of cold storage) [13]. After initiating NMP and observing evidence of good graft function including normalized lactate levels in the perfusate and robust bile production, the authors proceeded with transplantation. The recipient had an unremarkable posttransplant recovery and no evidence of ischemic-type biliary strictures at 15 months post transplant. In 2016, Watson and colleagues reported a similarly impressive clinical outcome using NMP to resuscitate a DCD graft from a 57-year-old donor with 160 minutes of warm ischemia time

(WIT) followed by 350 minutes of cold storage [14]. After establishing NMP, the assessment phase demonstrated decreasing lactate levels in the perfusate and bile production, and the graft was successfully transplanted. The recipient had an uncomplicated postoperative course and no evidence of ischemic-type biliary strictures at 6-month follow-up.

6. Conclusion

In the last decade, warm ex vivo liver perfusion has made tremendous progress and transitioned from animal studies to clinical use. It has demonstrated great potential to improve organ preservation, particularly for extended criteria grafts. As the portability and expense associated with perfusion technology improve, wider clinical application will become feasible and may facilitate expansion of the donor pool. The potential future benefit of warm machine perfusion may extend beyond rescuing marginal grafts. Due to the restoration of cellular metabolism facilitated by warm ex vivo perfusion, this technology provides an ideal platform for a variety of graft interventions including alteration of the graft response to hepatitis C infection, prevention of hepatocellular carcinoma recurrence, decreasing the graft immune response, and the application of stem cell and gene therapy. Further research in these exciting avenues has great potential to improve liver transplantation outcomes in the future.

Author details

Nicolas Goldaracena, Andrew S. Barbas and Markus Selzner*

*Address all correspondence to: markus.selzner@uhn.ca

University of Toronto, University Health Network, Toronto General Research Institute, Toronto, ON, Canada

References

[1] Reddy, S., et al., *Non-heart-beating donor porcine livers: the adverse effect of cooling.* Liver Transpl, 2005. 11(1): p. 35–8.

[2] Verran, D., et al., *Clinical experience gained from the use of 120 steatotic donor livers for orthotopic liver transplantation.* Liver Transpl, 2003. 9(5): p. 500–5.

[3] Knaak, J.M., et al., *Subnormothermic ex vivo liver perfusion reduces endothelial cell and bile duct injury after donation after cardiac death pig liver transplantation.* Liver Transpl, 2014. 20(11): p. 1296–305.

[4] Spetzler, V.N., et al., *Subnormothermic ex vivo liver perfusion is a safe alternative to cold static storage for preserving standard criteria grafts.* Liver Transpl, 2015. 22(1): p. 111–9.

[5] Fontes, P., et al., *Liver preservation with machine perfusion and a newly developed cell-free oxygen carrier solution under subnormothermic conditions.* Am J Transplant, 2015. 15(2): p. 381–94.

[6] Minor, T., et al., *Controlled oxygenated rewarming of cold stored liver grafts by thermally graduated machine perfusion prior to reperfusion.* Am J Transplant, 2013. 13(6): p. 1450–60.

[7] Bruinsma, B.G., et al., *Subnormothermic machine perfusion for ex vivo preservation and recovery of the human liver for transplantation.* Am J Transplant, 2014. 14(6): p. 1400–9.

[8] Schon, M.R., et al., *Liver transplantation after organ preservation with normothermic extracorporeal perfusion.* Ann Surg, 2001. 233(1): p. 114–23.

[9] Brockmann, J., et al., *Normothermic perfusion: a new paradigm for organ preservation.* Ann Surg, 2009. 250(1): p. 1–6.

[10] Boehnert, M.U., et al., *Normothermic acellular ex vivo liver perfusion reduces liver and bile duct injury of pig livers retrieved after cardiac death.* Am J Transplant, 2013. 13(6): p. 1441–9.

[11] Liu, Q., et al., *Sanguineous normothermic machine perfusion improves hemodynamics and biliary epithelial regeneration in donation after cardiac death porcine livers.* Liver Transpl, 2014. 20(8): p. 987–99.

[12] Ravikumar, R., et al., *Liver transplantation after ex vivo normothermic machine preservation: a Phase 1 (first-in-man) clinical trial.* Am J Transplant, 2016. 16(6): p. 1779–87.

[13] Perera, T., et al., *First human liver transplantation using a marginal allograft resuscitated by normothermic machine perfusion.* Liver Transpl, 2016. 22(1): p. 120–4.

[14] Watson, C.J., et al., *Preimplant normothermic liver perfusion of a suboptimal liver donated after circulatory death.* Am J Transplant, 2016. 16(1): p. 353–7.

Chapter 5

Pharmacogenetics of Immunosuppressants in Solid Organ Transplantation: Time to Implement in the Clinic

María José Herrero, Juan Eduardo Megías,
Virginia Bosó, Jesús Ruiz, Luis Rojas,
Ignacio Sánchez-Lázaro, Luis Amenar,
Julio Hernández, José Luis Poveda, Amparo Pastor,
Amparo Solé, Rafael López-Andújar and
Salvador F. Aliño

Additional information is available at the end of the chapter

http://dx.doi.org/10.5772/63071

Abstract

Our aim in this chapter is to present the state of the art, including our own group research, in the field of immunosuppressant pharmacogenetics in the four main types of solid organ transplantation: kidney, heart, lung, and liver. The main focus will be on those findings in the field that have been widely investigated and then in those that are close to clinical implementation, mainly CYP3A5 genotyping for the adjustment of the initial tacrolimus dose. This recommendation will be discussed in more detail, explaining its clinical potential as well as its limitations. To end, a short opinion about the feasibility of implementation in the health systems as well as discussion about private companies selling pharmacogenetic tests will be presented.

Keywords: SNP, tacrolimus, pharmacogenetic-guided therapy, CYP3A5, ABCB1, precision medicine

1. Introduction

Since the first successful kidney transplantation was performed in the 1950s, great advances have been achieved in the control of immunosuppression and graft outcome, improving drastically patient survival. Nowadays, the most common immunosupressant regimens in solid organ transplantation consist of a combination of a calcineurin inhibitor (CNI: cyclosporine [Cs] or tacrolimus [TAC]) with an antiproliferative agent such as mycophenolic acid (MPA: mycophenolate mofetil or mycophenolate sodium) or the less used azathioprine. Corticosteroids are also widely employed. Also, mTOR inhibitors [sirolimus (SIR) and everolimus (EVE)] have become common drugs in the prophylaxis of rejection after transplantation [1, 2]. Immunosuppressive agents have a narrow therapeutic index and substantial inter-patient variability, so achieving the optimal equilibrium between efficacy and an acceptable grade of toxicity is essential for the success of the treatment, and individualizing drug therapy has become an important goal.

Therapeutic drug monitoring (TDM) is indispensable for immunosuppressive agents dosing and reduces the pharmacokinetic component of variability by controlling drug blood concentrations. However, TDM is only possible after the drug is administered and steady state and patient's compliance are achieved; thus, complementary strategies are needed. The intra- and inter-patient differences in immunosuppressant dosage requirements and pharmacokinetics are attributable to several factors, such as kidney function, ethnicity, concomitant use of other drugs [3], and qualitative and quantitative changes of proteins whose activity plays key roles in the absorption, distribution, metabolism, and function of these drugs. In these last mentioned protein changes is where pharmacogenetics plays a crucial role: Functional changes of these proteins (transporters, metabolizing enzymes, target proteins, etc.) have been attributed to polymorphism in their coding genes [4, 5]. Single-nucleotide polymorphisms (SNPs) are the main type of polymorphisms involved in human genome variation. These are different alleles or variants that naturally occur at a determined position of a gene, the frequency of the less common allele in the population being not higher than 1%. For instance, in a concrete point of a determined gene, part of the population, let's say 80%, could have an adenine (A) or AA, and this would be the most frequent genotype at that genomic position, while 5% would have a thymine, being the variant and less frequent allele (TT genotype), and the rest 15% of the mentioned population would be heterozygous for the variant, AT genotype. Pharmacogenetics aims to determine the effect of those genetic variants regarding the efficacy and toxicity of drugs, and therefore, it may be able to predict patients' response to them. These genetic characteristics can be known for each single patient before the drug is administered, allowing the design of the best strategy to treat the patient, what we nowadays know as precision medicine.

In this scenario, it is also very important to take into account that in transplantation each patient actually contains two different genetic entities: the donor and the recipient. Therefore, the drugs administered to the recipient will be metabolized or excreted by the transplanted organ from the donor when we are talking about liver or kidney transplantation, respectively. But also in heart- or lung-transplanted patients, the effect of the donors' genotype could be seen if we find toxicities and/or efficacies directly related to these organs. This is the reason why more and more studies in transplantation pharmacogenetics consider both the donor and recipient genotypes to evaluate the response to treatment [6–9].

2. The genes related to the immunosuppressants

Cs and TAC are metabolized by CYP3A subfamily in both enterocytes and hepatocytes. Cs is primarily metabolized by *CYP3A4* and in a lesser extent by *CYP3A5*, while TAC is mainly metabolized by *CYP3A5*. Both enzymes are characterized by great variations in their expression and activity caused by genetic variability but also by concomitant administration of drugs that act as inhibitors or inducers [4, 5, 10–13]. P450 (cytochrome) oxidoreductase (*POR*) has been suggested as an element that also influences *CYP3A5* activity.

The *ABCB1* gene encodes the efflux transporter P-glycoprotein (P-gp), which is responsible for the active transport and expulsion of multiple substances across cell membranes and is present in several tissues but mainly in excretory organs [14].This pump plays a major role in the pharmacokinetics of TAC and Cs. P-gp has been found to be present at high concentrations in enterocytes, and it is present in hepatocytes, kidney cells, and lymphocytes [15]. A 17% of the variability in oral clearance of Cs depends on the P-gp accounts in intestinal enterocytes [16]. In TAC, the level of *ABCB1* intestinal expression showed a strong inverse correlation with the TAC concentration/dose ratio [17]. Genotypes associated with lower P-gp function have been associated with greater drug absorption and higher blood concentration. The three most frequent *ABCB1* gene polymorphisms studied are the synonymous SNPs 1236C<T (rs1128503) and 3435C<T (rs1045642), as well as the nonsynonymous SNP 2677G<T/A (rs2032582). The variant TT genotype of these SNPs is proposed to result in decreased levels of mRNA expression and P-gp activity, although this point is still controversial.

Following administration, mycophenolate mofetil (MMF) or enteric-coated mycophenolate sodium is hydrolyzed to MPA, the active metabolite. MPA is metabolized in the liver, gastrointestinal tract, and kidney by uridine diphosphate gluconosyltransferases (UGTs). MPAG, the main metabolite, is a phenolic glucuronide, which has no pharmacological activity and is excreted into the urine via active tubular secretion and into the bile by multidrug resistance protein 2 (*MRP-2* or *ABCC2*). MPAG is de-conjugated back to MPA by gut bacteria and then reabsorbed in the colon, the so-called enterohepatic circulation pathway [18–21]. MPA acts as a selective inhibitor of inosine 5′-monophosphate dehydrogenase (*IMPDH*). Two isoforms of *IMPDH* exist and MPA is more active against type II (expressed primarily in malignant and activated lymphocytes) than against type I (predominantly found in normal, resting leukocytes) [22–25]. SNPs in these genes might affect the efficacy of MPA and therefore acute rejection in transplant patients.

Azathioprine is employed in patients with intolerance to mycophenolate as an alternative antimetabolite. This prodrug is activated to 6-mercaptopurine in the erythrocytes, and thiopurine methyltransferase (*TPMT*) is the main enzyme for 6-mercaptopurine metabolism. Described *TPMT* polymorphisms produce a decreased enzyme function and a higher risk of side effects related to the 6-thioguanine formation such as bone marrow suppression. The Clinical Pharmacogenetics Implementation Consortium has published guidelines for the clinical implementation of *TPMT* genotype analysis in patients treated with azathioprine; likewise the US Food and Drug Administration label also recommends TPMT testing [26]. One study evaluated this association in liver transplantation, and aversely, its findings suggest that

TPMT, ITPA, and *MTHFR* genotypes do not predict adverse drug reactions, including bone marrow suppression [27].

Information about genetic variations affecting SIR and EVE response is still scarce. Both drugs are metabolized via *CYP3A4, CYP3A5,* and *CYP2C8* enzymes [28] and both are P-gp substrates. EVE is used as off-label immunosuppressive therapy in lung transplantation with CNI-associated renal insufficiency, skin neoplasms, and bronchiolitis obliterans syndrome [29, 30]. As the rest of immunosuppressive drugs, SIR and EVE have a narrow therapeutic index and a significant inter- and intra-individual pharmacokinetic variability.

Glucocorticoid-induced osteonecrosis is an important adverse event affecting transplant patients, leading to severe joint pain and limitations on physical activity. Numerous studies have reported that *ABCB1* polymorphisms are associated with glucocorticoid-induced osteonecrosis, as, for instance, in renal transplant patients [31]. A recent meta-analysis suggested that some *ABCB1* alleles may decrease the risks of corticoid-induced osteonecrosis [32].

Other clinical consequences, mainly long term, of immunosuppressants are being subject to really interesting pharmacogenetic studies: tumor development, fertility impairment, or hypertension [33–35].

3. Kidney transplantation

3.1. Calcineurin inhibitors

The expression of *ABCB1* in the kidney plays an important role in the renal elimination of metabolic waste products and toxins. It seems like after renal injury, *ABCB1* expression is upregulated, which may represent an adaptive response in the renal regeneration process. Also, it has been shown that treatment with CNI induces *ABCB1* expression both in vivo and in vitro, which could serve to protect the kidney from the injurious effects of CNIs by facilitating their extrusion [36]. A decrease in *ABCB1* levels of expression could lead to intrarenal accumulation of CNIs and predispose patients to the occurrence of CNI-related nephrotoxicity [37]. Capron et al. showed in a prospective study with 96 renal transplant recipients that *ABCB1* 1199G>A, 3435C>T, and 2677G>T/A (rs2229109, 1045642, 2032582, respectively) seemed to reduce the activity of P-gp increasing TAC peripheral blood mononuclear cell concentrations. Nevertheless, the impact of *ABCB1* SNPs on TAC blood concentrations was negligible [38]. In another study conducted in Asian renal transplant recipients, *ABCB1* C3435T was not an important factor in TAC pharmacokinetics [39]. The presence of *ABCB1* 3435T variant allele in the donor was related to a higher risk of histologic kidney damage [40], maybe due to a local drug accumulation.

In the meta-analysis conducted by Terrazzino et al. [41], no evidence of an effect of the *ABCB1* 3435C>T variant was detected on TAC Cmin/D, except for a modest effect limited to the first month after renal transplantation. In contrast, another meta-analysis conducted by Li et al. [42] showed that *ABCB1* 3435C>T could influence the TAC pharmacokinetics at different post-transplant times, so subjects with wild-type genotype showed lower Cmin/D than those carrying variant T allele. Results of a more recent meta-analysis published in 2015 in Cs-treated kidney transplant recipients indicated a significant difference of Cmin/D and Cmax/D between 3435CC and 3435TT genotype carriers (p = 0.03). Subgroup analysis by ethnicity demonstrated that in Asians, Cmin/D was lower in CC versus TT genotype carriers but did not vary for Caucasian recipients. This meta-analysis showed that patients with 3435CC genotype will require a higher dose of Cs to achieve target drug blood concentrations when compared with 3435TT carriers, especially in the Asian population and especially during the early and middle time periods after transplantation [43].

A polymorphism in intron 3 of *CYP3A5* (rs776746 or *CYP3A5**3) results in altered mRNA splicing that leads to a premature stop codon and hence a nonfunctional protein [11]. So, while *3/*3 carriers do not express the enzyme (nonexpressers), individuals carrying at least one functional *CYP3A5**1 allele express the enzyme (expressers) and are able to metabolize CNIs via *CYP3A5* [12]. Our studies in Spanish Caucasian population show that although *1/*1 genotype is rare and carried by only 1% of the population, 16% of transplanted patients and donors present *CYP3A5**1/*3 genotype and might have different dosage needs than *3/*3 carriers [13].

The first studies about the relationship between *CYP3A5* and CNI dosage in transplant recipients were published over 10 years ago. In 2003 Hesselink et al. [5] reported in kidney transplant recipients receiving Cs or TAC that TAC dose-adjusted trough levels were higher in *CYP3A5**3/*3 patients than in *1/*3 plus *1/*1 patients, but found no differences in Cs-treated patients. The same year, MacPhee et al. [44] also reported a reduced exposure to TAC in the first weeks after kidney transplantation in *CYP3A5* expressers, but found no difference in the rate of biopsy-confirmed acute rejection. Haufroid et al. [10] reported in 2004 that dose-adjusted trough concentrations were threefold and 1.6-fold higher in *CYP3A5**3/*3 patients than in *CYP3A5**1/*3 patients for TAC and Cs, respectively. Since then, several studies have shown that *CYP3A5* expressers require higher TAC doses than nonexpressers to achieve the same blood concentrations [45–50]. A pharmacogenetic substudy of a randomized-controlled trial where patients were treated with TAC, MPA, and corticosteroids compared *CYP3A5* expressers with *CYP3A5* nonexpressers. TAC doses were higher for expressers, whereas dose-corrected Cmin were lower for this group. This would mean that patients expressing *CYP3A5* need more TAC to reach target concentrations and have a lower TAC exposure. However, no differences in biopsy-proven acute rejection were found [51]. Regarding graft rejection, whereas some studies have found an association with *CYP3A5* genotype [52, 53], others have not shown this [54, 55]. In the case of nephrotoxicity, results are also controversial [47, 54, 56].

The first prospective randomized-controlled trial (by Thervet et al.) to compare the pharmacokinetic characteristics of TAC in patients receiving a fixed dose of the drug or a dose adapted according to the patient's *CYP3A5* genotype showed that, in the genotype-based group, a higher proportion of patients had values within the targeted Cmin at day 3 after initiation of TAC (43.2% vs. 29.1%; p = 0.03); they required fewer dose modifications and the targeted Cmin was achieved by 75% of these patients more rapidly [57]. No differences in clinical outcome were found, but the study population was at low immunological risk. A later randomized-controlled trial with similar pharmacogenetic-guided TAC starting dose found no differences between groups in the percent of patients having a TAC exposure within the target range or the incidence of acute rejection [58].

Other authors have studied the influence of donors' genotype. Opposite to liver transplantation, donors' *CYP3A5* genotype seems to have no influence in CNI dose requirements to achieve target drug concentrations [56].

Several meta-analyses have been performed. The results of a meta-analysis performed by our group suggest a significantly lower TAC dose-normalized Cmin among *CYP3A5*1* allele carriers compared with carriers of the *CYP3A5*3/*3* genotype at weeks 1 and 2 and months 1, 3, 6, and 12 after kidney transplantation. Also *CYP3A5* expressers might have higher risk of acute rejection and chronic nephrotoxicity [59]. Terrazzino et al. [41] conducted another meta-analysis in which random-effects model showed significantly higher TAC Cmin/D in *CYP3A5*3/*3* compared with *CYP3A5*1* allele carriers, either in the overall analysis and when stratifying for ethnicity or time of posttransplantation (≤1, 3–6, 12–24 months). In the meta-analysis conducted by Tang et al. [60], *CYP3A5* expressers required higher mean TAC daily doses [95% confidence interval (CI), 0.033–0.056] than nonexpressers. In Cs-treated patients, a meta-analysis also showed that *CYP3A5*3* polymorphism is associated with Cs dose-adjusted concentration in renal transplant recipients [50].

Regarding *CYP3A4*, different studies have explored the impact of *CYP3A4*1B* on CNI pharmacokinetics. Gervasini et al. found that carriers of the *CYP3A4*1B* variant allele showed TAC Cmin that were on average 59% lower than in patients with the *CYP3A4*1/*1* genotype. Furthermore, among *CYP3A5**1 carriers, those also carrying the *CYP3A4*1B* allele showed the lowest dose-corrected Cmin, as compared with *CYP3A4*1/CYP3A5*3* carriers [61]. Other studies have shown the influence of this variant in TAC and Cs pharmacokinetics [46, 62], but results are still inconsistent [63, 64]. This variant has been reported to lead, in vitro, to increased transcription of the gene [65], but several authors attribute its observed effects to the fact that *CYP3A4*1B* is in strong linkage disequilibrium (LD) with the *CYP3A5*1* active allele, meaning that very frequently they are carried together. This could explain the inconsistencies of the reported associations with Cs and TAC pharmacokinetics, if only one of those two SNPs is addressed [1, 2]. Another functional SNP, located in *CYP3A4* intron 6 (*CYP3A4*22*, rs35599367, C>T), has been found associated with decreased mRNA hepatic expression and therefore decreased enzymatic activity and has also been correlated with the statin dose requirement for lipid concentration control [66]. This SNP was associated with altered TAC and Cs metabolism and dose-adjusted Cmin were higher for *22 carriers in a study carried out in 99 stable renal transplant recipients [67]. This difference was even higher when combining *CYP3A4/CYP3A5* poor metabolizer genotypes, for both TAC and Cs, and was reproduced in 185 kidney transplant recipients treated with TAC [68].

POR has been suggested as an element that influences *CYP3A5* activity. Carrying *28 allele was associated with increased dose of TAC in kidney transplant recipients. And an association for a higher daily dose requirement was found only in *CYP3A5* expressers [69]. Another study showed that *POR*28* allele is associated with increased in vivo *CYP3A5* activity for TAC in *CYP3A5* expressers, whereas *POR*28* homozygosity was associated with a significant higher CYP3A4 activity in *CYP3A5* nonexpressers for both TAC and Cs [70]. But other studies have not replicated these results [71–73]. Also *POR*28* allele has been associated with increased risk of diabetes mellitus in patients treated with TAC [74].

Transplant patients receive a large number of drugs and the effect of concomitant drugs is important. Gastric protection is very common in transplant recipients. We conducted a study in 75 renal transplant recipients treated with TAC and omeprazole. This drug is mainly metabolized via *CYP2C19* and secondarily by *CYP3A4/5*. In patients carrying a nonfunctional *CYP2C19* variant, omeprazole inhibits TAC metabolism via *CYP3A5*, increasing TAC blood concentrations. The patients with *CYP2C19*2/*2* genotype showed a median posttransplantation hospital stay of 27.5 days (95%CI: 23–39), compared with 12 days (95%CI: 10–15) in patients with *CYP2C19*1/*1* or *1/*2* genotype. In the group of *CYP3A5* nonexpressers (expressers were excluded to avoid its influence), there was a direct correlation with an increase in Cmin/D TAC blood levels and *CYP2C19*2/*2* genotype, which also showed allograft delayed function (acute tubular necrosis in 3 out of 4 patients). So *CYP2C19*2/*2* variant indirectly elicits an increase of TAC blood levels in *CYP3A5* nonexpressers and may lead to adverse events [3].

3.2. mTOR inhibitors

CYP3A5 genotype might explain part of the variability in SIR drug levels. In a few studies, *CY3A5* expressers showed increased dose requirements to achieve adequate blood trough levels of SIR in people with kidney transplantation as compared to *CYP3A5*3/*3* genotype. Also, *CYP3A5*3/*3* was associated with decreased metabolism of SIR and higher blood levels [75–77].

A study also showed that *CYP3A4*1B* carriers may require an increased dose of SIR as compared to patients with the *1/*1 genotype [75]. Preliminary data demonstrated that human liver microsomes carrying *CYP3A4*22* metabolized SIR at a significantly slower rate than noncarriers [1]. *ABCB1* genotype does not seem to be of relevance for mTOR inhibitor therapy, although patients with the CC genotype in 3435C>T or 1236C>T may have decreased total and low-density lipoprotein cholesterol when treated with SIR, as was shown by Sam et al. [78].

3.3. Mycophenolic acid

Several studies have reported the role of SNPs in the promoter region of *UGT1A9* in MPA pharmacokinetics and the risk of rejection, including gain of function SNPs -275T>A (rs6714486) and -2152C>T (rs17868320) [79]. Van Schaik et al. [80] showed in a study including 338 kidney transplant recipients that *UGT1A9* -275T>A and -2152C>T SNPs were associated to lower MPA exposure in patients receiving TAC and corticosteroids plus MMF. Additionally, in this study *UGT1A9**3 was associated with higher MPA exposure when MMF was given in combination with CNIs. In another study including 133 stable Caucasian renal transplant recipients, promoter SNPs -275T>A and -2152C>T were associated with lower MPA exposure, and additionally the carriers of these SNPs had higher incidence of gastrointestinal side effects [81]. *UGT1A8**3 and *UGT1A9**3 might influence MPA pharmacokinetics but occur with a very low allele frequency (<5%), so their clinical impact is limited [82]. *UGT1A8*2* might also be associated to less adverse gastrointestinal adverse events. *UGT2B7* has also been postulated as a candidate biomarker of MPA pharmacokinetics, but no relevant results have been found yet.

Regarding *ABCC2*, MPAG is excreted in bile primarily by this transporter and this transport is essential for the enterohepatic circulation. *ABCC2* -24C>T (rs717620) has been associated with lower MPA clearance in patients with concomitant treatment with TAC [83]. *ABCC2* 1249G>A (rs2273697) was also related to higher MPA metabolite levels [84].

MPA is also substrate of organic anion-transporting polypeptides (OATPs), which are responsible for the entrance of MPA and MAPG into hepatocytes. This has been observed in vitro [85], but in vivo results are still contradictory [85–87]. Picard et al. [85] observed that the pharmacokinetics of both MPA and MPAG were significantly influenced by the *SLCO1B3* polymorphism 334T>G/699G>A in 70 renal transplant patients receiving combination treatment of MMF with either TAC or SIR, but not in 115 patients receiving MMF and Cs. Miura et al. [87] found a significant association between MPA excretion into bile and *SLCO1B3* 334T>G. The organic anion transporter polypeptide-1B1 (SLCO1B1) is involved in the liver uptake of MMF. In renal transplantation, the minor allele of SLCO1B1 (rs4149056) polymorphism was associated to lower MPA clearance than wild-type genotype, because this genotype reduces drug uptake [88].

The association of SNPs in IMPDH with MPA is not clear. *IMPDH1* rs2278294 allele T was found associated with decreased risk of biopsy-proven acute rejection [22, 89], but this was not found in other studies [23, 90]. Regarding *IMPDH2* rs11706052, allele G carriers who are treated with Cs and MMF may have an increased risk of biopsy-proven acute rejection and decreased response [82], but several other studies have not confirmed this association [24, 25].

4. Heart transplantation

Heart transplantation has experienced a great improvement in the last years. Survival among cardiac transplant recipients is estimated to be 83% 5 years posttransplantation as a result of improvements in immunosuppressant treatments, surgical technique, and reduction of adverse events [91, 92]. Nevertheless, still a considerable number of patients experience morbidity and mortality after transplantation. These outcomes could be related to genetic variability in genes that encodes transporters, metabolizers, or molecular targets of immunosuppressant therapy.

4.1. Calcineurin inhibitors

Most of the published studies analyzed the relationship between *ABCB1* polymorphisms and CNI pharmacokinetics. Regarding TAC, some studies found a relationship between wild-type *ABCB1* genotypes and reduced drug blood levels during the first 2 weeks after transplantation in adult patients [7] or after 6 and 12 months after transplantation in pediatric population [93]. However, several other studies did not find significant results [94–97]. Cs is also substrate of P-gp, and there are numerous reports of lesser cyclosporine blood concentrations with wild-

http://dx.doi.org/10.5772/63071

type *ABCB1* genotypes [7, 97–100], although again other authors did not obtain significant differences [96]. The inconsistent influence of *ABCB1* genotypes on CNI therapies may be due to unique genetic populations or small sample size.

High CNI levels are related to the appearance of nephrotoxicity. Most of the studies did not detect association between *ABCB1* variants and renal function [95, 100–104]. On the other hand, in one of our last works, we obtained lower renal function in patients with AG genotype of a rarely studied polymorphism of *ABCB1* (rs9282564), related to higher Cs blood concentrations [97]. Besides, *ABCB1* wild-type genotype of 1236C<T SNP was correlated to lower risk of serious infections and lower Cs blood levels. Wild-type homozygosity for the 3435C<T and 2677G<T/A SNPs has been associated to increased steroid dependency after 1 year of heart transplantation in pediatric patients treated with TAC [105, 106], but this effect was not reproduced in a larger adult cohort of 337 patients with Cs therapy [100]. Wild-type genotypes of 3435C<T and 2677G<T/A were also correlated to higher risk of graft rejection in a large cohort of 170 adult recipients [107], although in smaller cohorts these effects were not reproduced [94, 100]. Other outcomes studied with these SNPs were new-onset diabetes [95] and plasma lipid concentrations [108]. Of these outcomes only higher LDL cholesterol pretransplant values were related to variant alleles of *ABCB1,* but this association was lost after transplantation.

The differences in TAC blood levels regarding the already explained CYP3A5 variants *1 or *3 were clearly observed in adult heart transplantation [95, 96, 98, 109, 110] and also in children [93, 94, 111]. However with Cs it was only described in our small cohort of 25 adult heart transplant patients, in which the CYP3A5*3/3* variant was associated to an increase in trough blood levels corrected by dose and body weight [98]. These results were not reproduced in two other similar studies (30 and 45 adult heart recipients) [96, 99].

Age and *CYP3A5* genotype were related to TAC concentration/dose ratio and dosing requirements in pediatric cardiac transplant population [94]. This was reflected in *CYP3A5* expressers, because when they were older than 6, the dosing requirements were more than 1.5 times lower than in *CYP3A5* expressers younger than 6 years. Besides CNI clearance, *CYP3A5*1* carriers were associated to higher estimated glomerular filtration rate after heart transplantation in a cohort of 160 adult recipients treated with TAC or Cs [102]. Other studies in cohorts of 53 and 60 adult cardiac transplants and 39 and 453 pediatric cardiac recipients did not find significant relationships between *CYP3A5* genotypes and renal outcomes [94, 97, 101, 103]. A study in a large cohort of 115 adult heart recipients did not find associations between CNI nephrotoxicity and *CYP3A5* genotypes, but it showed significant relationship with posttransplant kidney function in *CYP3A5*3/3** and *CYP2A6* (rs28399433) variants in European Americans (subgroup of 99 recipients) [104]. Other outcomes as steroid dependency, graft rejection, and risk of developing new-onset diabetes after transplantation were studied without significant relationships [94, 95, 106].

A study in 60 pediatric heart transplant recipients investigated the combined effect of *CYP3A5* and *CYP3A4*22* (rs35599367) [111]. *CYP3A* poor metabolizers (*CYP3A5*3/3* and CYP3A4*1/*22) required 17% less TAC than intermediate (*CYP3A5*3/3* and CYP3A4*1/*1*) and 48% less than extensive metabolizers (*CYP3A5*1/1* or CYP3A5*1/3* and CYP3A4*1/*1*). This study also obtained similar effects with *CYP3A4*22* allele carriers alone in number of TAC doses to reach target concentrations, but not in TAC concentrations and the dose-adjusted concentration. However, a later study in adult cardiac transplant patients treated with TAC (52 patients) or Cs (45 patients) did not find significant associations with *CYP3A4*22* variants [96] but showed that *POR*28* variant carriers had higher dose-adjusted TAC concentrations 3 and 6 months posttransplantation. This variant had previously been studied in kidney transplantation combined with *CYP3A5* expressers [112–114], with a contradictory effect compared to this effect in heart transplant recipients. Another *CYP3A* modulator is the pregnane X receptor encoded by *NR1I2* gene, whose SNP rs3814055 was studied by Lesche without changes in TAC clearance [96].

Other different CYP enzymes were studied in heart transplantation. *CYP2C8* and *CYP2J2* are expressed in the kidney and are involved in the metabolism of arachidonic acid–promoting kidney homeostasis. The *CYP2C8*3* variant was associated with a higher risk of nephrotoxicity in liver recipients treated with TAC or Cs [115]. In heart transplantation, *CYP2C8* variants were studied in a small cohort of 30 patients treated with maintenance therapy (Cs, EVE, prednisolone) and there were no differences in EVE dose requirements between *CYP2C8* genotypes [116].

4.2. mTor inhibitors

A report in adult heart recipients suggested that EVE blood levels were not related to *ABCB1* genotypes. No significant associations between *CYP3A5* poor expressers and EVE pharmacokinetics were observed either [110, 117]. *CYP2C8* variants were also studied in a heart transplantation cohort of 30 recipients without significant differences in EVE pharmacokinetics [116].

4.3. Mycophenolic acid

In pediatric heart transplantation, the gastrointestinal intolerance was reproduced with variant allele of *ABCC2* rs717620, causing MMF discontinuation [118]. Other toxicities associated to *ABCC2* SNPs were anemia (rs3740066) and leucopenia (rs17222723) [119].

Regarding serum levels of MPA and their metabolites, a study did not obtain significant relationships with *ABCC2* polymorphisms (34Ting LSL 2010). In a large pediatric cohort of 290 heart recipients, wild-type *ABCC2* (rs717620) genotype was correlated to higher risk of graft rejection and late rejection, both with hemodynamic compromise [120].

The influence of *UGT* SNPs on MPA plasma concentrations is moderate and must be analyzed along with *ABCC2* and *ABCB1* polymorphisms. In a cohort of 68 thoracic transplant recipients (36 lung and 32 heart transplants), two variants of *UGT2B7* (rs7439366 and rs73823859) and acyl-MPA glucuronide levels were associated in both cohorts [119]. In this study, two variants of *UGT2B7* (rs7668258 and rs73823859) showed a significant influence in thoracic graft rejection, as well as *UGT1A7* variant rs11692021 with anemia and *UGT* 3′UTR T1813 variant with leucopenia.

The presence of polymorphisms in IMPDH1 and IMPDH2 genes does not result in lower activity in all cases [121]. In a cohort of 59 pediatric cardiac transplant, two variants of IMPDH1

http://dx.doi.org/10.5772/63071

(rs2278294 and rs2228075) were associated to greater gastrointestinal toxicity [122]. On the other hand, this study also found that variant G of IMPDH2 (rs11706052) polymorphism was related to neutropenia that required dose holding. A posterior haplotype analysis repeated the association of IMPDH1 to gastrointestinal intolerance but this was not greater than individual IMPDH1 polymorphisms [122].

4.4. Azathioprine

In heart transplantation, heterozygotes for TPMT SNPs (rs1142345, rs1800460, rs1800462) were shown lower enzyme activity and earlier and higher rejection than wild-type genotypes, although without changes in leukopenia incidence [123].

4.5. Other genes: the immunomodulatory pathway

The immune response and acute transplant rejection could be influenced by cytokines and growth factors; hence regulating cytokine production is a strategy to minimize rejection. Of these, the most studied in heart transplantation is the transforming growth factor- ß1 (*TGF-ß1*), because this inductor of the collagen has profibrotic activity during the progression of glomerulonephritis, consequence of CNI nephrotoxicity. Polymorphisms in the *TGF-ß1* promoter region produced a reduction of *TGF-ß1* level [124]. In a large cohort of 237 cardiac transplants, the presence of variants of two *TGF-ß1* polymorphisms (rs1800470 and rs1800471) was associated to CNI-induced end-stage renal failure [125]. However, in two smaller cohorts and a larger pediatric cohort, these two SNPs were not related to renal outcomes [101, 103, 126]. Other polymorphisms included in one of these studies an SNP in the protein kinase C-β gene (*PRKCB*; rs11074606), a gene implicated in the renin-angiotensin-aldosterone intracellular signaling, was related to posttransplant estimated glomerular filtration rate [126].

Polymorphisms in cytokine genes (*TNF-α, TGF-ß1, IL-10, IL-6, and INF-γ*) were also analyzed regarding steroid dependency. Of these SNPs, only *IL-10* polymorphisms (rs1800896, rs1800871, rs1800872) were associated as independent risk factor with steroid dependency at 1 year after heart transplantation [106]. In a large multiethnic cohort of 300 pediatric cardiac transplant patients, acute rejection at 5 years was related to the combination *VEGF* high (rs699947, rs833061, rs2010963), *IL-6* high (rs1800795), and IL-10 low (rs1800896, rs1800871, rs1800872) expression genotypes, but not with *TNF-α* (rs1800629) [127].

The nucleotide-binding oligomerization domain containing 2 (*NOD2/CARD15*) encodes a protein involved in intracellular pathogen recognition and lymphocyte activation. In our latest study we observed a tendency of association between CC genotype in NOD2/CARD15 (rs2066844) and increased graft rejection [97].

A new gene that was studied in heart transplantation was the connective tissue growth factor (*CTGF*), whose expression has been shown to be induced in in vitro models of chronic heart allograft rejection. Carriers of the C allele of rs6918698 SNP were associated to high risk for the development of cardiac allograft vasculopathy, a surrogate marker for chronic rejection [128].

5. Lung transplantation

Lung transplantation has become an alternative option for a variety of end-stage pulmonary diseases, including cystic fibrosis, idiopathic pulmonary fibrosis, pulmonary arterial hypertension, bronchiolitis, or advanced chronic obstructive pulmonary disease. Hardy performed the first human lung transplantation in 1963 but the recipient survived only 18 days. In the 1980s, the introduction of Cs generated renewed interest in this area, and in 1986, Dr Joel Cooper reported the first successful single lung transplant. Since the early 1990s, more than 30,000 lung transplants have been performed around the world.

The increasing success of thoracic transplantation is largely attributable to the development of effective immunosuppressive regimens. However, it remains as one of the solid organ transplant with the worst outcomes, with less than 80% 1-year survival and less than 70% after 3 years [129]. Several reasons for these poor results have been identified; some of them are shared with other solid organ transplants, including acute rejection and drug treatment toxicity. Lung-transplanted patients are a particularly difficult group to study: Immunosuppressive treatment variations and the way they are administered (intravenous and oral) during the first weeks post transplantation make changes in blood concentration difficult to evaluate. On the other hand, patients with cystic fibrosis, one of the main groups of lung transplantation patients, present high absorption variability, leading to lower immunosuppressive drugs blood levels [130]. It should be noticed that most of the lung transplant studies have not considered this variable in their analyses, potentially leading to erroneous results. This complexity has made this group of patients less studied than other groups such as heart, liver, or kidney transplantation. However, some relevant findings have been published.

Contradictory results have been reported regarding the effect of *ABCB1* polymorphisms on TAC disposition in lung transplantation. Wang et al. [131] reported an association between *ABCB1* haplotype and TAC blood concentration. This result has been replicated in subsequent studies [132]. However, other authors have not found this relationship [5, 45]. It should be noticed that these two studies did not considered the concomitant effect of *CYP3A5* genotype, which has shown to have important effects in this group of patients [133].

Initial studies have demonstrated a positive association between TAC dosing and the CYP3A5 gene polymorphism in heart and adult lung transplant patients [5, 131]. The CYP3A5 *3/*3 nonexpresser patients have a higher TAC level/dose than the CYP3A5 *1/*1 or *1/*3 enzyme expressers. Several authors have recommended that CYP3A5 expressers should initially get double dose of TAC than the administered to CYP3A5 nonexpressers [44], but this proposal should be tested thoroughly in lung transplantation before initiation in clinical practice.

No relevant information related to SNP variations and MPA concentrations in lung transplantation has been published. In a 51 patients study, we found that those patients with heterozygous at *ABCC2* rs3740066 had lower MPA blood concentrations than homozygotes [132]. However, large study sizes are needed to confirm these results.

Schoeppler et al. [134] in 65 lung transplant recipients did not find associations between several polymorphisms, in genes including *ABCB1, CYP3A5, CYP3A4, CYP2C8,* and EVE blood concentration. The author concluded that genotyping lung transplantation patients for these polymorphisms is unlikely to be helpful for clinicians in optimizing EVE therapy. However, the small number of patients included makes necessary new studies to confirm this hypothesis. In the last years, SIR has been introduced as an alternative immunosuppressive therapy for lung transplantation patients [135, 136], but still no information has been reported about pharmacogenetics of this drug in lung transplantation.

The process of chronic rejection is a pathologic process very different to acute rejection, and almost all lung transplant patients at 4 years posttransplantation have some evidence of chronic rejection [137]. Whether the chronic rejection process either directly or indirectly involves P-gp is unknown but is a possibility worth to be explored.

Budding et al. [138] found an association between complement regulatory gene *CD59* polymorphism and the pathogenesis of acute rejection in lung transplantation. *HLA-G* haplotypes have also been associated with increased graft survival and decreased rejection episodes in lung transplantation [139]. NOD/CARD15 has been related with graft organ survival outcomes of transplanted patients [140, 141], but information in lung transplantation is scarce.

6. Liver transplantation

The concept that a single gene polymorphism could affect patient survival in a complex patient population is difficult to conceive. However, a study by Hashida et al. [142] suggested that patients who had high amounts of *ABCB1* mRNA had a significantly poorer patient survival than the patients with low amounts of *ABCB1* mRNA. Patients with the *ABCB1* 2677GG, 1236 CC, and 3435CC genotypes would have greater function of the drug transporter associated with lower TAC bioavailability and level/dose ratio, but the evidence remains uncertain. Some studies in Caucasian patients [143, 144] have not reported association between both variables; however a meta- analysis reported a significative association between ABCB1 C3435T and C/D ratio TAC, although with a low quality of evidence [145]. Other *ABCB1* polymorphisms do not seem to relevantly influence TAC pharmacokinetics.

In summary, there is not sufficient information to support prospective clinical trials about TAC dosing based only in these polymorphisms, but they may be good candidates for combined analyses of polymorphisms affecting the inter-individual variability in TAC pharmacokinetics among *CYP3A5* expressers.

6.1. Influence of donor versus recipient genotype

Pharmacokinetic studies in liver transplant recipients are complex due to the fact that the recipient's intestinal genotype and the donor liver genotype may act together influencing the overall drug disposition. Several studies have evaluated the effect of donors and recipients *CYP3A5* 6986A>G. They had showed that nonexpresser recipients grafted with *CYP3A5* nonexpresser donors had the largest TAC C/D ratio and this genetic effect changed over time since transplantation [146–149]. These results suggest that the organ influencing TAC disposition may change from the native intestine (recipients) in the early phase following transplantation to the graft liver (donors) in the stable phase, when the transplanted organ has gained the recovery of metabolic function.

In view of this and many more studies published through the years, there is enough evidence to carry out studies to assess the prescription of TAC based on both the donor and the recipient *CYP3A5* genotype [150]. The recipient *ABCB1* and donor *CYP3A5* genotypes may also act together in overall drug disposition. Previous studies have evaluated the effect of recipients' *ABCB1* C3435T or G2677T/A genotype and graft *CYP3A5* genotype. We published a meta-analysis [151] showing that donors with *CYP3A5* nonexpresser genotype had a TAC blood C/D ratio (concentration normalized for daily dose received on a body weight basis) 1.3 to 2 times higher than *CYP3A5* expressers, during the first month after transplantation. When the C/D ratio was analyzed with regard to the recipient genotype, this polymorphism variant also affected the pharmacokinetics, although its effect was less pronounced (1.1 to 1.4 times higher). The quality of evidence was at least moderate.

Regarding *CYP3A4*, its association with the TAC dose requirement or trough dose-adjusted concentrations has not been demonstrated. Recently a study in renal transplantation reported that only a significant influence of *CYP3A4*22* on Cs pharmacokinetics was found, but this effect is not high enough to justify dose modification based on *CYP3A4*22* [152]. There are not similar studies in liver transplantation, and current knowledge about this polymorphism does not justify the genotyping of this SNP to assist in selecting the best initial dose.

Influence of the *CYP3A5* 6986A> G SNP on the pharmacokinetics of Cs also remains uncertain [153]. Monostory et al. evaluated the effect of donors' *CYP3A5* genotype and *CYP3A4* expression in the blood concentrations and dose requirements of CNIs in liver transplant recipients. They reported that recipients transplanted with liver grafts from *CYP3A4* low expresser donors carrying also *CYP3A5 *3 /*3* required about 50% lower dose of Cs or TAC than that of the patients with grafts from donors expressing *CYP3A4* at the normal level [154]. So, estimating a donor' s *CYP3A4* expression combined with *CYP3A5* can have predictive power regarding the recipient's medication options and may refine the immunosuppressant therapy facilitating the appropriate dosage for each individual recipient.

Influence of ABCB1 3435C> T, 1236C> T, and 2677G> T/ A SNPs on the pharmacokinetics of Cs remains uncertain, with inconsistent results to date. Higher Cs exposure at a given dose was found in liver transplant recipients with the 3435CT heterozygous variant genotype compared with the 3435CC wild-type genotype [155]. However, other studies reported contradictory results. Jiang et al. [156] conducted a meta-analysis and they failed to demonstrate a correlation between *ABCB1* C3435T and pharmacokinetics of cyclosporine.

Respect to the combined effect of CYP3A5 and ABCB1 polymorphism in donors and recipients regarding Cs, there are no studies published to date.

No relevant studies regarding mTor inhibitors or mycophenolate pharmacogenetics in liver transplantation have been found either.

6.2. Impact of pharmacogenetics on clinical outcomes

Acute rejection: Acute cellular rejection occurs in 20 to 35% patients during the first 2 weeks after liver transplantation. The impact of SNPs of drug transporter proteins and metabolizing enzymes needs to be further analyzed, as studies about the impact of *CYP3A5* showed controversial results [157] and no correlations have been found regarding *CYP3A4* and *ABCB1* polymorphism [158, 159]. Maybe, the efficiency on TAC routine TDM may partly abrogate the polymorphism clinical impact on drug exposure and acute graft rejection.

Acute nephrotoxicity occurs in 30 to 90% patients. It is due to vasoconstriction of the afferent arterioles, a dose-dependent and reversible effect. Its etiology had been associated with relatively higher systemic exposure to CIs, but recent studies could not confirm this association, which could explain why the evidence does not support an effect of *CYP3A4, CYP3A5,* and *ABCB1* on this clinical outcome.

The improvement of the outcome and survival of liver transplant patients has been associated with the occurrence of long-term chronic complication. One of them is chronic nephropathy, whose frequency is higher than in other solid organ transplants (5-year cumulative incidence of 20–37%) [160]. The main cause is local renal exposure of CNIs or their metabolites in kidney tissue, which is not necessarily associated to the CNI blood level [161]. Some studies have linked the inter-individual variability in kidney accumulation of CNIs to *ABCB1* and *CYP3A5* polymorphisms. There are two studies that detected significant association with *ABCB1* polymorphism in liver transplantation, but they have special characteristics. Hebert et al. [162] found a significant effect of *ABCB1* 2677, but the patients were treated with TAC and Cs, the latter with known increased risk of nephrotoxicity. Hawwa et al. [163, 164] found an association for the 3 *ABCB1* SNPs, albeit they studied children and did not evaluate potential confounding factors that could affect the creatinine clearance.

Respect to *CYP3A5*, Fukudo et al. [165] did not find a significant association in donors, although they only used changes in serum creatinine concentrations (and not creatinine clearance) for diagnosing chronic nephrotoxicity. Tapirdamaz et al. [166] reported that neither the *CYP3A5* 6989A>G nor *ABCB1* 3435C>T genotype of either donor or recipient was associated with risk of chronic kidney disease, but they did not consider as exclusion criteria other different causes of chronic kidney disease, so further studies are needed.

7. So, what can we actually do in the clinical practice?

After reviewing the state of the art with the most recent works published in each type of solid organ transplantation, which of all those findings does really have evidence enough to be implemented in the clinic? Currently, CYP3A5 association related to TAC dosage and metabolism is the only one classified with a level of evidence 1A by PharmGKB consortium (www.pharmgkb.org), with an actionable consequence: a dosing guideline proposed by the Clinical Pharmacogenetics Implementation Consortium (CPIC) [167]. The authors of this guideline underline that "…we are not recommending whether or not to test for CYP3A5 genotype in transplant, but we are providing recommendations on how to use CYP3A5 genotype information if it is known. Since it is typical clinical practice to achieve target blood concentrations as quickly as possible, we do recommend if CYP3A5 genotype is known, to individualize initial tacrolimus treatment using CYP3A5 genotype to guide tacrolimus dosing…" and also "Thus at present, there is no definitive evidence to indicate that genotype-guided dosing for tacrolimus affects long term clinical outcomes. However there is strong evidence to support its effect on achieving target trough whole blood concentrations, which is routine clinical practice for most centers…."

This considers that patients with at least one *1 allele (genotype GA or AA) being recipients of a kidney, heart, lung, or hematopoietic stem cell transplant and liver transplant patients where the donor and the recipient genotypes are identical, who are treated with TAC, would present lower dose-adjusted trough concentrations and decreased chance of achieving target concentrations, so they recommend to increase the starting dose 1.5 to 2 times the initially recommended starting dose (weight guided), not exceeding 0.3mg/kg/day, and then to use TDM to guide following dose adjustments. The same would apply for children and adolescents. Of course, other clinical factors influencing the treatment must be considered.

The association of *CYP3A5* rs776746 with Cs dosage and metabolism is classified with a level of evidence 2B by PharmGKB, with no further recommendations regarding genotype-guided dose adjustment.

7.1. And how can we have these analyses performed?

As in any field of knowledge that directly affects the improvement of health, even more if it deals with drug use, clinical applications arising from pharmacogenetics should be well regulated and should be given proper use. Both the patient and the doctor should be well informed of the scope and meaning of the data to be obtained. It is vital to know what we expect from pharmacogenetic analysis realistically, without creating false hopes.

In the last years, many private companies have developed "direct to consumer genetic analyses." Many of them analyze tens to hundreds of genetic variants and it seems like "the more, the better," but what can we do with that large amount of information? How do we interpret all those results? Is there enough knowledge about which is the biological meaning of each variant? And least but not last, what level of evidence does that knowledge have?

Regulatory agencies, academia, and industry agree in their worry about the alarm with regard to some proposals, which are clearly misleading for the consumer. Just a quick search on the Internet to realize that consumers can buy genotyping kits that offer scientifically implausible predictions, such as predicting vulnerability to sudden death in athletes, obesity, the ability to succeed in school, etc. The US committee SACGHS (the Secretary's Advisory Committee on Genetics, Health and Society) has issued several reports concerning this point, stressing the need to regulate this area of biomedicine to protect consumers. There are two excellent publications about Dr. J.P. Evans, illustrating the problem [168, 169].

Therefore, researchers still have a huge amount of work to do, to validate the associations proposed between certain SNPs and drug efficacy and toxicity and to discover new ones. These studies should finally be prospective and well designed and include the whole steps of the drug fate inside the organism, interactions, etc. and of course include accurate biostatistical and bioinformatic tools. The development of informatic tools to make pharmacogenetic results accessible and easy to interpret for clinicians is also a hot point. Only those associations with the highest level of evidence should be implemented in the clinical practice, as in our case *CYP3A5* rs776746 regarding TAC initial dosing.

8. Conclusions

The variability in solid organ transplantation therapy outcomes cannot be predicted only by clinical factors. Pharmacogenetics will help to implement personalized medicine based on patient data, clinical parameters, and genotypes. Evidences of the role of polymorphisms in some candidate genes have been established, as *CYP3A5* in pharmacokinetics of TAC, *TPMT* in clearance and toxicity of azathioprine, and possibly also *ABCB1* in CNI-associated nephrotoxicity. Besides, other genes related to immunosuppressant pathways are being studied, although their influence still has to be correctly validated. The relatively small size of some cohorts, the absence of ethnic subgroup analysis, or isolated analysis of some genes ignoring other genes that affect drug disposition could cause the inconsistent results obtained by different studies. These SNPs should be analyzed taking into consideration real biological pathways, as complete as possible, and the results should be validated in prospective studies involving larger groups of patients. Still, the biological consequences of many of the most studied SNPs seem to be the same, independently of the type of transplant studied. And also another consideration to keep in mind is the interest of studying both the donor and the recipient genotypes, again, in spite of the organ.

Certainly pharmacogenetics is already a reality in clinical application. To know about it and to understand its limits are unavoidable challenges that must be confronted by those who are responsible for the health of the population. Likewise, to establish the frames of cost-effectiveness for a feasible implementation is crucial for its real use in the clinical setting, in order to be used correctly and in a sustainable manner.

Author details

María José Herrero[1*], Juan Eduardo Megías[1,2], Virginia Bosó[1,2], Jesús Ruiz[1], Luis Rojas[1,3], Ignacio Sánchez-Lázaro[4], Luis Amenar[4], Julio Hernández[5], José Luis Poveda[1,2], Amparo Pastor[6], Amparo Solé[6], Rafael López-Andújar[7] and Salvador F. Aliño[1,8]

*Address all correspondence to: maria.jose.herrero@uv.es

1 Unidad de Farmacogenética, Instituto Investigación Sanitaria La Fe and Área Clínica del Medicamento Hospital Universitario y Politécnico La Fe (HUPLF), Valencia, Spain

2 Servicio de Farmacia, HUPLF

3 Dpto. Medicina Interna, Facultad de Medicina, Pontificia Universidad Católica de Chile, Santiago de Chile, Chile

4 Unidad de Insuficiencia Cardiaca y Trasplante Cardiaco, Servicio Cardiología, HUPLF, Spain

5 Servicio Nefrología, HUPLF, Spain

6 Unidad de Trasplante Pulmonar, HUPLF, Spain

7 Unidad de Cirugía Hepatobiliopancreática y Trasplante Hepático, HUPLF, Spain

8 Unidad Farmacología Clínica, HUPLF and Dpto. Farmacología, Fac. Medicina, Universidad de Valencia, Valencia, Spain

References

[1] Elens L, Hesselink DA, van Schaik RHN, van Gelder T. Pharmacogenetics in kidney transplantation: recent updates and potential clinical applications. Mol Diagn Ther. 2012;16:331–345.

[2] Elens L, Bouamar R, Shuker N, Hesselink D, van Gelder T, van Schaik RHN. Clinical implementation of pharmacogenetics in kidney transplantation: calcineurin inhibitors in the starting blocks. Br J Clin Pharmacol. 2014;77:715–28.

[3] Bosó V, Herrero MJ, Bea S, Galiana M, Marrero P, Marqués MR, et al. Increased hospital stay and allograft dysfunction in renal transplant recipients with Cyp2c19 AA variant in SNP rs4244285. Drug Metab Dispos. 2013;41:480–487.

[4] Dai Y, Iwanaga K, Lin YS, Hebert MF, Davis CL, Huang W, et al. In vitro metabolism of cyclosporine A by human kidney CYP3A5. Biochem Pharmacol. 2004;68:1889–1902.

[5] Hesselink DA, van Schaik RHN, van der Heiden IP, van der Werf M, Gregoor PJHS, Lindemans J, et al. Genetic polymorphisms of the CYP3A4, CYP3A5, and MDR-1 genes and pharmacokinetics of the calcineurin inhibitors cyclosporine and tacrolimus. Clin Pharmacol Ther. 2003;74:245–254.

[6] Provenzani A, et al. The effect of CYP3A5 and ABCB1 single nucleotide polymorphisms on tacrolimus dose requirements in Caucasian liver transplant patients. Ann Transplant. 2009;14:23–31.

[7] Herrero MJ, Almenar L, Jordán C, Sánchez I, Poveda JL, Aliño SF. Clinical interest of pharmacogenetic polymorphisms in the immunosuppressive treatment after heart transplantation. Transp Proc. 2010;42:3181–3182.

[8] Herrero MJ, Sánchez-Plumed J, Galiana M, Bea S, Marqués MR, Aliño SF. Influence of the pharmacogenetic polymorphisms in the routine immunosuppression therapy after renal transplantation. Transp Proc. 2010;42:3134–3136.

[9] Ran Jun K, Lee W, Jang M, et al. Tacrolimus concentrations in relations to CYP3A and ABCB1 polymorphisms in solid organ transplant recipients in Korea. Transplantation. 2009;87:1225–1231.

[10] Haufroid V, Mourad M, Van Kerckhove V, Wawrzyniak J, De Meyer M, Eddour DC, et al. The effect of CYP3A5 and MDR1 (ABCB1) polymorphisms on cyclosporine and tacrolimus dose requirements and trough blood levels in stable renal transplant patients. Pharmacogenetics. 2004;14:147–154.

[11] Kuehl P, Zhang J, Lin Y, Lamba J, Assem M, Schuetz J, et al. Sequence diversity in CYP3A promoters and characterization of the genetic basis of polymorphic CYP3A5 expression. Nat Genet. 2001;27:383–391.

[12] Kim I-W, Moon YJ, Ji E, Kim KI, Han N, Kim SJ, et al. Clinical and genetic factors affecting tacrolimus trough levels and drug-related outcomes in Korean kidney transplant recipients. Eur J Clin Pharmacol. 2012;68:657–669.

[13] Bosó V, Herrero MJ, Buso E, Galán J, Almenar L, Sánchez-Lázaro I, et al. Genotype and allele frequencies of drug-metabolizing enzymes and drug transporter genes affecting immunosuppressants in the spanish white population. Ther Drug Monit. 2014;36:159–168.

[14] Anglicheau D, Verstuyft C, Laurent-Puig P, Becquemont L, Schlageter M-H, Cassinat B, et al. Association of the multidrug resistance-1 gene single-nucleotide polymorphisms with the tacrolimus dose requirements in renal transplant recipients. J Am Soc Nephrol. 2003;14:1889–19610

[15] Barbarino JM, Staatz CE, Venkataramanan R, Klein TE, Altman RB. PharmGKB summary: cyclosporine and tacrolimus pathways. Pharmacogenet Genomics. 2013;23:563–585.

[16] Lown KS, Mayo RR, Leichtman AB, Hsiao HL, Turgeon DK, Schmiedlin-Ren P, Brown MB, Guo W, Rossi SJ, Benet LZ, Watkins PB. Role of intestinal P-glycoprotein (mdr1) in interpatient variation in the oral bioavailability of cyclosporine. Clin Pharmacol Ther. 1997;62:248–260.

[17] Masuda S, Goto M, Okuda M, Ogura Y, Oike F, Kiuchi T, Tanaka K, Inui K. Initial dosage adjustment for oral administration of tacrolimus using the intestinal MDR1 level in living-donor liver transplant recipients. Transplant Proc. 2005;37:1728–1729.

[18] Perez-aytes A, Ledo A, Bosó V, Carey JC, Castell M, Vento M. Immunosuppressive drugs and pregnancy: mycophenolate mofetil embryopathy. Neoreviews. 2010;11:e578–e578.

[19] Shaw LM, Figurski M, Milone MC, Trofe J, Bloom RD. Therapeutic drug monitoring of mycophenolic acid. Clin J Am Soc Nephrol. 2007;2:1062–1072.

[20] Staatz CE, Tett SE. Clinical pharmacokinetics and pharmacodynamics of mycophenolate in solid organ transplant recipients. Clin Pharmacokinet. 2007;46:13–58.

[21] Hesselink D, van Gelder T. Genetic and nongenetic determinants of between-patient variability in the pharmacokinetics of mycophenolic acid. Clin Pharmacol Ther. 2005;78:317–321.

[22] Gensburger O, Van Schaik RHN, Picard N, Le Meur Y, Rousseau A, Woillard J-B, et al. Polymorphisms in type I and II inosine monophosphate dehydrogenase genes and association with clinical outcome in patients on mycophenolate mofetil. Pharmacogenet Genomics. 2010;20:537–543.

[23] Kagaya H, Miura M, Saito M, Habuchi T, Satoh S. Correlation of IMPDH1 gene polymorphisms with subclinical acute rejection and mycophenolic acid exposure parameters on day 28 after renal transplantation. Basic Clin Pharmacol Toxicol. 2010;107:631–636.

[24] Shah S, Harwood SM, Döhler B, Opelz G, Yaqoob MM. Inosine monophosphate dehydrogenase polymorphisms and renal allograft outcome. Transplantation. 2012;94:486–491.

[25] Pazik J, Ołdak M, Podgórska M, Lewandowski Z, Sitarek E, Płoski R, et al. Lymphocyte counts in kidney allograft recipients are associated with IMPDH2 3757T>C gene polymorphism. Transplant Proc. 2011;43:2943–2945.

[26] Relling M V, Gardner EE, Sandborn WJ, Schmiegelow K, Pui C-H, Yee SW, et al. Clinical Pharmacogenetics Implementation Consortium guidelines for thiopurine methyltransferase genotype and thiopurine dosing. Clin Pharmacol Ther. 2011;89:387–391.

[27] Breen DP, Marinaki AM, Arenas M, Hayes PC. Pharmacogenetic association with adverse drug reactions to azathioprine immunosuppressive therapy following liver transplantation. Liver Transpl. 2005;11:826–833.

[28] Jacobsen W, Serkova N, Hausen B, Morris RE, Benet LZ, Christians U. Comparison of the in vitro metabolism of the macrolide immunosuppressants sirolimus and RAD. Transplant Proc. 2001;33:514–515.

[29] Gullestad L, Iversen M, Mortensen SA, Eiskjaer H, Riise GC, Mared L, et al. Everolimus with reduced calcineurin inhibitor in thoracic transplant recipients with renal dysfunction: a multicenter, randomized trial. Transplantation. 2010;89:864–872.

[30] Parada MT, Alba A, Sepúlveda C, Melo J. Long-term use of everolimus in lung transplant patients. Transplant Proc. 2011;43:2313–2315.

[31] Asano T, Takahashi KA, Fujioka M, Inoue S, Okamoto M, Sugioka N, et al. ABCB1 C3435T and G2677T/A polymorphism decreased the risk for steroid-induced osteo-

http://dx.doi.org/10.5772/63071

necrosis of the femoral head after kidney transplantation. Pharmacogenetics. 2003;13:675–682.

[32] Zhou Z, Hua Y, Liu J, Zuo D, Wang H, Chen Q, et al. Association of ABCB1/MDR1 polymorphisms in patients with glucocorticoid-induced osteonecrosis of the femoral head: evidence for a meta-analysis. Gene. 2015;569:34–40.

[33] Burke MT, Isbel N, Barraclough KA, Jung JW, Wells JW, Staatz CE. Genetics and nonmelanoma skin cancer in kidney transplant recipients. Pharmacogenomics. 2015;16:161–172.

[34] Leroy C, Rigot JM, Leroy M, Decanter C, Le Mapihan K, Parent AS, et al. Immunosuppressive drugs and fertility. Orphanet J Rare Dis. 2015;10:136.

[35] Moes AD, Hesselink DA, Zietse R, van Schaik RHN, van Gelder T, Hoorn EJ. "Calcineurin inhibitors and hypertension: a role for pharmacogenetics?" Pharmacogenomics. 2014;15:1243–1251.

[36] Huls M, van den Heuvel JJMW, Dijkman HBPM, Russel FGM, Masereeuw R. ABC transporter expression profiling after ischemic reperfusion injury in mouse kidney. Kidney Int. 2006;69:2186–2193.

[37] Hesselink DA, Bouamar R, van Gelder T. The pharmacogenetics of calcineurin inhibitor-related nephrotoxicity. Ther Drug Monit. 2010;32:387–393.

[38] Capron A, Mourad M, De Meyer M, De Pauw L, Eddour DC, Latinne D, et al. CYP3A5 and ABCB1 polymorphisms influence tacrolimus concentrations in peripheral blood mononuclear cells after renal transplantation. Pharmacogenomics. 2010;11:703–714.

[39] Rong G, Jing L, Deng-Qing L, Hong-Shan Z, Shai-Hong Z, Xin-Min N. Influence of CYP3A5 and MDR1(ABCB1) polymorphisms on the pharmacokinetics of tacrolimus in Chinese renal transplant recipients. Transplant Proc. 2010;42:3455–3458.

[40] Naesens M, Lerut E, de Jonge H, Van Damme B, Vanrenterghem Y, Kuypers DRJ. Donor age and renal P-glycoprotein expression associate with chronic histological damage in renal allografts. J Am Soc Nephrol. 2009;20:2468–2480.

[41] Terrazzino S, Quaglia M, Stratta P, Canonico PL, Genazzani AA. The effect of CYP3A5 6986A>G and ABCB1 3435C>T on tacrolimus dose-adjusted trough levels and acute rejection rates in renal transplant patients: a systematic review and meta-analysis. Pharmacogenet Genomics. 2012;22:642–645.

[42] Li Y, Hu X, Cai B, Chen J, Bai Y, Tang J, et al. Meta-analysis of the effect of MDR1 C3435 polymorphism on tacrolimus pharmacokinetics in renal transplant recipients. Transpl Immunol. 2012;27:12–18.

[43] Lee J, Wang R, Yang Y, Lu X, Zhang X, Wang L, et al. The effect of ABCB1 C3435T polymorphism on cyclosporine dose requirements in kidney transplant recipients: a meta-analysis. Basic Clin Pharmacol Toxicol. 2015;117:117–125.

[44] MacPhee IAM, Fredericks S, Tai T, Syrris P, Carter ND, Johnston A, et al. The influence of pharmacogenetics on the time to achieve target tacrolimus concentrations after kidney transplantation. Am J Transplant. 2004;4:914–919.

[45] Haufroid V, Wallemacq P, VanKerckhove V, Elens L, De Meyer M, Eddour DC, et al. CYP3A5 and ABCB1 polymorphisms and tacrolimus pharmacokinetics in renal transplant candidates: guidelines from an experimental study. Am J Transplant. 2006;6:2706–2713.

[46] Hesselink DA, van Gelder T, van Schaik RHN, Balk AHMM, van der Heiden IP, van Dam T, et al. Population pharmacokinetics of cyclosporine in kidney and heart transplant recipients and the influence of ethnicity and genetic polymorphisms in the MDR-1, CYP3A4, and CYP3A5 genes. Clin Pharmacol Ther. 2004;76:545–556.

[47] Kuypers DRJ, de Jonge H, Naesens M, Lerut E, Verbeke K, Vanrenterghem Y. CYP3A5 and CYP3A4 but not MDR1 single-nucleotide polymorphisms determine long-term tacrolimus disposition and drug-related nephrotoxicity in renal recipients. Clin Pharmacol Ther. 2007;82:711–725.

[48] Kuypers DRJ, de Jonge H, Naesens M, Vanrenterghem Y. A prospective, open-label, observational clinical cohort study of the association between delayed renal allograft function, tacrolimus exposure, and CYP3A5 genotype in adult recipients. Clin Ther. 2010;32:2012–2023.

[49] Zhang X, Liu Z, Zheng J, Chen Z, Tang Z, Chen J, et al. Influence of CYP3A5 and MDR1 polymorphisms on tacrolimus concentration in the early stage after renal transplantation. Clin Transplant. 2005;19:638–643.

[50] Zhu HJ, Yuan SH, Fang Y, Sun XZ, Kong H, Ge WH. The effect of CYP3A5 polymorphism on dose-adjusted cyclosporine concentration in renal transplant recipients: a meta-analysis. Pharmacogenomics J. 2011;11:237–246.

[51] Hesselink DA, van Schaik RHN, van Agteren M, de Fijter JW, Hartmann A, Zeier M, et al. CYP3A5 genotype is not associated with a higher risk of acute rejection in tacrolimus-treated renal transplant recipients. Pharmacogenet Genomics. 2008;18:339–348.

[52] Quteineh L, Verstuyft C, Furlan V, Durrbach A, Letierce A, Ferlicot S, et al. Influence of CYP3A5 genetic polymorphism on tacrolimus daily dose requirements and acute rejection in renal graft recipients. Basic Clin Pharmacol Toxicol. 2008;103:546–552.

[53] Min S-I, Kim SY, Ahn SH, Min S-K, Kim SH, Kim YS, et al. CYP3A5 *1 allele: impacts on early acute rejection and graft function in tacrolimus-based renal transplant recipients. Transplantation. 2010;90:1394–1400.

[54] Satoh S, Saito M, Inoue T, Kagaya H, Miura M, Inoue K, et al. CYP3A5 *1 allele associated with tacrolimus trough concentrations but not subclinical acute rejection or

chronic allograft nephropathy in Japanese renal transplant recipients. Eur J Clin Pharmacol. 2009;65:473–481.

[55] Cho J-H, Yoon Y-D, Park J-Y, Song E-J, Choi J-Y, Yoon S-H, et al. Impact of cytochrome P450 3A and ATP-binding cassette subfamily B member 1 polymorphisms on tacrolimus dose-adjusted trough concentrations among Korean renal transplant recipients. Transplant Proc. 2012;44:109–114.

[56] Glowacki F, Lionet A, Buob D, Labalette M, Allorge D, Provôt F, et al. CYP3A5 and ABCB1 polymorphisms in donor and recipient: impact on tacrolimus dose requirements and clinical outcome after renal transplantation. Nephrol Dial Transplant. 2011;26:3046–3050

[57] Thervet E, Loriot MA, Barbier S, Buchler M, Ficheux M, Choukroun G, et al. Optimization of initial tacrolimus dose using pharmacogenetic testing. Clin Pharmacol Ther. 2010;87:721–726.

[58] Shuker N, Bouamar R, van Schaik RHN, Clahsen-van Groningen MC, Damman J, Baan CC, et al. A Randomized controlled trial comparing the efficacy of CYP3A5 genotype-based with bodyweight-based tacrolimus dosing after living donor kidney transplantation. Am J Transplant. 2015; Epub ahead of print doi:10.1111/ajt.13691.Epub ahead of print

[59] Rojas L, Neumann I, Herrero MJ, Bosó V, Reig J, Poveda JL, et al. Effect of CYP3A5*3 on kidney transplant recipients treated with tacrolimus: a systematic review and meta-analysis of observational studies. Pharmacogenomics J. 2015;15:38–48.

[60] Tang H, Xie H, Yao Y, Hu Y. Lower tacrolimus daily dose requirements and acute rejection rates in the CYP3A5 nonexpressers than expressers. Pharmacogenet Genomics. 2011;21:713–720.

[61] Gervasini G, Garcia M, Macias RM, Cubero JJ, Caravaca F, Benitez J. Impact of genetic polymorphisms on tacrolimus pharmacokinetics and the clinical outcome of renal transplantation. Transpl Int. 2012;25:471–480.

[62] Birdwell KA, Grady B, Choi L, Xu H, Bian A, Denny JC, et al. The use of a DNA biobank linked to electronic medical records to characterize pharmacogenomic predictors of tacrolimus dose requirement in kidney transplant recipients. Pharmacogenet Genomics. 2012;22:32–42.

[63] Singh R, Srivastava A, Kapoor R, Sharma R, Mittal R. Impact of CYP3A5 and CYP3A4 gene polymorphisms on dose requirement of calcineurin inhibitors, cyclosporine and tacrolimus, in renal allograft recipients of North India. Naunyn Schmiedebergs Arch Pharmacol. 2009;380:169–177.

[64] Santoro AB, Struchiner CJ, Felipe CR, Tedesco-Silva H, Medina-Pestana JO, Suarez-Kurtz G. CYP3A5 genotype, but not CYP3A4*1b, CYP3A4*22, or hematocrit, predicts

tacrolimus dose requirements in Brazilian renal transplant patients. Clin Pharmacol Ther. 2013;94:201–202.

[65] Amirimani B, Ning B, Deitz AC, Weber BL, Kadlubar FF, Rebbeck TR. Increased transcriptional activity of the CYP3A4*1B promoter variant. Environ Mol Mutagen. 2003;42:299–305.

[66] Wang D, Guo Y, Wrighton SA, Cooke GE, Sadee W. Intronic polymorphism in CYP3A4 affects hepatic expression and response to statin drugs. Pharmacogenomics J. 2011;11:274–286.

[67] Elens L, van Schaik RH, Panin N, de Meyer M, Wallemacq P, Lison D, et al. Effect of a new functional CYP3A4 polymorphism on calcineurin inhibitors' dose requirements and trough blood levels in stable renal transplant patients. Pharmacogenomics. 2011;12:1383–1396.

[68] Elens L, Bouamar R, Hesselink DA, Haufroid V, van der Heiden IP, van Gelder T, et al. A new functional CYP3A4 intron 6 polymorphism significantly affects tacrolimus pharmacokinetics in kidney transplant recipients. Clin Chem. 2011;57:1574–1583.

[69] de Jonge H, Metalidis C, Naesens M, Lambrechts D, Kuypers DRJ. The P450 oxidoreductase *28 SNP is associated with low initial tacrolimus exposure and increased dose requirements in CYP3A5-expressing renal recipients. Pharmacogenomics. 2011;12:1281–1291.

[70] Elens L, Hesselink DA, Bouamar R, Budde K, de Fijter JW, De Meyer M, et al. Impact of POR*28 on the pharmacokinetics of tacrolimus and cyclosporine A in renal transplant patients. Ther Drug Monit. 2013;0:1–9.

[71] Li C-J, Li L, Lin L, Jiang H-X, Zhong Z-Y, Li W-M, et al. Impact of the CYP3A5, CYP3A4, COMT, IL-10 and POR genetic polymorphisms on tacrolimus metabolism in Chinese renal transplant recipients. PLoS One. 2014;9:e86206.

[72] Kurzawski M, Malinowski D, Dziewanowski K, Droździk M. Impact of PPARA and POR polymorphisms on tacrolimus pharmacokinetics and new-onset diabetes in kidney transplant recipients. Pharmacogenet Genomics. 2014;24:397–400.

[73] Bruckmueller H, Werk AN, Renders L, Feldkamp T, Tepel M, Borst C, et al. Which genetic determinants should be considered for tacrolimus dose optimization in kidney transplantation? A combined analysis of genes affecting the CYP3A locus. Ther Drug Monit. 2015;37:288–295.

[74] Elens L, Sombogaard F, Hesselink DA, van Schaik RHN, van Gelder T. Single-nucleotide polymorphisms in P450 oxidoreductase and peroxisome proliferator-activated receptor-α are associated with the development of new-onset diabetes after transplantation in kidney transplant recipients treated with tacrolimus. Pharmacogenet Genomics. 2013;23:649–657.

[75] Anglicheau D, Le Corre D, Lechaton S, Laurent-Puig P, Kreis H, Beaune P, et al. Consequences of genetic polymorphisms for sirolimus requirements after renal transplant in patients on primary sirolimus therapy. Am J Transplant. 2005;5:595–603.

[76] Le Meur Y, Djebli N, Szelag J-C, Hoizey G, Toupance O, Rérolle JP, et al. CYP3A5*3 influences sirolimus oral clearance in de novo and stable renal transplant recipients. Clin Pharmacol Ther. 2006;80:51–60.

[77] Li Y, Yan L, Shi Y, Bai Y, Tang J, Wang L. CYP3A5 and ABCB1 genotype influence tacrolimus and sirolimus pharmacokinetics in renal transplant recipients. Springerplus. 2015;4:637.

[78] Sam W-J, Chamberlain CE, Lee S-J, Goldstein JA, Hale DA, Mannon RB, et al. Associations of ABCB1 and IL-10 genetic polymorphisms with sirolimus-induced dyslipidemia in renal transplant recipients. Transplantation. 2012;94:971–977.

[79] Girard H, Court MH, Bernard O, Fortier L-C, Villeneuve L, Hao Q, et al. Identification of common polymorphisms in the promoter of the UGT1A9 gene: evidence that UGT1A9 protein and activity levels are strongly genetically controlled in the liver. Pharmacogenetics. 2004;14:501–515.

[80] van Schaik RHN, van Agteren M, de Fijter JW, Hartmann A, Schmidt J, Budde K, et al. UGT1A9 -275T>A/-2152C>T polymorphisms correlate with low MPA exposure and acute rejection in MMF/tacrolimus-treated kidney transplant patients. Clin Pharmacol Ther. 2009;86:319–327.

[81] Sánchez-Fructuoso AI, Maestro ML, Calvo N, Viudarreta M, Pérez-Flores I, Veganzone S, et al. The prevalence of uridine diphosphate-glucuronosyltransferase 1A9 (UGT1A9) gene promoter region single-nucleotide polymorphisms T-275A and C-2152T and its influence on mycophenolic acid pharmacokinetics in stable renal transplant patients. Transplant Proc. 2009;41:2313–2316.

[82] Whirl-Carrillo M, McDonagh EM, Hebert JM, Gong L, Sangkuhl K, Thorn CF, et al. Pharmacogenomics knowledge for personalized medicine. Clin Pharmacol Ther. 2012;92:414–417.

[83] Naesens M, Kuypers DRJ, Verbeke K, Vanrenterghem Y. Multidrug resistance protein 2 genetic polymorphisms influence mycophenolic acid exposure in renal allograft recipients. Transplantation. 2006;82:1074–1084.

[84] Zhang W-X, Chen B, Jin Z, Yu Z, Wang X, Chen H, et al. Influence of uridine diphosphate (UDP)-glucuronosyltransferases and ABCC2 genetic polymorphisms on the pharmacokinetics of mycophenolic acid and its metabolites in Chinese renal transplant recipients. Xenobiotica. 2008;38:1422–1436.

[85] Picard N, Yee SW, Woillard J-B, Lebranchu Y, Le Meur Y, Giacomini KM, et al. The role of organic anion-transporting polypeptides and their common genetic variants in mycophenolic acid pharmacokinetics. Clin Pharmacol Ther. 2010;87:100–108.

[86] Geng F, Jiao Z, Dao Y-J, Qiu X-Y, Ding J-J, Shi X-J, et al. The association of the UGT1A8, SLCO1B3 and ABCC2/ABCG2 genetic polymorphisms with the pharmacokinetics of mycophenolic acid and its phenolic glucuronide metabolite in Chinese individuals. Clin Chim Acta. 2012;413:683–690.

[87] Miura M, Satoh S, Inoue K, Kagaya H, Saito M, Inoue T, et al. Influence of SLCO1B1, 1B3, 2B1 and ABCC2 genetic polymorphisms on mycophenolic acid pharmacokinetics in Japanese renal transplant recipients. Eur J Clin Pharmacol. 2007;63:1161–1169.

[88] Han N, Yun HY, Kim IW, Oh YJ, Kim YS, Oh JM. Population pharmacogenetic pharmacokinetic modeling for flip-flop phenomenon of enteric-coated mycophenolate sodium in kidney transplant recipients. Eur J Clin Pharmacol. 2014;70:1211–1219.

[89] Wang J, Yang JW, Zeevi A, Webber SA, Girnita DM, Selby R, et al. IMPDH1 gene polymorphisms and association with acute rejection in renal transplant patients. Clin Pharmacol Ther. 2008;83:711–717.

[90] Michelon H, König J, Durrbach A, Quteineh L, Verstuyft C, Furlan V, et al. SLCO1B1 genetic polymorphism influences mycophenolic acid tolerance in renal transplant recipients. Pharmacogenomics. 2010;11:1703–1713.

[91] Nilsson J, Ohlsson M, Höglund P, Ekmehag B, Koul B, Andersson B. The international heart transplant survival algorithm (IHTSA): a new model to improve organ sharing and survival. PLoS One. 2015;10:e0118644.

[92] Lund LH, Edwards LB, Kucheryavaya AY, Dipchand AI, Benden C, Christie JD, Dobbels F, Kirk R, Rahmel AO, Yusen RD, Stehlik J; International Society for Heart and Lung Transplantation. The registry of the international society for heart and lung transplantation: thirtieth official adult heart transplant report—2013; focus theme: age. J Heart Lung Transplant. 2013;32:951–964.

[93] Zheng H, Webber S, Zeevi A, Schuetz E, Zhang J, Bowman P, Boyle G, Law Y, Miller S, Lamba J, Burckart GJ. Tacrolimus dosing in pediatric heart transplant patients is related to CYP3A5 and MDR1 gene polymorphisms. Am J Transplant. 2003;3:477–483.

[94] Gijsen V, Mital S, van Schaik RH, Soldin OP, Soldin SJ, van der Heiden IP, Nulman I, Koren G, de Wildt SN. Age and CYP3A5 genotype affect tacrolimus dosing requirements after transplant in pediatric heart recipients. J Heart Lung Transplant. 2011;30:1352–1359.

[95] Díaz-Molina B, Tavira B, Lambert JL, Bernardo MJ, Alvarez V, Coto E. Effect of CYP3A5, CYP3A4, and ABCB1 genotypes as determinants of tacrolimus dose and clinical outcomes after heart transplantation. Transplant Proc. 2012;44:2635–2638.

[96] Lesche D, Sigurdardottir V, Setoud R, Oberhänsli M, Carrel T, Fiedler GM, Largiadèr CR, Mohacsi P, Sistonen J. CYP3A5*3 and POR*28 genetic variants influence the required dose of tacrolimus in heart transplant recipients. Ther Drug Monit. 2014;36:710–715.

[97] Sánchez-Lázaro I, Herrero MJ, Jordán-De Luna C, Bosó V, Almenar L, Rojas L, Martínez-Dolz L, Megías-Vericat JE, Sendra L, Miguel A, Poveda JL, Aliño SF. Association of SNPs with the efficacy and safety of immunosuppressant therapy after heart transplantation. Pharmacogenomics. 2015;16:971–979.

[98] Jordán de Luna C, Herrero Cervera MJ, Sánchez-Lázaro I, Almenar Bonet L, Poveda Andrés JL, Aliño Pellicer SF. Pharmacogenetic study of ABCB1 and CYP3A5 genes during the first year following heart transplantation regarding tacrolimus or cyclosporine levels. Transplant Proc. 2011;43:2241–2243.

[99] Isla Tejera B, Aumente Rubio MD, Martínez-Moreno J, Reyes Malia M, Arizón JM, Suárez García A. Pharmacogenetic analysis of the absorption kinetics of cyclosporine in a population of Spanish cardiac transplant patients. Farm Hosp. 2009;33:324–329.

[100] Taegtmeyer AB, Breen JB, Smith J, Burke M, Leaver N, Pantelidis P, Lyster H, Yacoub MH, Barton PJ, Banner NR. ATP-binding cassette subfamily B member 1 polymorphisms do not determine cyclosporin exposure, acute rejection or nephrotoxicity after heart transplantation. Transplantation. 2010;89:75–82.

[101] Klauke B, Wirth A, Zittermann A, Bohms B, Tenderich G, Körfer R, Milting H. No association between single nucleotide polymorphisms and the development of nephrotoxicity after orthotopic heart transplantation. J Heart Lung Transplant. 2008;27:741–745.

[102] de Denus S, Zakrzewski M, Barhdadi A, Leblanc MH, Racine N, Bélanger F, Carrier M, Ducharme A, Dubé MP, Turgeon J, White M. Association between renal function and CYP3A5 genotype in heart transplant recipients treated with calcineurin inhibitors. J Heart Lung Transplant. 2011;30:326–331.

[103] Feingold B, Brooks MM, Zeevi A, Ohmann EL, Burckart GJ, Ferrell RE, Chinnock R, Canter C, Addonizio L, Bernstein D, Kirklin JK, Naftel DC, Webber SA. Renal function and genetic polymorphisms in pediatric heart transplant recipients. J Heart Lung Transplant. 2012;31:1003–1008.

[104] Oetjens M, Bush WS, Birdwell KA, Dilks HH, Bowton EA, Denny JC, Wilke RA, Roden DM, Crawford DC. Utilization of an EMR-biorepository to identify the genetic predictors of calcineurin-inhibitor toxicity in heart transplant recipients. Pac Symp Biocomput. 2014;2014:253–264.

[105] Zheng H, Webber S, Zeevi A, Schuetz E, Zhang J, Lamba J, Bowman P, Burckart GJ. The MDR1 polymorphisms at exons 21 and 26 predict steroid weaning in pediatric heart transplant patients. Hum Immunol. 2002;63:765–770.

[106] Zheng HX, Webber SA, Zeevi A, Schuetz E, Zhang J, Lamba J, Boyle GJ, Wilson JW, Burckart GJ. The impact of pharmacogenomic factors on steroid dependency in pediatric heart transplant patients using logistic regression analysis. Pediatr Transplant. 2004;8:551–557.

[107] Barnard JB, Richardson S, Sheldon S, Fildes J, Pravica V, Hutchinson IV, Leonard CT, Yonan N. The MDR1/ABCB1 gene, a high-impact risk factor for cardiac transplant rejection. Transplantation. 2006;82:1677–1682.

[108] Taegtmeyer AB, Breen JB, Smith J, Rogers P, Kullak-Ublick GA, Yacoub MH, Banner NR, Barton PJ. Effect of ABCB1 genotype on pre- and post-cardiac transplantation plasma lipid concentrations. J Cardiovasc Transl Res. 2011;4:304–312.

[109] Staatz CE, Goodman LK, Tett SE. Effect of CYP3A and ABCB1 single nucleotide polymorphisms on the pharmacokinetics and pharmacodynamics of calcineurin inhibitors: part I. Clin Pharmacokinet. 2010;49:141–175.

[110] Kniepeiss D, Renner W, Trummer O, Wagner D, Wasler A, Khoschsorur GA, Truschnig-Wilders M, Tscheliessnigg KH. The role of CYP3A5 genotypes in dose requirements of tacrolimus and everolimus after heart transplantation. Clin Transplant. 2011;25:146–150.

[111] Gijsen VM, van Schaik RH, Elens L, Soldin OP, Soldin SJ, Koren G, de Wildt SN. CYP3A4*22 and CYP3A combined genotypes both correlate with tacrolimus disposition in pediatric heart transplant recipients. Pharmacogenomics. 2013;14:1027–1036.

[112] Miller WL, Agrawal V, Sandee D, et al. Consequences of POR mutations and polymorphisms. Mol Cell Endocrinol. 2011;336:174–179.

[113] Gijsen VM, van Schaik RH, Soldin OP, et al. P450 oxidoreductase *28 (POR*28) and tacrolimus disposition in pediatric kidney transplant recipients—a pilot study. Ther Drug Monit. 2014;36:152–158.

[114] Zhang JJ, Zhang H, Ding XL, et al. Effect of the P450 oxidoreductase *28 polymorphism on the pharmacokinetics of tacrolimus in Chinese healthy male volunteers. Eur J Clin Pharmacol. 2013;69:807–812.

[115] Smith HE, Jones JP, 3rd, Kalhorn TF, Farin FM, Stapleton PL, Davis CL, Perkins JD, Blough DK, Hebert MF, Thummel KE, Totah RA. Role of cytochrome P450 2C8 and 2J2 genotypes in calcineurin inhibitor-induced chronic kidney disease. Pharmacogenet Genomics. 2008;18:943–953.

[116] Kniepeiss D, Wagner D, Wasler A, Tscheliessnigg KH, Renner W. The role of CYP2C8 genotypes in dose requirement and levels of everolimus after heart transplantation. Wien Klin Wochenschr. 2013;125:393–395.

[117] Lemaitre F, Bezian E, Goldwirt L, Fernandez C, Farinotti R, Varnous S, Urien S, Antignac M. Population pharmacokinetics of everolimus in cardiac recipients: comedications, ABCB1, and CYP3A5 polymorphisms. Ther Drug Monit. 2012;34:686–694.

[118] Ohmann EL, Burckart GJ, Brooks MM, Chen Y, Pravica V, Girnita DM, Zeevi A, Webber SA. Genetic polymorphisms influence mycophenolate mofetil-related adverse events in pediatric heart transplant patients. J Heart Lung Transplant. 2010;29:509–516.

[119] Ting LSL, Benoit-Biancamano M-O, Bernard O, Riggs KW, Guillemette C, Ensom MHH. Pharmacogenetic impact of UDP-glucuronosyltransferase metabolic pathway and multidrug resistance-associated protein 2 transport pathway on mycophenolic acid in thoracic transplant recipients: an exploratory study. Pharmacotherapy. 2010;30:1097–108.

[120] Burckart GJ, Figg WD, 2nd, Brooks MM, Green DJ, Troutman SM, Ferrell R, Chinnock R, Canter C, Addonizio L, Bernstein D, Kirklin JK, Naftel D, Price DK, Sissung TM, Girnita DM, Zeevi A, Webber SA. Multiinstitutional study of outcomes after pediatric heart transplantation: candidate gene polymorphism analysis of ABCC2. J Pediatr Pharmacol The. 2014;19:16–24.

[121] Sombogaard F, van Schaik RH, Mathot RA, Budde K, van der Werf M, Vulto AG, Weimar W, Glander P, Essioux L, van Gelder T. Interpatient variability in IMPDH activity in MMF-treated renal transplant patients is correlated with IMPDH type II 3757T > C polymorphism. Pharmacogenet Genomics. 2009;19:626–634.

[122] Ohmann EL, Burckart GJ, Chen Y, Pravica V, Brooks MM, Zeevi A, Webber SA. Inosine 5'-monophosphate dehydrogenase 1 haplotypes and association with mycophenolate mofetil gastrointestinal intolerance in pediatric heart transplant patients. Pediatr Transplant. 2010;14:891–895.

[123] Liang JJ, Geske JR, Boilson BA, Frantz RP, Edwards BS, Kushwaha SS, Kremers WK, Weinshilboum RM, Pereira NL. TPMT genetic variants are associated with increased rejection with azathioprine use in heart transplantation. Pharmacogenet Genomics. 2013;23:658–665.

[124] Baan CC, Balk AH, Holweg CT, van Riemsdijk IC, Maat LP, Vantrimpont PJ, Niesters HG, Weimar W. Renal failure after clinical heart transplantation is associated with the TGF-beta 1 codon 10 gene polymorphism. J Heart Lung Transplant. 2000;19:866–872.

[125] van de Wetering J, Weimar CHE, Balk AHMM, Roodnat JI, Holweg CT, Baan CC, van Domburg RT, Weimar W. The impact of transforming growth factorbeta1 gene polymorphism on end-stage renal failure after heart transplantation. Transplantation. 2006;82:1744–1748.

[126] Lachance K, Barhdadi A, Mongrain I, Normand V, Zakrzewski M, Leblanc MH, Racine N, Carrier M, Ducharme A, Turgeon J, Dubé MP, Phillips MS, White M, de Denus S. PRKCB is associated with calcineurin inhibitor-induced renal dysfunction in heart transplant recipients. Pharmacogenet Genomics. 2012;22:336–343.

[127] Girnita DM, Brooks MM, Webber SA, Burckart GJ, Ferrell R, Zdanowicz G, DeCroo S, Smith L, Chinnock R, Canter C, Addonizio L, Bernstein D, Kirklin JK, Ranganathan S, Naftel D, Girnita AL, Zeevi A. Genetic polymorphisms impact the risk of acute rejection in pediatric heart transplantation: a multi-institutional study. Transplantation. 2008;85:1632–1639.

[128] Pantou MP, Manginas A, Alivizatos PA, Degiannis D. Connective tissue growth factor (CTGF/CCN2): a protagonist in cardiac allograft vasculopathy development? J Heart Lung Transplant. 2012;31:881–887.

[129] ISHLT Transplant Registry Quarterly Reports for Lung in Europe. Available at: https://www.ishlt.org/registries/quarterlyDataReportResults.asp?organ=LU&rptType=recip_p_surv&continent=3. Date accessed: Dec 20, 2015.

[130] Saint-Marcoux F, Knoop C, Debord J, Thiry P, Rousseau A, Estenne M, et al. Pharmacokinetic study of tacrolimus in cystic fibrosis and non-cystic fibrosis lung transplant patients and design of Bayesian estimators using limited sampling strategies. Clin Pharmacokinet. 2005;44:1317–28.

[131] Wang J, Zeevi A, McCurry K, Schuetz E, Zheng H, Iacono A, et al. Impact of ABCB1 (MDR1) haplotypes on tacrolimus dosing in adult lung transplant patients who are CYP3A5 *3/*3 non-expressors. Transpl Immunol. 2006;15:235–240.

[132] Ruiz J, Herrero MJ, Bosó V, Megías JE, Hervás D, Poveda JL, et al. Impact of single nucleotide polymorphisms (SNPs) on immunosuppressive therapy in lung transplantation. Int J Mol Sci. 2015;16:20168–20182.

[133] Zheng H, Zeevi A, Schuetz E, Lamba J, McCurry K, Griffith BP, et al. Tacrolimus dosing in adult lung transplant patients is related to cytochrome P4503A5 gene polymorphism. J Clin Pharmacol. 2004;44:135–140.

[134] Schoeppler KE, Aquilante CL, Kiser TH, Fish DN, Zamora MR. The impact of genetic polymorphisms, diltiazem, and demographic variables on everolimus trough concentrations in lung transplant recipients. Clin Transplant. 2014;28:590–7.

[135] Villanueva J, Boukhamseen A, Bhorade SM. Successful use in lung transplantation of an immunosuppressive regimen aimed at reducing target blood levels of sirolimus and tacrolimus. J Heart Lung Transplant. 2005;24:421–425.

[136] Shitrit D, Rahamimov R, Gidon S, Bakal I, Bargil-Shitrit A, Milton S, et al. Use of sirolimus and low-dose calcineurin inhibitor in lung transplant recipients with renal impairment: results of a controlled pilot study. Kidney Int. 2005;67:1471–1475.

[137] Woodrow JP, Shlobin OA, Barnett SD, Burton N, Nathan SD. Comparison of bronchiolitis obliterans syndrome to other forms of chronic lung allograft dysfunction after lung transplantation. J Heart Lung Transplant. 2010;29:1159–1164.

[138] Budding K, van de Graaf EA, Kardol-Hoefnagel T, Broen JCA, Kwakkel-van Erp JM, Oudijk E-JD, et al. A promoter polymorphism in the CD59 complement regulatory protein gene in donor lungs correlates with a higher risk for chronic rejection after lung transplantation. Am J Transplant. 2016;16(3):987–998.

[139] Di Cristofaro J, Reynaud-Gaubert M, Carlini F, Roubertoux P, Loundou A, Basire A, et al. HLA-G*01:04~UTR3 recipient correlates with lower survival and higher frequency

of chronic rejection after lung transplantation. Am J Transplant Off J Am Soc Transplant Am Soc Transpl Surg. 2015;15:2413–2420.

[140] Ningappa M, Higgs BW, Weeks DE, Ashokkumar C, Duerr RH, Sun Q, et al. NOD2 gene polymorphism rs2066844 associates with need for combined liver-intestine transplantation in children with short-gut syndrome. Am J Gastroenterol. 2011;106:157–65.

[141] Saner FH, Nowak K, Hoyer D, Rath P, Canbay A, Paul A, et al. A non-interventional study of the genetic polymorphisms of NOD2 associated with increased mortality in non-alcoholic liver transplant patients. BMC Gastroenterol. 2014;14:4.

[142] Hashida T, Masuda S, Uemoto S, Saito H, Tanaka K, Inui K. Pharmacokinetic and prognostic significance of intestinal MDR1 expression in recipients of living-donor liver transplantation. Clin Pharmacol Ther. 2001;69:308–316.

[143] Barrera-Pulido L, Aguilera-Garcia I, Docobo-Perez F, Alamo-Martinez J, Pareja-Ciuro F, Nunez-Roldan A, et al. Clinical relevance and prevalence of polymorphisms in CYP3A5 and MDR1 genes that encode tacrolimus biotransformation enzymes in liver transplant recipients. Transplant Proc. 2008;40:2949–2951.

[144] Gomez-Bravo MA, Salcedo M, Fondevila C, Suarez F, Castellote J, Rufian S, et al. Impact of donor and recipient CYP3A5 and ABCB1 genetic polymorphisms on tacrolimus dosage requirements and rejection in Caucasian Spanish liver transplant patients. J Clin Pharmacol. 2013;53:1146–1154.

[145] Liu YY, Li C, Cui Z, Fu X, Zhang S, Fan LL, et al. The effect of ABCB1 C3435T polymorphism on pharmacokinetics of tacrolimus in liver transplantation: a meta-analysis. Gene. 2013;531:476–488.

[146] Ji E, Choi L, Suh KS, Cho JY, Han N, Oh JM. Combinational effect of intestinal and hepatic CYP3A5 genotypes on tacrolimus pharmacokinetics in recipients of living donor liver transplantation. Transplantation. 2012 Oct 1 94:866–872.

[147] Uesugi M, Masuda S, Katsura T, Oike F, Takada Y, Inui K. Effect of intestinal CYP3A5 on postoperative tacrolimus trough levels in living-donor liver transplant recipients. Pharmacogenet Genomics. 2006;16:119–127.

[148] Fukudo M, Yano I, Yoshimura A, Masuda S, Uesugi M, Hosohata K, et al. Impact of MDR1 and CYP3A5 on the oral clearance of tacrolimus and tacrolimus-related renal dysfunction in adult living-donor liver transplant patients. Pharmacogenet Genomics. 2008;18:413–423.

[149] Muraki Y, Usui M, Isaji S, Mizuno S, Nakatani K, Yamada T, et al. Impact of CYP3A5 genotype of recipients as well as donors on the tacrolimus pharmacokinetics and infectious complications after living-donor liver transplantation for Japanese adult recipients. Ann Transplant. 2011;16:55–62.

[150] Goto M, Masuda S, Kiuchi T, Ogura Y, Oike F, Okuda M, et al. CYP3A5*1-carrying graft liver reduces the concentration/oral dose ratio of tacrolimus in recipients of living-donor liver transplantation. Pharmacogenetics. 2004;14:471–478.

[151] Rojas LE, Herrero MJ, Boso V, Garcia-Eliz M, Poveda JL, Librero J, et al. Meta-analysis and systematic review of the effect of the donor and recipient CYP3A5 6986A>G genotype on tacrolimus dose requirements in liver transplantation. Pharmacogenet Genomics. 2013;23:509–517.

[152] Moes DJ, Swen JJ, den Hartigh J, van der Straaten T, van der Heide JJ, Sanders JS, et al. Effect of CYP3A4*22, CYP3A5*3, and CYP3A Combined genotypes on cyclosporine, everolimus, and tacrolimus pharmacokinetics in renal transplantation. CPT Pharmacometrics Syst Pharmacol. 2014;3:e100.

[153] Fredericks S, Jorga AM, Macphee IAM, Reboux S, Shiferaw E, Moreton M, et al. Multidrug resistance gene-1 (MDR-1) haplotypes and the CYP3A5*1 genotype have no influence on ciclosporin dose requirements as assessed by C0 or C2 measurements. Clin Transplant. 2007;21:252–257.

[154] Monostory K, Toth K, Kiss A, Hafra E, Csikany N, Paulik J, et al. Personalizing initial calcineurin inhibitor dosing by adjusting to donor CYP3A-status in liver transplant patients. Br J Clin Pharmacol. 2015;80:1429–1437.

[155] Bonhomme-Faivre L, Devocelle A, Saliba F, Chatled S, Maccario J, Farinotti R, et al. MDR-1 C3435T polymorphism influences cyclosporine a dose requirement in liver-transplant recipients. Transplantation. 2004;78:21–25.

[156] Jiang ZP, Wang YR, Xu P, Liu RR, Zhao XL, Chen FP. Meta-analysis of the effect of MDR1 C3435T polymorphism on cyclosporine pharmacokinetics. Basic Clin Pharmacol Toxicol. 2008;103:433–444.

[157] Uesugi M, Kikuchi M, Shinke H, Omura T, Yonezawa A, Matsubara K, et al. Impact of cytochrome P450 3A5 polymorphism in graft livers on the frequency of acute cellular rejection in living-donor liver transplantation. Pharmacogenet Genomics. 2014;24:356–366.

[158] Uesugi M, Hosokawa M, Shinke H, Hashimoto E, Takahashi T, Kawai T, et al. Influence of cytochrome P450 (CYP) 3A4*1G polymorphism on the pharmacokinetics of tacrolimus, probability of acute cellular rejection, and mRNA expression level of CYP3A5 rather than CYP3A4 in living-donor liver transplant patients. Biol Pharm Bull. 2013;36:1814–1821.

[159] Masuda S, Goto M, Fukatsu S, Uesugi M, Ogura Y, Oike F, et al. Intestinal MDR1/ABCB1 level at surgery as a risk factor of acute cellular rejection in living-donor liver transplant patients. Clin Pharmacol Ther. 2006;79:90–102.

[160] Sharma P, Schaubel DE, Guidinger MK, Merion RM. Effect of pretransplant serum creatinine on the survival benefit of liver transplantation. Liver Transpl. 2009;15:1808–1813.

[161] Ojo AO, Held PJ, Port FK, Wolfe RA, Leichtman AB, Young EW, et al. Chronic renal failure after transplantation of a nonrenal organ. N Engl J Med. 2003;349:931–940.

[162] Hebert MF, Dowling AL, Gierwatowski C, Lin YS, Edwards KL, Davis CL, et al. Association between ABCB1 (multidrug resistance transporter) genotype and post-liver transplantation renal dysfunction in patients receiving calcineurin inhibitors. Pharmacogenetics. 2003;13:661–674.

[163] Hawwa AF, McElnay JC. Impact of ATP-binding cassette, subfamily B, member 1 pharmacogenetics on tacrolimus-associated nephrotoxicity and dosage requirements in paediatric patients with liver transplant. Expert Opin Drug Saf. 2011;10:9–22.

[164] Hawwa AF, McKiernan PJ, Shields M, Millership JS, McElnay JC. Influence of ABCB1 polymorphisms and haplotypes on tacrolimus nephrotoxicity and dosage requirements in children with liver transplant. Brit J Clin Pharmacol. 2009;68:413–421.

[165] Fukudo M, Yano I, Yoshimura A, Masuda S, Uesugi M, Hosohata K, et al. Impact of MDR1 and CYP3A5 on the oral clearance of tacrolimus and tacrolimus-related renal dysfunction in adult living-donor liver transplant patients. Pharmacogenet Genomics. 2008;18:413–423.

[166] Tapirdamaz O, Hesselink DA, el Bouazzaoui S, Azimpour M, Hansen B, van der Laan LJ, et al. Genetic variance in ABCB1 and CYP3A5 does not contribute toward the development of chronic kidney disease after liver transplantation. Pharmacogenet Genomics. 2014;24:427–435.

[167] Birdwell KA, Decker B, Barbarino JM, et al. Clinical Pharmacogenetics implementation. Consortium (CPIC) guidelines for CYP3A5 genotype and tacrolimus dosing. Clin Pharmacol Ther. 2015;98:19–24.

[168] Evans JP, Green RC. Direct to consumer genetic testing: avoiding a culture war. Genet Med. 2009;11:568–569.

[169] Evans JP, Dale DC, Fomous C. Preparing for a consumer-driven genomic age. N Engl J Med. 2010;363:1099.

Chapter 6

Viral Transmission in Organ Transplantation: The Importance of Risk Assessment

Cristina Baleriola and William D Rawlinson

Additional information is available at the end of the chapter

http://dx.doi.org/10.5772/62737

Abstract

Organ transplantation presents a low but extant risk of allograft transmission of blood-borne viruses (BBV) including human immunodeficiency virus (HIV), hepatitis B virus (HBV), and hepatitis C virus (HCV). Other infections temporarily present in blood are also transmissible from donor to recipient, such as cytomegalovirus (CMV), polyomavirus (BK), Epstein-Barr virus (EBV), and others, where the donor has acute infection at the time of donation. Decisions about accepting organs for transplantation involve a trade-off between the acquisition of good-quality organs, which can confer longer survival time for the recipient, but at the risk of dying from waiting too long from the underlying condition, versus accepting an organ of less quality, but at the risk of potentially acquiring a donor-derived infection (DDI), unless such infection can be ruled out in the donated organ. In this chapter, we describe the different factors contributing to the overall risk of acquiring a BBV infection through the allograft, mechanisms for assessing risk of the donor and the different strategies available to minimize or mitigate the risk. The process is one of risk assessments and risk ameliorations through optimum laboratory and clinical assessment processes, so that transplantation professionals can balance the overall risk against the life-saving and life-enhancing benefits of organ transplantation.

Keywords: blood-borne virus infection through transplantation, donor-derived infections, risk assessment, risk management, risk mitigation

1. Introduction

Organ transplantation currently provides definitive therapy for individuals with end-organ failure. Despite the enormous therapeutic advances in this area, donor-derived infections (DDI)

in the recipient from the donated organ, although rare, have been associated with significant morbidity and mortality [1,2]. These unexpected DDI are often with blood-borne viruses (BBV), including hepatitis B virus (HBV), hepatitis C virus (HCV), and less frequently human immunodeficiency virus (HIV) [3–5]. There are few data available to ascertain the risk of infection in organ transplantation for known and emerging pathogens, as most information comes from events of transmission, which are rare and not always well characterized, with few countries having well-established post-transplant surveillance systems with universal recipient assessment [6].

Due to the scarcity of donor organs, the safety paradigm in solid organ transplantation (SOT) should be based on a risk-benefit trade-off and the decision-making strategy for organ allocation be based on risk management. In this context, it is important to consider that most often the benefits of transplanting the organ outweigh the risk of DDI. Therefore, care should be taken to find the appropriate balance between minimizing the risk of transmission and organ wastage or recipient illness progression [7].

This chapter describes the different factors contributing to the overall risk of acquiring a BBV infection through the allograft, the risk assessment of the donor, and the different strategies available to minimize or mitigate the risk.

2. Donor assessment

Donor assessment often uses a questionnaire based on review of medical and social history to identify donor risks, including those associated with infection with blood-borne pathogens. In Australia, a standard questionnaire is available nationwide to streamline the assessment criteria [8]. The organ donor coordinator must review all potential donor's available medical records to identify evidence of an infectious disease or documentation of established risk behaviors associated with BBV infection. The information should be obtained from a next of kin and/or other person who has an established relationship with the donor (e.g. the donor's general practitioner). Attention to travel history is critical to identify donors at risk of endemic infections [9,10].

- Men who have had sex with another man in the preceding 5 years.
- Intravenous, intramuscular, or subcutaneous injection of drugs in the preceding 5 years.
- Incarceration in the previous 12 months.
- Persons who have had sex in the preceding 12 months with any of the above persons or a person known or suspected to have HIV, HCV, or HBV infection.
- Persons who have engaged in sex in exchange for money or drugs in the preceding 5 years.
- Exposure in preceding 12 months through percutaneous inoculation or open wound.
- Nonsterile tattooing, piercings in the past 12 months.
- Unexplained fever/weight loss/LAD/cough.
- Cocaine snorting.
- Physical concern.

Table 1. Donors with identified risk factors.

Careful physical assessment of the donor's body is conducted by both the organ procurement team and the procuring surgeon. The examination also searches for evidence of underlying disease, such as cirrhosis or other surface manifestations of infections, malignancies or of recent drug use [11]. In the acute donation situation, the appropriate person is not always available to question regarding the donor's risk, and manifestations of BBV can be minimal or non-existent. Thus, optimal donor screening testing is of paramount importance.

3. Prevalence of infection

The prevalence of BBV infection on a given population is particularly important as donor history may fail to uncover donor risk factors and, especially in the case of HBV or HCV, the rate of prevalent disease remains relatively high in 2016 in many countries, even in donors without identified risks. BBV potentially transmitted from donor organ to recipient are prevalent at 2% of the Australian population (**Table 2**) [12], whereas cytomegalovirus (CMV), Epstein–Barr virus (EBV), and polyomavirus (BK) virus are far more common, with prevalence rates of 50–70%, 95% [13], and ~60% [14], respectively.

Virus estimated	Infected population	Prevalence rate (%)	Prevalence rate in high-risk population (%)
HIV	25,700	0.10	2.8
HBV	218,000	0.87	50
HCV	233,525	0.93	50
Total	468,525	1.9	80*

* Some individuals are infected with both HCV and HBV.

Table 2. Prevalence of BBV (HIV-1, HBV, and HCV) in the Australian population.

The prevalence of BBV among potential increased-risk organ donors in our laboratory in the Serology and Virology Division (SAVID), providing testing services to the NSW Organ and Tissue Donation Service was 50% for HBV, 10% for HCV, and 0.1% for HIV-1 [15]. In the United States, the prevalence of HIV and HCV in average-risk donors was reported to be 0.10 and 3.45%, respectively, whereas the prevalence of HIV and HCV among increased risk donors (IRDs) was 0.50 and 18.20%, respectively [16]. Viruses endemic to certain geographical areas or population groups including human T-cell lymphotropic virus 1 (HTLV-1) in the Australian Aboriginal population and HBV in Mediterranean and Asian Countries may be one reason for unexpected positive screening results of average-risk donors or donors without apparent risk factors [17]. The WHO publishes updated prevalence figures of BBV worldwide, which could assist in ascertaining the probability of BBV latent infections [18] and hence background risk of donor infection.

4. Serology/nucleic acid testing results

Donors are routinely screened to identify viral or bacterial infection using serology and nucleic acid testing (NAT) assays. NAT assays detect the presence of specific viral or bacterial RNA/DNA in a patient's blood. The latter is a marker of infectivity of the organ donor when compared with antibody tests, which show previous infection without distinguishing current infection. All BBV serological tests have a 'window period' (WP), which is a time after infection during which the antibody response cannot be detected by the usual testing methods (**Figure 1**). The serological WP varies with the sensitivity of the assay, but generally are 17–22 days for HIV, 38–60 days for HBV, and 70 days for HCV.

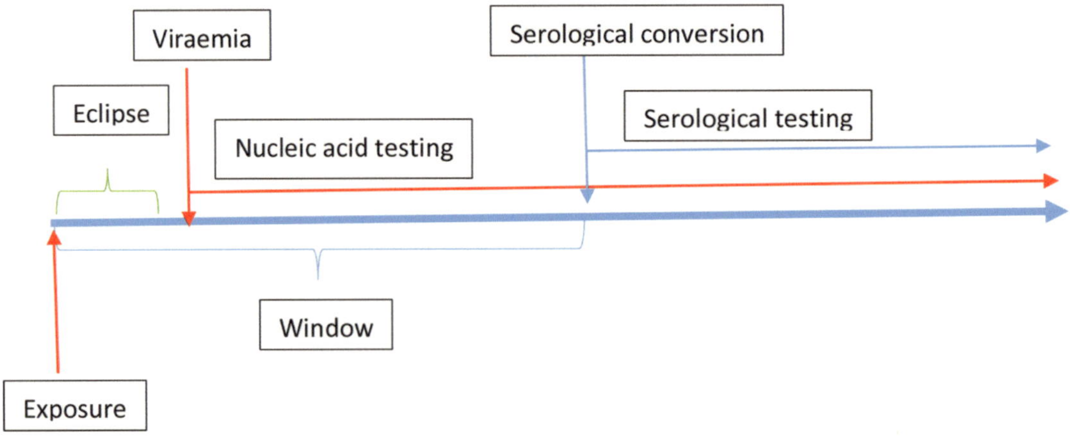

Figure 1. Events taking place after viral exposure.

NAT assays significantly reduce the WP between infection and detection compared with serological testing (6–7 days for HIV, 30–40 days for HBV, and 4–6 days for HCV) (**Figure 2**). Thus, NAT assays also have WP when they are negative following acute infection, therefore a negative NAT assay result does not completely eliminate the possibility of recent infection. In practice, the risk of infection from screened donors has been extremely low, but no screening test that is performed on a donor is entirely capable of reducing risk of transmission to nil, although all efforts are taken to reduce risk of BBV transmission and effectively resulting in extremely low risk.

All potential organ donors (living or deceased) should be tested for antibodies to HIV (anti-HIV 1/2 antigen/antibody combo assay), HCV and HBV. Donors should also be tested for HIV, HCV, and HBV RNA/DNA, whereas increased-risk organ donors should be tested by NAT for HIV, HCV, and HBV prospectively (**Table 3**).

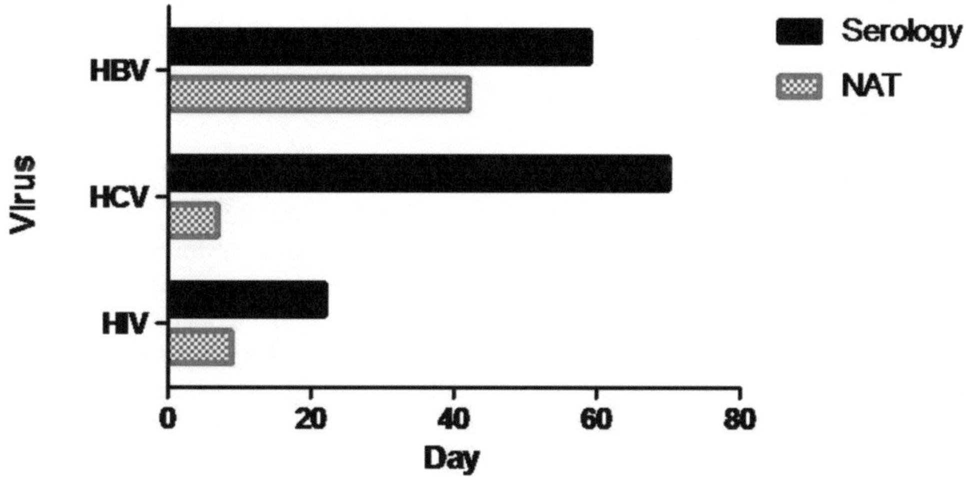

Figure 2. Differences in window periods for serology and NAT for HIV, HCV, and HBV (Data from SAVID).

Serology:	NAT:
• Anti-HIV-1/2	• HIV-1 RNA
• Anti-HCV	• HCV RNA
• Anti-HTLV-I/II	• HBV DNA
• HBsAg	• Prospective in increased risk donors
• Anti-HBc	• Retrospective in average-risk donors
• Anti-HBs	
• Anti-EBV	
• Anti-CMV	
• Syphilis antibody (TPHA)	

Table 3. Mandatory testing for prospective organ donors in Australia.

The WP of an assay has important implications for the risk assessment of a particular donor. The definition of IRD as per the Transplantation Society of Australia and New Zealand guidelines [11] is "where there is concern regarding the donor's risk behavior and it cannot be reliably determined or the behavior may have occurred within the last 2 months". These 2 months cover the NAT WPs for HIV, HCV, and HBV (**Figure 2**).

The arrival of fully automated platforms for triple viral NAT currently in 2016 in Australia by at least two manufacturers opens the possibility of 24-hour access to HBV, HCV, and HIV NAT testing. New technologies, such as the Cobas 6800 system [19] from Roche Molecular Systems and the Panther system [20] from Hologic, are now available with shorter turnaround time (TAT = 3.5 hours), and the possibility of confirmatory testing of initially positive results.

5. Conduct of donor testing

If the specimen sample used for testing has unusual characteristics, such as where donors have had massive blood and/or blood product transfusion, it is essential to indicate to the testing laboratory and the transplanting team the underlying condition of the donor. If the donor has received greater than 50% of blood volume in blood product transfusion, the sample is unsuitable for serology and NAT testing due to dilution of native antibodies by transfused fluids [21]. A pre-transfusion sample should be provided to the laboratory. If this is not possible, NAT-enhanced sensitivity may reduce the frequency of false-negative test results when donor specimens are haemodiluted.

There are significant concerns that the use of assays with higher sensitivity for pathogen detection—such as NAT assays—will result in net organ loss. This is because the majority of positive tests in low-prevalence populations will be false positives [22], and time constrains do not allow confirmatory testing with certain testing platforms. The NAT laboratory at SAVID, Prince of Wales Hospital in Sydney, Australia, has developed screening algorithms using three NAT assays run in parallel for prospective screening of IRD to maximize organ availability by effectively eliminating false-positive results (FPR) [15]. The availability of a 24-hour NAT screening service for organ donors provided diagnosis within 8 hours and enabled the use of organs from donors with positive serology but negative NAT results or donors with false-positive serology results. This algorithm allowed us to perform real-time discrimination of initially reactive results and the use of 35 IRD, which resulted in transplantation of 102 additional organs with safer expansion of the donor pool.

Positive serology or NAT results should be interpreted consistent with current guidelines [10,16] by the accepting teams in consultation with an Infectious Disease Physician.

6. Risk of transmission

The risk of acquisition of a BBV through organ transplantation is related to the efficiency of virus transmission and replication after contact with blood and tissues. Not all BBV are transmitted in the same way, and the result may be related to the type and size of the inoculum, the titre of virus and the immunization status of the recipient. Most of the well-documented transmissions are from blood transfusions but this may correlate with similar level of infectivity from donated organs. In humans, HBV transmission has been reported to be from blood donors in the WP or from donors with occult hepatitis B (OBI) with HBV viral loads of >20 IU/ml [23], whereas donors with an anti-HBs titre of >100 seem to have a protective role to prevent de novo HBV infection [24]. In terms of HIV, a pre-seroconversion donation with a viral load of ≤150 copies of RNA/ml went undetected and resulted in an HIV transmission [25]. Finally, HCV-infected recipients have been reported from donors with a viral load of as low as 182 cp/

ml and even from a donor with undetectable levels of RNA in the transcription-mediated amplification (TMA) assay (limit of detection (LOD) = 9.6 IU/ml)) [26].

In a report by the Canadian Society for Transplantation and Canadian National Transplant Research Program [27], the residual risk to acquire a HIV or HCV infection from transplanted organs of IRD after screening with serology and NAT was calculated (**Table 4**). The group concluded that these donors should screened by serological testing in conjunction with NAT testing for HCV and HIV and hepatitis B surface antigen (HBsAg) or NAT for HBV.

Virus	Risk of WP infection for NAT and ELISA per 10,000	Risk of WP infection for NAT and ELISA expressed as ratio
HIV	0.71	1:14,923
HCV	3.79	1:2,637

Table 4. Risk per 10,000 donors of an HIV or HCV infection occurring during the WP, by enzyme-linked immunosorbent assay (ELISA) and NAT. Assumes a WP of 21 days for ELISA and 7 days for NAT.

7. Organ-specific risks

HBV- and HCV-infected livers produce universally infected HBV- or HCV-naïve recipients, with outcomes determined by factors, such as the viral genotype, the presence or absence of previous immunity and the response to antiviral therapy. On the other hand, a HCV- or HBV-infected donor may be able to donate other organs rather than the liver. As both HBV and HCV can be transmitted via organ donation, especially through liver grafts, a thorough approach is needed for successful management of the recipient, and an emphasis on aggressive immunization and risk mitigation of transplant candidates prior to transplant should be pursued.

Allografts from HBV-infected donors should preferentially be given to recipients who are HBsAg positive, hepatitis B core antibody (anti-HBc) positive, or hepatitis B surface antibody (HBsAb) positive [28]. Transmission of de novo HBV infection to liver grafts recipients from anti-HBc–positive donors has been detected since 1992; however, further studies demonstrated that non-liver allografts from these donors can be safely used [29,30]. Several studies have clearly shown that non-liver organs and tissues from donors who are anti-HBc positive and HBsAg negative can be used with negligible risk, especially if the recipient is protected through vaccination or prior exposure to HBV [31,32].

A different scenario is that of donors with OBI, characterized by persistence of HBV DNA in the liver tissue (and in some cases also in serum) of HBsAg-negative individuals [33], therefore exhibiting undetectable HBsAg in serum and low-level HBV DNA (<200 IU/ml). In HBV, low-prevalence countries, the prevalence of OBI is low (0.1–2.4%) [34], whereas in HBV, high-prevalence countries, the prevalence can range from 7.5 to 16% [35,36].

The molecular bases of OBI appear to be related to the long-lasting persistence in the nuclei of the hepatocytes of the HBV cccDNA, an intermediate form of the virus life cycle that serves as a template for gene transcription [37,38]. The risk of OBI being associated with anti-HBc seropositivity has been demonstrated [39,40], and one of the best sentinel markers for OBI is a positive anti-HBc serology result [41]. Long-standing abnormal results of liver function tests of unknown aetiology in the absence of HBV serological markers and serum HBV DNA may also indicate the presence of HBV DNA in the liver and peripheral blood mononuclear cells [42]. Donors with OBI may transmit HBV infection, especially in orthotopic liver transplantation (OLT), because the hepatocytes are the reservoir of the viral cccDNA. These recipients may develop de novo hepatitis B, particularly when they are HBV naïve [43,44]. Prevention measures include anti-HBV prophylaxis, based on anti-HBs immunoglobulin alone or in combination with lamivudine. These measures, however, cannot completely eliminate HBV transmission because there have been documented reports on the development of OBI in recipients who received an organ from an OBI carrier [44], exhibiting the same viral genomes (including HBV cccDNA) in the transplanted liver.

As already mentioned, HBV-infected donors can be safely used for potential HBV-infected recipients [28] with the use of post-transplantation prophylaxis (hepatitis B immune globulin (HBIg) and nucleoside/nucleotide polymerase inhibitors, such as lamivudine in combination with adefovir, entecavir, or tenofovir) [45–47]. It has also been reported that a titre of HBsAb greater than 100 in the donor has a protective effect [48]. Recipient sero-protection through prior exposure or vaccination is a highly effective way to prevent transmission of HBV through organ transplantation [49]. As some potential organ recipients do not respond well to vaccination and remain unprotected, a priority area is to devise new ways to enhance vaccination responses.

HCV-positive donor organs can also be used in HCV-positive recipients with minimal impact on clinical outcomes [50,51]. Clinical studies have shown that there is no significant difference in survival in HCV-positive recipients who receive either HCV-positive or HCV-negative livers or kidneys [51–55]. Therefore, there needs to be education to enhance uptake of HCV-positive organs in HCV-positive recipients. As first-generation direct acting antivirals (DAAs) offer a significant therapeutic improvement when compared with previous therapies, particularly for patients with HCV genotype-1 infection, this may lead to the use of more HCV-infected organ donors for HCV-infected recipients treated with this highly effective post-transplant prophylaxis [56,57].

8. Use of IRDs

In the United States alone, almost 10,000 individuals die annually while awaiting organ transplantation [58], whereas in Australia, there are almost 3000 individuals in the waiting list. Due to organ scarcity, attempts at expanding the pool of potential donors are necessary, and the criteria for donation are under continuous scrutiny. Recent campaigns globally from organ procurement agencies to expand the donor pool have resulted in use of organs from IRD, who

http://dx.doi.org/10.5772/62737

are at greater risk of infection with BBV, including HBV, HCV, and HIV. The use of NAT to screen such IRD has been associated with increased utilization of these organs [10,11,16,27].

The key to using these IRD is to maximize the measures to identify risk factors; particularly ensuring that infectious diseases are not transmitted from donor to recipient in the allograft. A successful strategy to mitigate the overall risk has been to match the allograft to the most appropriate recipient by improved selection and monitoring. In such scenarios, additional consent and recipient screening at regular intervals during the first year after transplant should be performed [10,11,16,27].

We documented in one study that with the use of prospective NAT, 102 additional organs from IRD were used in Australia. These organs would otherwise have been discarded or used with restrictions [15]. This represents 18.8% of all organs transplanted during the study period. Furthermore, the utilization of parallel NAT assays combined with mathematical modeling enabled us to estimate the probability that the combination of results were predictive of true-positive results. Thus, we piloted a methodology for effectively minimizing FPR. This resulted in higher confidence in the NAT results and minimizing the loss of organs secondary to FPR to negligible.

In a Canadian study of 3746 transplants using deceased liver donors [59], it was concluded that over the last decade, there was an increase in the use of older donors and donation after cardiac death (DCD) organs, but recipient survival was not compromised. In Australia, IRDs are routinely used, and this strategy has substantially contributed to an increased use of organs [15]. Furthermore, the acceptance of these organs by the transplantation community has been increased over the years, and from 2013 onwards, the same number of organs was retrieved from IRD and from average-risk donors (**Figure 3**).

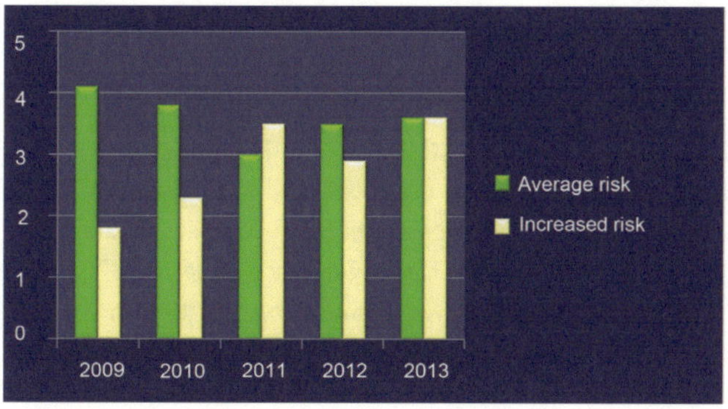

Figure 3. Number of organs retrieved from increased-risk donors vs average-risk donors over the years (data from SA-VID).

Final decisions in individual cases about using organs of IRD must acknowledge the recommendations from national and international guidelines, the risk-benefit trade-off in the context of the gravity of recipient's prognosis without transplantation, consideration of all clinical and laboratory assessment parameters and a fully informed consent and risk acceptance by the recipient.

9. Scoring the risk

Decision aids are increasingly being developed to support transplantation teams in making difficult treatment decisions involving trade-offs between provision of a good quality organ with longer survival but longer wait pre-transplant versus accepting an organ of less quality with earlier transplantation but higher risk of shorter survival post-transplantation or post-transplant infections. Furthermore, transplant providers who are helping patients to make treatment decisions may find it difficult to communicate the risks associated with each option in a clear, understandable fashion, particularly for IRD organs, given the complexities of risk assessment.

Scoring systems to indicate recipient's gravity include the Model for End-Stage Liver Disease (MELD) score, which is a scoring system for assessing the severity of chronic liver disease. It was found to be useful in determining prognosis and prioritizing for receipt of a liver transplant [60]. The score was developed by the Organ Procurement and Transplantation network (OPTN)/United Network for Organ Sharing (UNOS) and implemented in February 2002. MELD uses the patient's values for serum bilirubin, serum creatinine, and the international normalized ratio for prothrombin time (INR) to predict survival. It is calculated according to formula [61]. On the other hand, the donor risk index (DRI) by Feng et al. [62] using Organ Procurement and Transplantation Network (OPTN) data was developed as a continuous scoring system that includes donor and transplant parameters that significantly influence outcomes after liver transplantation (LTx). The author undertook a multivariate analysis of a large cohort (20,023 transplants) from the Scientific Registry of Transplant Recipients database. The parameters used were the donor's age, race, height, and cause of death (COD); the split liver donation status; the donation after cardiac death (DCD) status; the type of allocation (local, regional, or national); and the cold ischaemia time.

The DRI was validated in a study conducted by the Eurotransplant region, which aimed to identify its potential use [63]. The study was a database analysis of all 5939 liver transplants involving deceased donors and adult recipients from January 1, 2003, to December 31, 2007, in the Eurotransplant region. Follow-up data were available for 5723 patients with a median follow-up of 2.5 years. The mean DRI was remarkably higher in the Eurotransplant region versus OPTN (1.71 versus 1.45). The results demonstrated that Kaplan-Meier curves per DRI category showed a significant correlation between the DRI and outcomes ($p < 0.001$). A multivariate analysis demonstrated that the DRI was the most significant factor influencing outcomes ($p < 0.001$). Among all donor, transplant, and recipient variables, the DRI was the strongest predictor of outcomes.

In another study [64], it was investigated the impact of the DRI on the outcome of HCV-infected patients undergoing LTx, where the median DRI was 1.3 (range, 0.77–4.27). Increasing DRI was associated with a statistically significant increase in the relative risk (RR) of graft failure and patient death for both HCV (+) and HCV (−) recipients. Finally, Rosemberg et al. [65] using a prospectively collected infection data set, matched liver transplant recipients (and the respective allograft DRI scores) with their specific post-transplant infectious complications. All transplant recipients were organized by DRI score and divided into groups with low-DRI and high-DRI scores. Three hundred and seventy-eight liver transplants were identified, with 189 recipients each in the low-DRI and high-DRI groups. The mean MELD scores were 26.25–0.53 and 24.76–0.55, respectively ($p = 0.052$), and the mean number of infectious complications per patient were 1.60–0.19 and 1.94–0.24, respectively ($p = 0.26$). Logistic regression showed only length of hospital stay and a history of vascular disease as being associated independently with infection, with a trend toward significance for MELD score ($p = 0.13$). The study concluded that although DRI score predicts liver graft survival, infectious complications depended more heavily on recipient factors.

Even though organs from donors with high DRI score correlate with poorer post-transplant survival, the overall contribution of high-DRI grafts to the donor pool and the resultant reduction in wait list mortality make them cost-effective [66].

10. Clinical guidelines

Deciding how to allocate organs for transplantation is a very complex process and raises a number of clinical and ethical issues. Up-to-date guidelines provide an overarching framework to facilitate the decision-making process in clinical robust ways based on previous evidence. In general, transplantation guidelines follow many of the recommendations in place for the selection and microbiological testing of blood donors. However, as in organ donation and transplantation, the logistics are greatly influenced by the need to retain organ viability, the testing of potential donors will be conducted under severe time constraints. In these situations, the testing that needs to be carried out, and the general principles for balancing the risks and benefits are unique to this field.

Some of the most important transplantation guidelines published recently are as follows:

- *PHS Guideline for Reducing Human Immunodeficiency Virus, Hepatitis B Virus, and Hepatitis C Virus Transmission Through Organ Transplantation* was published in the United States in August 2013 [16]. The aim of the guide was to improve organ transplant recipient outcomes by reducing the risk of HIV, HBV, and HCV transmission. The guide is truly comprehensive and based on systematic reviews. It is extremely detailed and specialized and not very practical for the daily use of transplantation professionals.
- Advisory Committee on the Safety of Blood Tissues and Organs (SaBTO) published the *Guidance on the Microbiological Safety of Human Organs, Tissues and Cells Used for Transplantation* in February 2011 in the United Kingdom [67]. The guidance was written by a working group after extensive consultation and is extremely clear, accurate, and user friendly. However, as professionals involved in transplantation need to take real-time decisions that could be life saving for patients, most of the information given in the guidance could have been summarized and presented on tables to facilitate the information to readers.

- The Council of Europe in 2013 published the 5th edition of *the Guide to the Quality and Safety of Organs for Transplantation* [68]. This guideline collates updated information to provide professionals in transplantation with a useful overview of the most recent advancements in the field. The guide has a very comprehensive section on risk of transmission of infectious diseases. However, as pointed out before, the information is too comprehensive and should have been summarized.

- Transplantation Society of Australia and New Zealand (TSANZ) published version 1.4 of the guideline *Organ Transplantation from Deceased Donors: Consensus Statement on Eligibility Criteria and Allocation Protocols* in April 2015 [11]. The guide has only one section related to transmission of infectious agents from donor to recipient with data from HCV and HBV infection risks alone. The information is insufficient as many other real-life situations are not contemplated. Within Australia, the NSW Ministry of Health published the guide *Organ Donation and Transplantation—Managing Risks of Transmission of HIV, HCV and HBV* in 2013 [10]. This is a very useful guide for transplantation professionals.

Ideally, guidelines for transplantation should be comprehensive but presented in a concise manner to facilitate its use to readers, as shown in **Table 5** [69].

Donor status	Advice	References
Antibody to HIV (+)	Exclude from organ donation	[11,67]
Antibody to HCV (+)	Exclude from organ donation for HCV (−) recipients If used, usually reserve organ for recipient HCV (+) or severely ill recipient. HCV RNA testing should be done and allocated to a donor with a higher HCV viral load	[11,67]
Hepatitis B surface antigen HBsAg (+)	Exclude from organ donation. Use in life-threatening situations with recipient antiviral prophylaxis against HBV	[11,67]
Hepatitis B core antibody IgG (anti-HBc) (+)	Indicates past HBV infection. Organs from anti-HBc (+) of anti-HBs (−) may still be infectious. High risk for transmission with liver donation—generally used with intensive prophylaxis. Non-hepatic organs—small risk of transmission of HBV, and generally used for immunized HBsAb (+) recipients	[11,67,70,71]
Hepatitis B surface antibody Anti-HBs (+)	Anti-HBs >100 IU/l and anti-HBc (+) donations unlikely to be infectious and donation is permitted with the potential exception of livers (see above). HBV DNA NAT should be done and available prior to organ donation HBV DNA (−) indicates suitability for donation, though does not exclude risk of infection from liver. Use in vaccinated recipients and with negative NAT testing if donor vaccination unknown	[11,67,70,71]
Antibody to CMV (+)	Donation permitted. Post-transplant CMV monitoring and preventive strategy based on risk to the recipient	[67]
Antibody to EBV (+)	PCR monitoring of the seronegative or paediatric recipient	[67]

Donor status	Advice	References
RPR (+)	Not a contraindication to donation. Recipients receive standard prophylaxis (benzathine penicillin or ceftriaxone). Ensure administration of adequate antimicrobial therapy and the patient should be monitored for serological evidence of syphilis infection	[11,67,70,71]
Antibody to HTLV I/II (+)	High rate of false-positive results and consistent strategy not available. Some centers exclude from organ donation or use for life-threatening situations, with informed consent	[11,67,71]
Antibody to Toxoplasma IgG (+)	Not a contraindication to donation. Seronegative recipients with a seropositive donor should receive prophylaxis. Cardiac recipients particularly prone to transplant-associated toxoplasmosis	[11,67,71]
Viral encephalitis	Unknown etiology in donor is a contraindication to transplantation (risk of rabies, West Nile Virus or other exotic neurotropic infections). HSV or VZV CNS infection is a contraindication as it may cause systemic infection. HSV encephalitis without evidence of systemic infection treated with antivirals may be used, and antiviral prophylaxis should be used for the recipient. Local HSV/VZV infection treated with adequate antiviral therapy for >7 days organs can be used; if treated <7 days, recipient should receive antiviral prophylaxis (the serological status of the recipient must be known)	[67]

Anti-HBs, hepatitis B surface antibody; IgG, immunoglobulin G; RPR, rapid plasma reagin; VZV, Varicella Zoster virus.

Table 5. Recommendations for organ allocation based on screening data as at 2015 – subject to change with changes in policy.

This kind of format is how the Scandinavian guidelines have been presented and this could be a very useful resource for professionals identifying organ donors, transplant co-ordinators managing the donation process, and transplant physicians responsible for organ allocation [72].

11. Risk stratification and management

Currently, there are two ways in which organ donors are risk stratified in Australia: donors are dichotomized as being either at increased risk (IRD) or without identified risk factors for transmission of infectious diseases. **Figure 4** shows the flowchart for BBV testing and risk stratification in New South Wales (NSW), Australia [10].

In principle, any reactivity in one or more of the mandatory marker assays used for screening donors renders the donor ineligible. However, in life-preserving situations, it is possible to waive this exclusion. The risk-benefit trade-off means that using an IRD should only be considered when the donation is life-preserving. In this situation, the transplant surgeon with the informed consent of the potential recipient should balance the risk of infection against the risk of dying while waiting for another graft. Heart, lung, and liver transplants will almost always fit within this definition because the clinical situation of the recipient is likely to be terminal. However, short-term or intermediate support measures can be employed to avoid the immediate need for transplantation with an organ from an IRD.

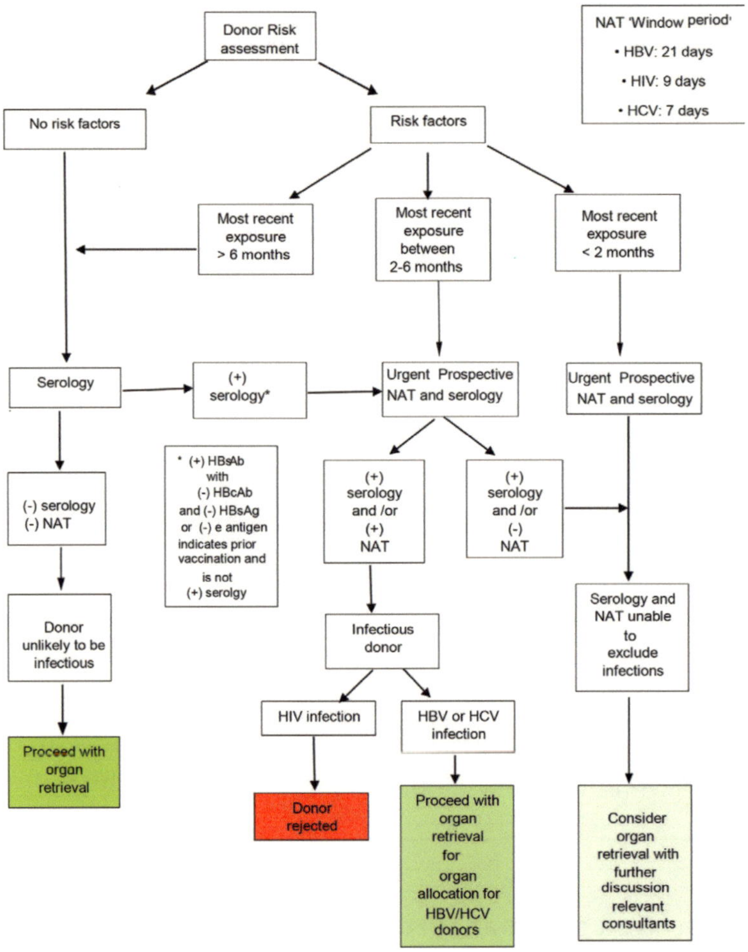

Figure 4. Blood-borne virus testing and risk stratification flowchart (from Organ Donation and Transplantation – Managing Risks of Transmission of HIV, HCV, and HBV). Reproduced with permission from NSW Ministry of Health, 2015.

One strategy when using IRD is matching infection status of donor and recipient. Previous infection, current infection, or immunization may decrease or remove the risk of infection following the use of a transplant from a donor who is known to be infected. Thus, it is appropriate to consider the use of an organ from a donor who is known to be infected, or who is potentially infected with HCV or HBV or a recipient who is also infected with HCV or HBV (i.e. infection match). Another approach involves matching of the immune status of the recipient to the infection status of the donor. For example, a recipient shown to be immune to hepatitis B, naturally or by immunization, is unlikely to suffer re-infection from an HBV-infected donor. In this type of matching, it is essential that the status of the recipient is known with certainty.

Matching the status will also include an assessment of the likelihood of transmitting viral genotypes, which may pose an additional hazard to the already infected recipient, such as using an organ infected with HCV genotype 1 for a non-1 genotype–infected recipient; drug-resistant variants, and immune escape variants. Infectious Disease specialist support should be sought to ensure that appropriate testing has been undertaken to inform the risk assessment and to confirm the recipient's status.

Risk mitigation measures include the use of prophylaxis with antiviral drugs or antibiotics; counseling and discussing with the recipient the potential infection risk and the possibility of disease arising from infection. In addition, a full informed consent and post-transplant surveillance for infection of the recipient with planned interventions should they become necessary in the case of infection transmission should be undertaken.

12. Post-transplant surveillance

The final verification of risk estimates for DDI is carried out using post-transplant surveillance aiming to identify possible donor-derived events and clusters of transmissions. These procedures require careful post-transplant follow-up, diligent clinicians to suspect and report cases and reporting systems to accept and inform investigation of potential transmission reports in a proactive manner. These systems, if universally instituted, could improve investigation of potential clusters of infection, with enhanced rapid detection and improved advice to clinicians. Furthermore, they can be valuable resources for examination of clinical data to establish evidence-based guidelines.

Recent biovigilance initiatives in the United States and Europe have occurred with the aim of developing national surveillance systems for cells, tissues, and organs. In Europe, the Eustite project [73] initiated in 2008 focused especially on inspection, training, and vigilance for tissue banks. The project developed special tools and a system for the classification and reporting of adverse events to all European countries that could be used internationally for biovigilance and surveillance. Subsequently, the tools developed by the Eustite project were streamlined by the WHO, resulting in an educational program designed for organs and tissues through the NOTIFY Project. The vigilance information database collected by the Notify Project is available on the WHO/CNT Global NOTIFY Library website [74]. The library aims to be a comprehensive reference of different types of adverse events and reactions identifying their underlying root causes. The library is regularly maintained and updated and serves as a communication hub for transplantation institutions with international vigilance and surveillance data to enhance donor and recipient safety and for greater public transparency in transplantation. The project also aims to be a reference of internationally terminology for biovigilance of organs, tissues, and cells.

The US program monitoring DDI (the UNOS and the Disease Transmission Advisory Committee (DTAC)) [75] undertakes data collection and dissemination on pre-transplant and post-transplant events and examines and classifies potential donor-derived transmission through transplantation of infection or malignancy. These aim to educate the transplant community and help change policy and improve processes. The membership includes CDC, FDA, transplant centers, transplant infectious disease professionals, laboratory testing personnel, and organ procurement organizations. The OPTN currently requires reporting of donor-derived events. All potential donor-derived transmission events (PDDTE) reported to OPTN/UNOS are reviewed by the DTAC, and real-time reports are available for transplantation professionals.

The ANZDATA [76] registry in Australia and New Zealand is a retrospective reporting system to evaluate data from donors and recipients. Attempts are recently made for timely data collection of key events and the creation of a real-time Web-based system utilization, including historical data for all years and real-time data for the current year grouped by country and state with interactive reports that can be generated at any point of time.

Most of the established surveillance systems are passive, that is laboratories notify positive test results to public health regulators. Thus, only recipients tested are notified. This system is far from ideal as most infections with a BBV do not have symptoms at the time of infection and an infected recipient may not be tested for some time post-transplant. Furthermore, not all notifications are followed up, so a recently infected organ recipient may not be detected even if tested and notified.

Despite the efforts in many countries to gather transplantation data, the main difficulty seems to lie in the absence of dedicated organ donation and transplantation surveillance registries, as usually the transplant team reports back to the organ donation agency and the data are not shared. The transplantation community requires a real-time worldwide surveillance system to identify possible clusters of infections worldwide. This could be achieved through data linkage from already established biovigilance programs. An important aspect of biovigilance systems is to develop data linkages with public health regulators and healthcare providers, so that the integration of databases can be conducted to strengthen responses to potential BBV threats worldwide.

13. Conclusions

The development of national policies for risk assessment and definition of acceptable levels of risk for BBV infection—including specific risk-benefit assessments—is increasing safety, equity and transparency in organ allocation. All decisions related to virological risk assessment need to be supported by up-to-date guidelines, optimal diagnostic testing and ongoing surveillance for DDI post-transplantation. This will continue to result in additional use of organs and continuous improvement of transplantation outcomes.

Acknowledgements

The authors thank the NSW Ministry of Health and the NSW Organ and Tissue Donation Service for the initial establishment and the ongoing support of the NAT organ donor screening program at SAVID.

Author details

Cristina Baleriola[1] and William D Rawlinson[2*]

*Address all correspondence to: w.rawlinson@unsw.edu.au

1 South Eastern Area Laboratory Service, Prince of Wales Hospital, Sydney, Australia

2 South Eastern Area Laboratory Services, Microbiology, Prince of Wales Hospital, Sydney, Australia

References

[1] Palacios G, Druce J, Du L,Tran T, Birch C, Briese T, et al. A new arenavirus in a cluster of fatal transplant associated diseases. N Engl J Med. 2008;358(10):991–998. DOI: 10.1056/NEJMoa073785.

[2] Smith JM, Mcdonald RA. Emerging viral infections in transplantation. Pediatr Transplant. 2006;10(7):838–843. DOI: 10.1111/j.1399-3046.2005.00481.x.

[3] Su WJ, Ho MC, Ni YH, Wu JF, Jeng YM, Chen HL, et al. Clinical course of de novo hepatitis B infection after paediatric liver transplantation. Liver Transpl. 2010;16(2): 215–221. DOI: 10.1002/lt.21980.

[4] Ison MG, Llata E, Conover CS, Friedewald JJ, Gerber SI, Grigoryan A, et al. Transmission of human immunodeficiency virus and hepatitis C virus from an organ donor to four transplant recipients. Am J Transplant. 2011;11(6):1218–1225. DOI: 10.1111/j.1600-6143.2011.03597.x.

[5] Suryaprasad A, Basavaraju SV, Hocevar SN, Theodoropoulos N, Zuckerman RA, Hayden T, et al. Transmission of hepatitis C virus from organ donors despite nucleic acid test screening. Am J Transplant. 2015;15(7):1827–1835. DOI: 10.1111/ajt.13283.

[6] Weikert BC, Blumberg EA. Viral infection after renal transplantation: surveillance and management. CJASN. 2008;3(Suppl 2):S76–S86. DOI: 10.2215/CJN.02900707.

[7] Duana KI, Englesbeb MJ, Volk ML. Centers for disease control 'high-risk' donors and kidney utilization. Am J Transplant. 2010;10(2):416–420. DOI: 10.1111/j.1600-6143.2009.02931.x.

[8] TSANZ. Confidential Organ Donation Referral Form [Internet]. 2013. Available from: http://www.tsanz.com.au/downloads/Protocols_Appendix1.pdf [Accessed: December 10, 2015.]

[9] Ison MG, Grossi P, the AST Infectious Disease Community of Practice. Donor-derived infections in solid organ transplantation. Am J Transplant. 2013;13(Suppl 4):22–30. DOI: 10.1111/ajt.12095.

[10] NSW Ministry of Health. Organ Donation and Transplantation—Managing the Risk of Transmission of HIV, HCV, and HBV [Internet]. 2013. Available from: http://wwwo.health.nsw.gov.au/policies/pd/2013/pdf/PD2013_029.pdf [Accessed: December 12, 2015].

[11] Donatelife. Consensus Statement on Eligibility Criteria and Allocation Protocols Version 1.4 – 15 April 2015. [Internet]. 2015. Available from: http://www.donatelife.gov.au/sites/default/files/Version%201.4_April%202015.pdf [Accessed: December 13, 2015].

[12] Kirby Institute. HIV/AIDS, Viral Hepatitis and Sexually Transmissible Infections in Australia. Annual Surveillance Report 2013 [Internet]. 2014. Available from: http://kirby.unsw.edu.au/sites/default/files/hiv/resources/2013AnnualSurvReport.pdf [Accessed: December 10, 2015].

[13] Watzinger F, Suda A, Preuner S, Baumgartinger R, Ebner K, Baskova L, et al. Real-time quantitative PCR assays for detection and monitoring of pathogenic human viruses in immunosuppressed pediatric patients. J Clin Microbiol. 2004;42(11):5189–5198. DOI: 10.1128/JCM.42.11.5189-5198.2004.

[14] Druce J, Catton M, Chibo D, Minerds K, Tyssen D, Kostecki R, et al. Utility of a multiplex PCR assay for detecting herpesvirus DNA in clinical samples. J Clin Microbiol. 2002;40(5):1728–1732. DOI: 10.1128/JCM.40.5.1728-1732.2002.

[15] Baleriola C, Tu E, Johal H, Gillis J, Ison M, Law M, et al. Organ donor screening using parallel nucleic acid testing allows assessment of transmission risk and assay results in real time. Transpl Infect Dis. 2012;14(3):278–287. DOI: 10.1111/j.1399-3062.2012.00734.x.

[16] Public Health Service US. PHS Guideline for Reducing Human Immunodeficiency Virus, Hepatitis B Virus and Hepatitis C Virus [Internet]. 2013. Available from: http://www.publichealthreports.org/issueopen.cfm?articleID=2975 [Accessed: December 8, 2015].

[17] Einsiede LI, Spelman T, Goeman E, Cassar O, Arundell M, Gessain A. Clinical associations of human T-lymphotropic virus type 1 infection in an indigenous Australian population. PLOS Negl Trop Dis. 2014;8(1):e2643. DOI: 10.1371/journal.pntd.0002643.

[18] WHO. Global Health Observatory (GHO) Data [Internet]. 2015. Available from: http://www.who.int/gho/en [Accessed: December 4, 2015].

[19] Roche Molecular Systems. Cobas 6800/880 Systems [Internet]. 2015. Available from: http://molecular.roche.com/instruments/Pages/cobas_6800_8800_Systems.aspx [Accessed: December 6, 2015].

[20] Hologic. Panther System [Internet]. 2015. Available from: http://www.hologic.com/products/clinical-diagnostics-and-blood-screening/instrument-systems/panther-system [Accessed: December 3, 2015].

[21] Eastlund T. Hemodilution due to blood loss and transfusion and reliability of cadaver tissue donor infectious disease testing. Cell Tissue Bank. 2000;1(Issue 2):121–127. DOI: 10.1023/A:1010120115451.

[22] Humar A, Morris M, Blumberg E, Freeman R, Preiksaitis J, Kiberd B, et al. Nucleic acid testing (NAT) of organ donors: is the 'best' test the right test? A consensus conference report. Am J Transplant. 2010;10(4):889–899. DOI: 10.1111/j.1600-6143.2009.02992.x.

[23] Gonzalez R, Torres P, Castro E, Barbolla L, Candotti D, Koppelman M, et al. Efficacy of hepatitis B virus (HBV) DNA screening and characterization of acute and occult HBV infections among blood donors from Madrid (Spain). Transfusion. 2010;50(1):221–230. DOI: 10.1111./j.1537-2995.2009.02343.x.

[24] Park JB, Kwon CH, Lee KW, Choi GS, Kim DJ, Seo JM, et al. Hepatitis B virus vaccine switch program for prevention of de novo hepatitis B virus infection in paediatric patients. Transplant Int. 2008;21(4):346–352. DOI: 10.1111/j.1432-2277.2007.00618.x.

[25] Delwart EL, Kalmin ND, Jones TS, Ladd DJ, Foley B, Tobler LH, et al. First report of human immunodeficiency virus transmission via an RNA screened blood donation. Vox Sang. 2004;86(3):171–177. DOI: 10.1111/j.0042-9007.2004.00416.x.

[26] Operskalski EA, Mosley JW, Tobler LH, Feibig EW, Nowicki MJ, Mimms LT, et al. Transfusion-transmitted viruses study. Retrovirus epidemiology donor study. HCV viral load in anti-HCV reactive donors and infectivity in their recipients. Transfusion. 2003;43(10):1433–1441. DOI: 10.1046/j.1537-2995.2003.00475.x.

[27] The CST/CNTRP increased risk donor working group. Guidance on the use of increased risk donors for organ transplantation. Transplantation. 2014;00(00):00. DOI: 10.1097/TP.0000000000000251.

[28] Chung RT, Feng S, Delmonico FL. Approach to the management of allograft recipients following the detection of hepatitis B virus in the prospective organ donor.. Am J Transplant. 2001;1(2):185/191. DOI: 10.1034/ j.1600-6143.2001.10214.x.

[29] Chazouilleres O, Mamish D, Kim M, Carey K, Farrell L, Roberts JP, et al. "Occult" hepatitis B virus as source of infection in liver transplant recipients. Lancet. 1994;343(8890):142–146. DOI: 10.1016/S0140-6736(94)90934-2

[30] Uemoto S, Sugiyama K, Marusawa H, Inomata Y, Asonuma K, Egawa H, et al. Transmission of hepatitis B virus from hepatitis B core antibody-positive donors in living related liver transplants. Transplantation. 1998;65(4):494–499. DOI: 10.1097/00007890-199802270-00007.

[31] Cholongitas E, Papatheodoridis GV, Burroughs AK. Liver grafts from anti-hepatitis B core positive donors: a systematic review. J Hepatol. 2010;52(2):272–279. DOI: 10.1111/j.1477-2574.2011.00399.x.

[32] Ouseph R, Eng M, Ravindra K, Brock GN, Buell JF, Marvin MR. Review of the use of hepatitis B core antibody-positive donors. Transplant Rev (Orlando). 2010;24(4):167–171. DOI: 10.1016/j.trre.2010.05.001.

[33] Raimondo G, Allain J, Brunetto MR, Buendia MA, Chen DS, Colombo M, et al. Statements from the Taormina expert meeting on occult hepatitis B virus infection. J Hepatol. 2008;49(4):652–657. DOI: 10.1016/j.jhep.2008.07.014.

[34] Allain JP. Occult hepatitis B virus infection: implications in transfusion. Vox Sang. 2004;86(2):83–91. DOI: 10.1111/j.0042-9007.2004.00406.x.

[35] Fang Y, Shang QL, Liu JY, Li D, Xu WZ, Teng X, et al. Prevalence of occult hepatitis B virus infection among hepatopathy patients and healthy people in China. J Infect. 2009;58(8):383–388. DOI: 10.1016/j.jinf.2009.02.013.

[36] Kim SM, Lee KS, Park CJ, Lee JY, Kim KH, Park JI, et al. Prevalence of occult HBV infection among subjects with normal serum ALT levels in Korea. J Infect. 2007;54(2): 185–191. DOI: http://dx.doi:org/10.1016/j.jinf.2006.02.002.

[37] Levrero M, Pollicino T, Petersen J, Belloni L, Raimondo G, Dandri M. Control of cccDNA function in hepatitis B virus infection. J Hepatol. 2009;51(3):581–592. DOI: 10.1016/j.jhep.2009.05.022.

[38] Zoulim F. New insight on hepatitis B virus persistence from the study of intrahepatic viral cccDNA. J Hepatol. 2005;42(3):302–308. DOI: http://dx.doi.org/10.1016/j.jhep.2004.12.015.

[39] Ramia S, Mokhbat J, Ramlawi F, El-Zaatari M. Occult hepatitis B virus infection in HIV infected Lebanese patients with isolated antibodies to hepatitis B core antigen. Int J STD AIDS. 2008;19(3):197–199. DOI: 10.1258/ijsa.2007.007200.

[40] Tseliou P, Spiliotakara A, Dimitracopoulos GO, Christofidou M. Detection of hepatitis B virus DNA in blood units with anti-HBc as the only positive serological marker. Haematologia (Budap). 2000;30(3):159–165. DOI: 10.1163/156855900300109152.

[41] Mei SD, Yatsuhashi H, Parquet MC, Hamada R, Fujino T, Matsumoto T, et al. Detection of HBV RNA in peripheral blood mononuclear cells in patients with and without HBsAg by reverse transcription polymerase chain reaction. Hepatol Res. 2000;18(1):19–28. DOI: 10.1016/S1386-6346(99)00081-9.

[42] Zaghloul H, El-Sherbiny W. Detection of occult hepatitis C and hepatitis B virus infections from peripheral blood mononuclear cells. Immunol Invest. 2010;39(3):284–291. DOI: 10.3109/08820131003605820.

[43] Raimondo G, Caccamo G, Filomia R, Pollicino T. Occult hepatitis B infection. Semin Immunopathol. 2013;35(1):39–52. DOI: 10.1007/s00281-012-0327-7.

[44] Cheung CK, Lo CM, Man K, Lau GK. Occult hepatitis B virus infection of donor and recipient origin after liver transplantation despite nucleoside analogue prophylaxis. Liver Transplant. 2010;16(11):1314–1323. DOI: 10.1002/lt.22169.

[45] MacConmara MP, Vachharajani N, Ellen JR, Anderson CD, Lowell JA, Shenoy S, et al. Utilization of hepatitis B core antibody-positive donor liver grafts. HPB (Oxford). 2012;14(1):42–48. DOI: 10.1111/j.1477-2574.2011.00399.x.

[46] Terrault N, Roche B, Samuel D. Management of the hepatitis B virus in the liver transplantation setting: a European and an American perspective. Liver Transpl. 2005;11(7):716–732. DOI: 10.1002/lt.20492.

[47] Suehiro T, Shimada M, Kishikawa K, Shimura T, Soejima Y, Yoshizumi T, et al. Prevention of hepatitis B virus infection from hepatitis B core antibody-positive donor graft using hepatitis B immune globulin and lamivudine in living donor liver transplantation. Liver Int. 2005;25(6):1169–1174. DOI: 10.1111/j.1478-3231.2005.01165.x.

[48] Candotti D, Allain J-P. Transfusion-transmitted hepatitis B infection. J Hepatol. 2009;51(4):798–809. DOI: 10.1016/j.jhep.2009.05.020.

[49] Saab S, Waterman B, Chi AC, Tong MJ. Comparison of different immunoprophylaxis regimens after liver transplantation with hepatitis B core antibody-positive donors: a systematic review. Liver Transpl. 2010;16(3):300–307. DOI: 10.1002/lt.21998.

[50] Northup PG, Argo CK, Nguyen DT, McBride MA, Kumer SC, Schmitt TM, et al. Liver allografts from hepatitis C positive donors can offer good outcomes in hepatitis C positive recipients: a US National Transplant Registry analysis. Transplant Int. 2010;23(10):1038-1044. DOI: 10.1111/j.1432-2277.2010.01092.x.

[51] Kasprzyk T, Kwiatkowski A, Wszola M, Ostrowski K, Danielewicz R, Domagala P, et al. Long-term results of kidney transplantation from HCV-positive donors. Transplant Proc. 2007;39(9):2701–2703. DOI: http://dx.doi.org/10.1016/j.transproceed.2007.09.021.

[52] Fabrizi F, Messa P, Martin P. Current status of renal transplantation from HCV-positive donors. Int J Artif Organs. 2009;32(5):251–261.

[53] Prieto M, Berenguer M, Rayon JM, Cordova J, Arguello L, Carrasco D, et al. High incidence of allograft cirrhosis in hepatitis C virus genotype 1b infection following transplantation: relationship with rejection episodes. Hepatology. 1999;29(1):250–256. DOI: 10.1002/hep.510290122.

[54] Saab S, Ghobrial RM, Ibrahim AB, Kunder G, Durazo F, Han S, et al. Hepatitis C positive grafts may be used in orthotopic liver transplantation: a matched analysis. Am J Transplant. 2003;3(9):1167–1172. DOI: 10.1034/j.1600-6143.2003.00189.x.

[55] Khapra AP, Agarwal K, Fiel MI, Kontorinis N, Hossain S, Emre S, et al. Impact of donor age on survival and fibrosis progression in patients with hepatitis C undergoing liver transplantation using HCV + allografts. Liver Transpl. 2006;12(10):1496–1503. DOI: 10.1002/lt.20849.

[56] Jacobson IM, McHutchinson JG, Dusheiko G, Di Bisceglie AM, Reddy KR, Bzowej NH, et al. Telaprevir for previously untreated chronic hepatitis C virus infection. N Eng J Med. 2011;364(25):2405–2416. DOI: 10.1056/NEJMoa1012912.

[57] Poordad F, McCone JJ, Bacon BR, Bruno S, Manns MP, Sulkowski MS, et al. Boceprevir for untreated chronic HCV genotype 1 infection. N Eng J Med. 2011;364(13):1195–1206. DOI: 10.1056/NEJMoa1010494.

[58] OPTN. Organ Procurement and Transplantation Network [Internet]. 2016 . Available from: http://optn.transplant.hrsa.gov/ [Accessed: January 1, 2016].

[59] Sela N, Croome KP, Chando N, Marotta P, Wall W, Hernandez-Alejandro R. Changing donor characteristics in liver transplantation over the last 10 years in Canada. Liver Transpl. 2013;19(11):1236–1244. DOI: 10.1002/lt.23718.

[60] Kamath PS, Kim WR. The model for end-stage liver disease (MELD). Hepatology. 2007;45(3):797–805. DOI: 10.1002/hep.21563.

[61] UNOS. PELD/MELD Calculator [Internet]. 2015. Available from: https://www.unos.org/wp-content/uploads/unos/MELD_PELD_Calculator_Documentation.pdf [Accessed: December 12, 2015].

[62] Feng S, Goodrich NP, Bragg-Gresham JL, Dykstra DM, Punch JD, DebRoy MA, et al. Characteristics associated with liver graft failure: the concept of a donor risk index. Am J Transplant. 2006;6(4):783–790. DOI: 10.1111/j.1600-6143.2006.01242.x.

[63] Blok JJ, Braat AE, Adam R, Burroughs AK, Putter H, Kooreman NG, et al. Validation of the donor risk index in orthotopic liver transplantation within the Eurotransplant Region. Liver Transpl. 2012;18(1):113–120. DOI: 10.1002/lt.22447.

[64] Maluf DG, Edwards EB, Stravitz RT, Kauffman HM. Impact of the donor risk index on the outcome of hepatitis C virus-positive liver transplant recipients. Liver Transpl. 2009;15(6):592–599. DOI: 10.1002/lt.21699.

[65] Rosemberg LH, Guillen JG, Hranjec T, Stokes JB, Brayman KL, Kumer SC, et al. Donor risk index predicts graft failure reliably but not post-transplant infections. Surg Infect. 2014;15(2):94–98. DOI: 10.1089/sur.2013.035.

[66] Schaubela DE, Guidingerb MK, Bigginsd SW, Kalbfleischa JD, Pomfrete EA, Sharmaf P, et al. Survival benefit-based deceased-donor liver allocation. Am J Transplant. 2009;9(4 Pt 2):970–981. DOI: 10.1111/j.1600-6143.2009.02571.x.

[67] UK Government. Guidance on the Microbiological Safety of human Organs, Tissues and Cells used in Transplantation [Internet]. 2011. Available from: https://www.gov.uk/government/uploads/system/uploads/attachment_data/file/215959/dh_130515.pdf [Accessed: December 3, 2015].

[68] EDQM. Guide to the Quality and Safety of Organs for Transplantation [Internet]. 2013. Available from: https://www.edqm.eu/medias/fichiers/leaflet_on_organ_transplantation_guide_5th_edition.pdf [Accessed: December 5, 2015].

[69] Baleriola C, Webster AC, Rawlinson WD. Characterization and risk of bloodborne virus transmission in organ transplantation: what are the priorities? Future Virol. 2014;9(12): 1049–1060. DOI: 10.2217/FVL.14.94.

[70] Grossi PA, Fishman JA, AST Infectious Disease Community of Practice. Donor-derived infections in solid organ transplant recipients. Am J Transplant. 2009;9(Suppl 4):S19–S26. DOI: 10.1111/j.1600-6143.2009.02889.x.

[71] Fischer SA, Avery RK, AST infectious disease community of practice. Screening of donor and recipient prior to solid organ transplantation. Am J Transplant. 2009;9(Suppl 4):S7–S18. DOI: 10.1111/j.1600-6143.2009.02888.x.

[72] Scandia Transplant. Guidelines for the Prevention of Transmission of Infectious Diseases from Organ Donors to Recipients [Internet]. 2015. Available from: http://www.scandiatransplant.org/organ-allocation/ScandtxInfGuidelines2015incEbola_5.pdf [Accessed: November 15, 2015].

[73] Europa EC. The Eustite Project [Internet]. 2013. Available from: http://ec.europa.eu/chafea/documents/health/conference_27-28_06_2013/EUSTITE [Accessed: November 6, 2015].

[74] Notify Project. Notify Library [Internet]. 2013. Available from: http://www.notifylibrary.org [Accessed: December 12, 2015].

[75] OPTN. Ad Hoc Disease Transmission Advisory Committee (DTAC) [Internet]. 2015. Available from: http://optn.transplant.hrsa.gov/converge/members/committeesDetail.asp?ID=95 [Accessed: December 23, 2015].

[76] ANZOD & ANZDATA. ANZDATA [Internet]. 2015. Available from: http://anzdata.org.au/ [Accessed: December 20, 2015].

Section 3

Liver Transplantation

Chapter 7

Split Liver Transplantation

Ahmed Zidan and Wei-Chen Lee

Additional information is available at the end of the chapter

http://dx.doi.org/10.5772/62450

Abstract

Liver transplantation is the most effective treatment for the patients with acute liver failure or end-stage liver diseases. Liver transplantation is also indicated for patients with hepatocellular carcinoma to yield a best result if the tumor/tumors meet Milan criteria, University of California San Francisco(UCSF) criteria, or up-to-seven criteria. It is no doubt that more and more people need liver transplantation to save their lives. However, liver donation is always short to match the demand of liver transplantation. Therefore, how to expand the donor pool to increase the opportunities of liver transplantation is paramount. Splitting liver is one of the ways to expand the donor pool and offers an additional chance of liver transplantation. At the beginning of split liver transplantation (SLT), the liver was split and transplanted to an adult and a child. Now, the liver can be split into full right and left lobes and transplanted to two adults. When split liver transplantation is to be performed, there are many considerations that should be clarified. With the improvement of surgical skill, the outcomes of split liver transplantation are similar to that of deceased whole liver transplantation. It is worth to promote the policy of split liver transplantation.

Keywords: split liver transplantation, deceased liver transplantation, liver splitting, Lee's formula, donor pool increase

1. Introduction

Liver transplantation is considered to be the most effective treatment for acute and chronic liver failure patients as well as the only definitive treatment for hepatocellular carcinoma(HCC). With increased demand for liver transplantation, a big gap and discrepancy have been developed between the demand for liver transplantation and donation of liver. This increases the waiting time in the waiting list, which carries the hazards of progression of the disease to be out of curability spectrum. This encourages those who work in the transplantation field to find new ways to increase the donor pool. Split liver transplant (SLT) is one of these methods for expanding the donor pool and giving another chance for transplant candidates, in which either one cadaver liver is split between one pediatric patient and an adult or between two adults.

SLT is considered to be a magic bullet, which gives the possibility to duplicate the numbers of transplanted patients using the same donor pool capacity.

2. Historical background

The concept of partial liver allograft was first advocated by Smith [1] in 1969 who proposed left lateral segments suitable for children. In 1988, Pichlmayr was the first surgeon who split the liver into two grafts, one for child (left lateral segment) and the other for adult (extended right trisegments) [2]. In 1989, Bismuth et al. [3] reported another case of split liver transplant for two patients with acute liver failure, and in 1990, Emond from the University of Chicago reported the first series of nine SLT procedures in 18 pediatric and adult recipients [4]. Although splitting of the liver between pediatric and adult patients has a good impact on the donor pool expansion for pediatric patients, it has little impact on the donor pool for adult patients, as only one adult patient will benefit from the splitting of the liver. Because most of the patients in the waiting list for liver transplantation are adults, this encouraged Bismuth and Paul Brousse hospital group in 1996 to publish a series of 26 adult patients receiving full left and right lobe split grafts [5]. In 1997, the first split liver transplant in Asia was performed in Taiwan, followed by the other Asian countries which need to augment the cadaveric donor pool, which is already low due to some cultural reasons [6].

Although the early experience of SLT was not encouraging as the results revealed higher rate of complications and graft loss, a European workshop held in 1993, analyzing data from different centers, published its findings in 1995, which reported 20% of the graft was lost due to complications including hepatic artery thrombosis (11%), portal vein thrombosis (4%), and biliary complications (19%). This report also revealed that the patient and graft survival were correlated to medical acuity at the time of transplantation. In transplantation due to acute emergency like fulminant liver failure, the 6-month pediatric graft and recipient survival were 61%, and adult recipient and graft survival were 67 and 55%, respectively. Contrarily, in elective liver transplantation, adult recipient and graft survival were 80 and 72%, respectively, and pediatric patient and graft survival were 89 and 80%, respectively [7].

So, it was clear that there was a learning curve to this technique, which contributed to higher incidence of complications and graft loss [8]. Another important factor was the recipient selection; high-risk recipient was unable to tolerate the technical complications, which contributed to the suboptimal results [9]. With the improvement in recipient selection and refinement of the surgical technique, significant improvement of the outcome was noticed. Azoulay et al. [5] described 27 split grafts with 1-year recipient and graft survival of 79 and 78%, respectively.

Our results from Chang Gung Memorial Hospital at Linkou were published in 2013 for 21 split liver transplants for 42 patients, which showed that 5-year recipient survival for right and left hemiliver were 70.1 and 61.5%, respectively, with no reported vascular complications of either hepatic artery or portal vein thrombosis [10].

3. Donor criteria

Donor selection is one of the crucial determinants in the splitting liver transplant procedure. The key is to be able to predict the potential graft function and the graft weight. Regarding graft function and quality, donors less than 50 years are defined to be suitable for splitting. Minimal to mild fatty liver (10–20%) may be suitable, if the cold ischemia time is maintained as short as possible. Donors with slightly elevated liver enzymes (less than three times the normal range), with intensive care stay of less than 7 days, and without significant vasopressor use with absent or short arrest time could be considered as potential donors [10–14]. Short warm and cold ischemia time is a determinant factor, as early graft dysfunction is usually associated with prolonged warm and cold ischemia time (**Table 1**).

Determinant factors in graft function and quality in SLT
1. Donor age <50 years
2. Steatosis (minimal to mild)
3. ICU stay <7 days
4. Vasopressor support
5. Arrest and its duration
6. Warm and cold ischemia time
7. Liver enzymes less than three times the normal range

Table 1. Determinant factors in graft function and quality.

The gross picture and the intraoperative assessments play a major rule in splitting decision, although the liver biopsy and microscopic examination are the ideal determinants [11]. There is no big difference regarding the graft quality between right and left hemiliver splitting (two adult recipients) and extended right graft and left latter segment (one adult and one pediatric recipient), except that in the former it is safer to have a better graft quality in the form of less steatosis, shorter warm and cold ischemia time, and younger donor age.

3.1. Determination of graft weight

Regarding graft weight, some centers correlate the graft weight with the donor weight, as liver weight constitutes about 2–2.7% of body weight. Donor weight gives an idea about the whole graft weight, but cannot predict each hemiliver graft weight. Furthermore, application of donor weight in clinical practice is limited as obese donors are considered to be a risk factor for splitting liver transplantation as significant steatosis increases the possibility of primary graft dysfunction.

Some donors may have computed tomography or MRI scan of the abdomen, especially if the cause of death is trauma, and the graft volume of each split liver graft can be obtained easily from these scans. However, not every donor has computed tomography or MRI scan of the abdomen. For splitting the liver, transporting a potential organ donor from an intensive care unit to a CT facility to enable measurements of the sizes of hemilivers is controversial. In addition, the relevant technical expertise required to measure liver volumes by CT may not be readily available.

We introduced a simple formula and procedure to determine each split graft weight using only bedside ultrasound scans to measure right and left portal vein diameters. This formula, known as Lee's formula, consisted of standard liver volume (SLV) and portal vein diameters. The standard liver volume (SLV) is calculated by Urata's formula to determine the whole liver weight. The weight of each split liver graft is determined as follows: right hemiliver volume (RHLV) = SLV × $[R^2/(R^2 + L^2)]$ and left hemiliver volume (LHLV) = SLV × $[L^2/(R^2 + L^2)]$, where (R) is maximal right portal vein diameter and (L) is maximal left portal vein diameter [15]. Lee's formula can be used in two adult split liver transplants to determine the weight of each graft and subsequently the graft-to-recipient weight ratio (GRWR).

4. Recipient criteria

As we mentioned earlier, improper recipient selection was one of the causes of the unfavorable outcome of split liver transplant at the beginning of the procedure development. Two important determinants in the recipient may act as keys for favorable outcome: the first is the patient's general condition and acuity of the disease; the second is the correlation between the graft weight and recipient weight. Regarding patient's condition and acuity of the disease, the early experience of considering high-risk patient with high MELD score or acute liver failure for SLT was associated with low outcome with high incidence of graft dysfunction, graft loss, and re-transplantation [16]. Generally, critically ill patients with high MELD score, with severe portal hypertension, are not good candidates for split liver transplantation, which should be preserved for low-risk patients with low MELD score. Also, urgency is considered to be a determinant factor for outcome in SLT, as patient survival in urgent liver transplant is lower than that for elective causes [7, 17]. Nevertheless, in countries with low cadaveric liver donor pool, as most of Asian countries, SLT is the only treatment in such an acute fatal condition and must be offered to high urgent patients [10, 18].

The other important key for favorable outcome after SLT is the correlation between graft weight and recipient weight (GRWR). In extended right/left lateral split, the effect of this factor is not prominent, as left lateral segment is suitable for all children with acute or chronic liver disease with good patient and graft survival. In right/left hemiliver split, GRWR plays an important rule, especially in patients who will receive left hemiliver. As mentioned earlier, graft weight can be roughly estimated using Lee's formula; this helps in the determination of the ideal recipient weight.

Most of the results published using GRWR <0.8% show inferior outcome than those with ≥0.8%, in spite of the results of living donor liver transplantation (LDLT) with GRWR < 0.8% being accepted. There are more risk factors and stresses on the SLT graft more than LDLT graft, as in the former, graft from deceased donor may suffer from hemodynamic instability of the donor and prolonged cold ischemia time, which have more injurious effect on the split graft [19]. Although most of the centers consider GRWR > 0.8% is the cutoff of safe SLT, our published data show that GRWR > 1% is the most optimal cutoff point to predict early graft and patient survival [10, 13].

5. Surgical techniques

5.1. Left lateral/extended right split

In the left lateral split, the liver is split into left lateral segment graft and extended right liver graft; left lateral segment is allocated to a child and the extended right graft is allocated to an adult recipient. The ex situ split technique was performed by Pichlmayr et al. [2]. Rogiers et al. introduced a technical modification in 1995, named in situ split technique in which split procedure is performed during procurement before aortic cross-clamp [20, 21].

5.1.1. Ex situ split

After retrieval and perfusion, the liver is split on back table while maintained in preservation solution at a temperature below 4°C. At first, the vascular inflow (portal vein and hepatic artery), outflow (hepatic veins), and biliary structures are assessed.

- Dissection of the left hepatic artery (LHA) from bifurcation of the hepatic artery proper is performed with the identification of segment IV artery, which may arise from right or left hepatic arteries; preservation of segment IV artery is important to maintain perfusion to segment IV and to avoid segment IV ischemia and necrosis. If segment IV artery arises from right hepatic artery, left hepatic artery could be cut at the bifurcation of hepatic artery proper (HAP) safely. If segment IV artery arises from left hepatic artery, some prefer to cut LHA distal to the origin of segment IV artery and others cut LHA at the bifurcation, with the reconstruction of segment IV artery later in the recipient. Actually, it depends on the experience of the transplant team and size matching with the child's recipient artery.
- Regarding biliary system, some prefer to do cholangiogram to identify segment IV duct and caudate ducts, but using a metallic probe only looks to be enough in left lateral split. Role of intraoperative cholangiogram may be more effective in right and left splits, which will be discussed later. Dissection of left hepatic duct should be avoided to maintain the periductal vascular plexus and avoid any injury to the caudate bile ducts. Then, the bile duct drain in the left lateral segment is cut at the level of hilar plate behind the junction of the transverse and longitudinal part of left portal vein, just proximal to segment IV duct, and its orifice in extended right graft is sutured.

- Then, left portal vein (LPV) is dissected from its bifurcation, and tributaries from the caudate and segment IV are isolated and ligated, Then, LPV is cut at the bifurcation, and its orifice in the main portal vein is sutured.
- After completing inflow and biliary duct division, liver parenchymal dissection is started 1 cm to the right of falciform ligament, using Kelly's clamp-crushing technique, with clipping or suturing any vascular structure.
- Left hepatic vein (LHV) is isolated during liver parenchymal transection, hanged with vascular loop, and then LHV is cut, and its orifice at the confluence of left and middle hepatic veins (LHV/MHV) is sutured.

Then, flushing of both grafts with preservation solution is done through portal veins; left lateral segment graft is prepared for implantation in a pediatric recipient, based on left hepatic vein, left portal vein, left hepatic artery, and left bile duct. Extended right graft is prepared for implantation in an adult recipient, based on IVC containing right and middle hepatic veins, main portal vein, main hepatic artery with aortic patch, and main bile duct. The main disadvantages of ex situ split is failure of assessment of segment IV perfusion and viability, prolonged cold ischemia time, and repeated rewarming during liver parenchymal transection, which may affect the graft survival (**Table 1**).

5.1.2. In situ split

Splitting is performed during organ retrieval before aortic cross-clamping.

- The liver parenchyma is divided at first 1 cm to the right of falciform ligament; transection of liver parenchyma is performed using clamp-crushing technique or cavitron ultrasonic surgical aspirator (CUSA), with the identification and ligation or clipping of vascular and biliary structures at the transection line.
- Segment IV perfusion is assessed, and hemostasis is performed on both cut surfaces of the liver. Once parenchymal transection is completed, retrieval procedure is continued as usual, and perfusion of the preservation solution is started.
- On back table, vascular and biliary structures are isolated as in ex situ technique.

In situ split has several advantages on ex situ split, as it decreases the total cold ischemia time by 1–2 h and reduces the possibility of rewarming in the back table split, which may have negative impact on the outcome. Also, the two liver grafts can be assessed for significant ischemia at the cut surface and margin, especially in segment IV. During parenchymal transection, hemostasis and vascular control may help in decreasing bleeding from cut surface after reperfusion.

On the other hand, there are some disadvantages of in situ split technique, as increased retrieval time may not only affect the liver itself but also the other retrieved organ, which makes this technique not a suitable option in hemodynamically unstable donors (**Table 2**).

Advantages	Disadvantages
1. Assessment of perfusion and viability of segment IV	1. Increase retrieval time
2. Better hemostasis on both liver cut surfaces	2. Not suitable in hemodynamic unstable donor
3. Decrease cold ischemia time	

Table 2. Advantages and disadvantages of in situ split over ex situ split technique.

5.2. Right/left split

There is no standard splitting technique in left/right split. Each center has its own technique with many modifications. We will try to present some of these modifications and techniques with our comments on each.

5.2.1. Ex situ split

- After retrieval of the whole liver with IVC, cholangiogram is performed on back table to detect any biliary anomaly.
- Then, transection line is identified in the midplane along Cantlie's line. Liver parenchyma transection is performed as described earlier with clamp-crushing technique and identification of large tributaries of veins from segment V and VIII. Caudate lobe is preserved to left hemiliver, in spite of some centers excising it completely from the graft.
- Many centers, including our center, preserve the middle hepatic vein (MHV) in the left hemiliver to guarantee good drainage of segment IV. If there is sizable segment V or VIII veins, they should be reconstructed either using vascular allograft, portal vein of the explanted liver, or synthetic (Gortex) vascular graft (**Figure 1**). Some authors describe MHV split in which the transection line passes through MHV, which is reconstructed by vascular patch on each side.
- The stump of LHV/MHV is hanged and cut near IVC, and its opening is closed.
- IVC is better to be maintained in the right hemiliver to allow better outflow through retrohepatic veins. Some centers describe IVC split technique in which IVC is split into two halves longitudinally, one with each graft, and then reconstructed using vascular patch on each side. Both MHV split and IVC split carry the hazards of suture leakage and bleeding due to the long reconstruction line.
- Hepatic artery and portal vein are dissected, and it is better to preserve the main branches (main portal vein and main hepatic artery) with the left hemiliver graft, as the size of its vessels is relatively smaller.
- Segment IV artery is isolated, and if it arises from RHA, RHA is cut distal to the origin of segment IV artery.
- The main bile duct is preserved with the right hemiliver, as the left hepatic duct has longer extrahepatic course, and possibility to have more than one duct is more frequent at the right side.

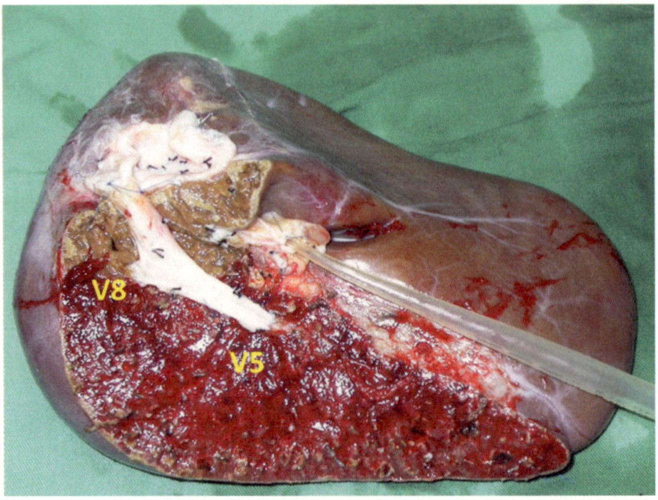

Figure 1. Reconstruction of the tributaries of segments V and VIII with a vein graft. Because the middle hepatic vein was preserved in left hemiliver graft, the tributaries of segments V and VIII were severed. When the diameters of tributaries were more than 5 mm, the tributaries were reconstructed with a vein graft into IVC.

Now we have two grafts: right hemiliver based on IVC, common bile duct, right hepatic artery (RHA), and right portal vein (RPV); and left hemiliver based on MHV/LHV confluence, main portal vein (MPV), hepatic artery proper (HAP), and left hepatic duct (LHD) (**Figure 2**).

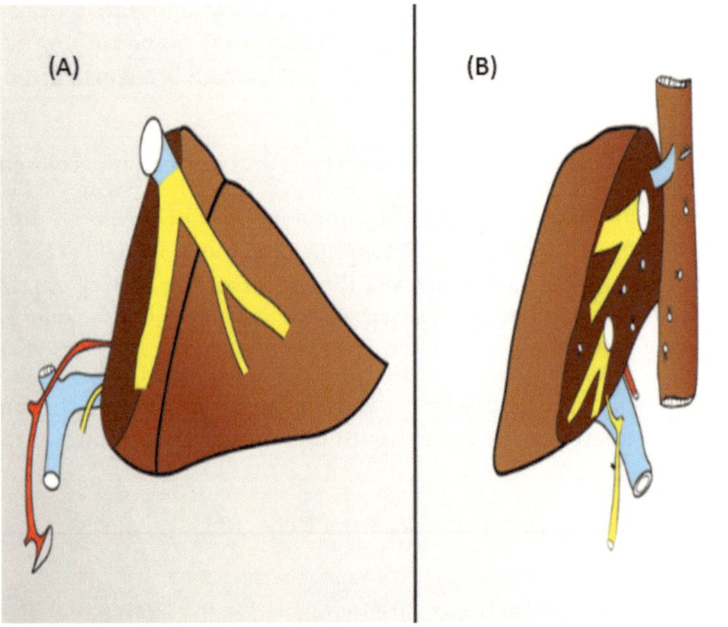

Figure 2. Diagram showing (**A**) left and (**B**) right split grafts with attached inflow and outflow structures.

5.2.1.1. Implantation of the right hemiliver

Vascular graft from reconstructed segments V and VIII branches can be anastomosed directly in donor IVC through a separate cavotomy. During implantation of the graft, IVC can be implanted by caval interposition technique, conventional piggyback (end-to-side) technique, or modified piggyback technique (side-to-side). RPV of the graft is anastomosed to RPV or MPV of the recipient; RHA of the graft is anastomosed to RHA of the recipient; and biliary reconstruction is achieved by duct-to-duct or Roux-en-Y technique (**Figure 3**).

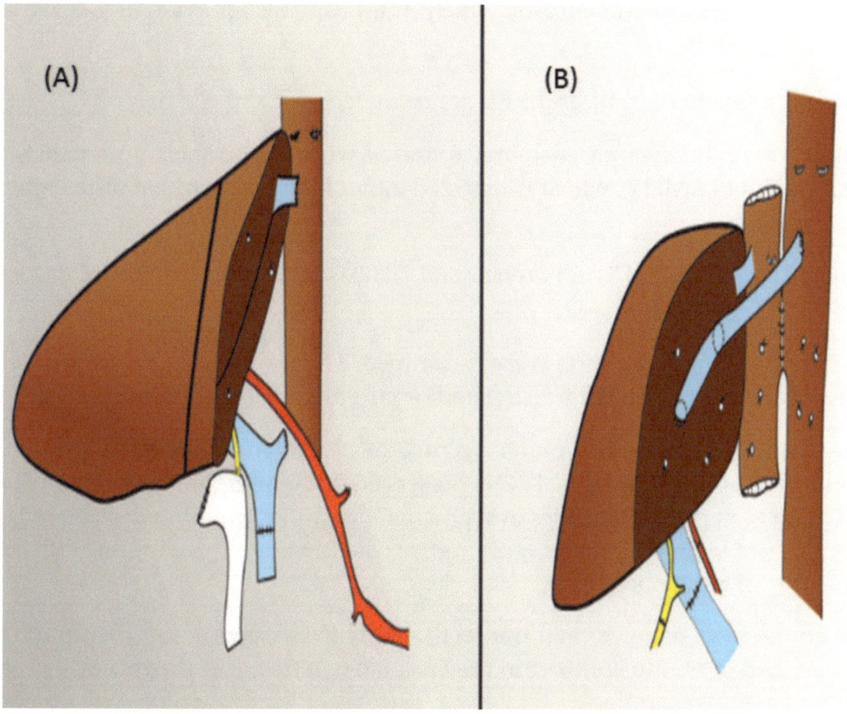

Figure 3. Diagram showing implantation of (**A**) left and (**B**) right hemiliver (left hemiliver was implanted by left at right technique).

5.2.1.2. Implantation of the left hemiliver

The left lobe could be implanted as usual in the left upper abdomen, but we have a new modification, published and innovated by Chang Gung Memorial hospital—Linkou, called left at right implantation [22], in which the left lobe is placed in the right upper quadrant to facilitate inflow and outflow reconstruction and avoid any compression of IVC or kinking of hepatic vein by the growing liver graft. Donor MHV/LHV confluence is anastomosed by separate cavotomy in recipient IVC; donor MPV is anastomosed to recipient RPV or MPV according to size-matching; donor HAP is anastomosed to recipient HAP; and biliary reconstruction is achieved by duct-to-duct or Roux-en-Y technique (**Figure 3**).

5.2.2. In situ split

In this technique, split is performed during retrieval procedure before aortic cross-clamping.

- First of all, careful examination of the liver with visual assessment of liver quality and size is performed.
- Then, intraoperative cholangiogram is performed to detect biliary anatomy and any anomaly in biliary system.
- The liver is mobilized from its attachment to diaphragm and retroperitoneum, but without interruption of the short hepatic veins which drain directly into IVC to keep reasonable outflow of the right lobe.
- Porta hepatis is examined. RHA and RPV are encircled.
- Then, transection of the liver parenchyma is started with CUSA or clamp-crushing technique, just to the right of MHV, which is detected either by intraoperative ultrasound or just through Cantlie's line.
- After complete transection of liver parenchyma, LHD is divided in the hilar plate just before the carina.
- Then, the infradiaphragmatic aorta is cross-clamped. The visceral organs are perfused with cooled preservation solution. All the donated organs are retrieved subsequently.
- Finally, two hemiliver grafts are separated completely by diving RHA, RPV, and confluence of MHV and LHV at the back table. IVC is preserved with the right hemiliver graft most of the time. The large venous tributaries of segments V and VIII are reconstructed to IVC with venous grafts. The two liver grafts now are kept in cold preservative solution, with irrigation of the grafts through the portal vein.

We prefer to do the liver parenchymal transection only in the donor and keep porta hepatis division as described in ex situ splitting in the back table to decrease the retrieval time.

6. SLT outcomes

On reviewing graft and patient survival of SLT, it is apparent that there is prominent improvement across the time since 1988 till now; this improvement can be attributed to the learning curve and the improvement of patient selection as we mentioned before.

6.1. Pediatric recipient

Data from U.S. Scientific Registry of Transplant Recipient and Organ Procurement showed that recipient survival after year 2000 ranged between 76 and 100%, while Broering reported that recipient survival before 2000 was 50–92%. The graft survival is also improved after 2000 from 50–80% to 66–100%. The incidence of complications is 32%, which is comparable with

LDLT. This improvement in outcome is associated with better surgical technique and better recipient selection [11, 12].

6.2. Adult recipient

Similar to pediatric data, there is significant improvement regarding adult recipient, either in extended right liver graft or right and left liver grafts. Recipient survival ranges from 79 to 100%, and graft survival is 69–100% after year 2000, with 26% of complications [12, 23, 24]. Our published data showed that 3-month and 1-year survival rates were 76.2 and 71.4% for SLT and 89.3 and 79.9% for living donor recipients, respectively. This result shows no significant difference in patient outcomes between SLT and LDLT [9, 10].

7. Ethical considerations

Since the introduction of SLT, there are many ethical considerations, and debates have evolved. As SLT is introduced as one of the solutions of the gap between liver demands and liver donor pool, SLT helps in decreasing the waiting list time, as about 15–20% of the deceased livers are eligible to be split from medical point of view. This increases the number of recipients to receive liver transplantation. On the other hand, it is clear that the outcomes of SLT are relatively lower than whole liver transplant, with relative increase in morbidities and complications. So, the ethical debate is to increase the number of patients receiving LT, decrease the waiting time list, and decrease dropouts from waiting list by splitting the liver, or increase the patient survival, outcomes, and decrease the number of patients receiving LT without splitting the liver.

Although the importance of this question is fading down with time, with improvement in the splitting techniques and outcome, still there are different morbidities and complications between whole organ transplant and SLT. When the donated liver graft is suitable for splitting, the primary recipient who is on the top of waiting list should be asked for his consent and agreement to receive a liver splitting graft and sharing with another recipient. Transplant coordinator and team are obliged to supply the recipient with full data about the possible morbidities of split liver graft and the benefits regarding sharing this organ with another recipient. However, the patients have the full right to accept the splitting or receiving the whole organ depending on the medical data given by the transplant coordinator. If the primary recipient has not consented to split a liver which is ideally suited for splitting, the liver should be offered to the next person on the list who consents to splitting the liver. But, the primary recipient would maintain their position based on the MELD score and wait for the next opportunity of whole liver transplantation [25].

Another important ethical issue is that all parties involved in the transplantation process must understand a stewardship rather than an ownership of an organ by a potential recipient, transplant center/program, or transplant surgeon. To maximize the opportunities of liver transplantation, high-quality organs such as young deceased donors with low BMI and related stable hemodynamics are used for splitting, and the suboptimal organs are kept as whole liver grafts.

Again, this confliction between maximizing the number of transplanted recipients and maximizing the recipient survival could fade down with the improvement of the outcome of SLT, which is based primarily on choosing the right donor livers for splitting and improvement in split techniques.

Author details

Ahmed Zidan and Wei-Chen Lee*

*Address all correspondence to: weichen@cgmh.org.tw

Division of Liver and Transplantation Surgery, Departments of General Surgery, Chang Gung Memorial Hospital at Linkou, Chang Gung University College of Medicine, Taoyuan, Taiwan

References

[1] Smith B. Segmental liver transplantation from a living donor. J Pediatr Surg 1969;4:126–132.

[2] Pichlmayr R, Ringe B, Gubernatis G, Hauss J, Bunzendahl H. Transplantation of a donor liver to 2 recipients (splitting transplantation)--a new method in the further development of segmental liver transplantation. Langenbecks Arch Chir 1988;373:127–130.

[3] Bismuth H, Morino M, Castaing D, Gillon MC, Descorps Declere A, Saliba F, et al. Emergency orthotopic liver transplantation in two patients using one donor liver. Br J Surg 1989;76:722–724.

[4] Emond JC, Whitington PF, Thistlethwaite JR, Cherqui D, Alonso EA, Woodle IS, et al. Transplantation of two patients with one liver. Analysis of a preliminary experience with 'split-liver' grafting. Ann Surg 1990;212:14–22.

[5] Azoulay D, Astarcioglu I, Bismuth H, Castaing D, Majno P, Adam R, et al. Split-liver transplantation. The Paul Brousse policy. Ann Surg 1996;224:737–746; discussion 746–738.

[6] de Villa VH, Chen CL, Chen YS, Wang CC, Tan KC, Suh KS, et al. Split liver transplantation in Asia. Transplant Proc 2001;33:1502–1503.

[7] de Ville de Goyet J. Split liver transplantation in Europe--1988 to 1993. Transplantation 1995;59:1371–1376.

[8] Schrem H, Kleine M, Lankisch TO, Kaltenborn A, Kousoulas L, Zachau L, et al. Long-term results after adult ex situ split liver transplantation since its introduction in 1987. World J Surg 2014;38:1795–1806.

[9] Lauterio A, Di Sandro S, Concone G, De Carlis R, Giacomoni A, De Carlis L. Current status and perspectives in split liver transplantation. World J Gastroenterol 2015;21:11003–11015.

[10] Lee WC, Chan KM, Chou HS, Wu TJ, Lee CF, Soong RS, et al. Feasibility of split liver transplantation for 2 adults in the model of end-stage liver disease era. Ann Surg 2013;258:306–311.

[11] Broering DC, Schulte am Esch J, Fischer L, Rogiers X. Split liver transplantation. HPB (Oxford) 2004;6:76–82.

[12] Renz JF, Yersiz H, Reichert PR, Hisatake GM, Farmer DG, Emond JC, et al. Split-liver transplantation: a review. Am J Transplant 2003;3:1323–1335.

[13] Ferla F, Lauterio A, Di Sandro S, Mangoni I, Poli C, Concone G, et al. Split-liver full-left full-right: proposal for an operative protocol. Transplant Proc 2014;46:2279–2282.

[14] Abradelo M, Sanabria R, Caso O, Alvaro E, Moreno E, Jimenez C. Split liver transplantation: where? when? how? Transplant Proc 2012;44:1513–1516.

[15] Wang F, Pan KT, Chu SY, Chan KM, Chou HS, Wu TJ, et al. Preoperative estimation of the liver graft weight in adult right lobe living donor liver transplantation using maximal portal vein diameters. Liver Transpl 2011;17:373–380.

[16] Broelsch CE, Emond JC, Whitington PF, Thistlethwaite JR, Baker AL, Lichtor JL. Application of reduced-size liver transplants as split grafts, auxiliary orthotopic grafts, and living related segmental transplants. Ann Surg 1990;212:368–375; discussion 375–367.

[17] Hashimoto K, Quintini C, Aucejo FN, Fujiki M, Diago T, Watson MJ, et al. Split liver transplantation using Hemiliver graft in the MELD era: a single center experience in the United States. Am J Transplant 2014;14:2072–2080.

[18] Maggi U, De Feo TM, Andorno E, Cillo U, De Carlis L, Colledan M, et al. Fifteen years and 382 extended right grafts from in situ split livers in a multicenter study: are these still extended criteria liver grafts? Liver Transpl 2015;21:500–511.

[19] Hill MJ, Hughes M, Jie T, Cohen M, Lake J, Payne WD, et al. Graft weight/recipient weight ratio: how well does it predict outcome after partial liver transplants? Liver Transpl 2009;15:1056–1062.

[20] Kilic M, Seu P, Stribling RJ, Ghalib R, Goss JA. In situ splitting of the cadaveric liver for two adult recipients. Transplantation 2001;72:1853–1858.

[21] Rogiers X, Malago M, Habib N, Knoefel WT, Pothmann W, Burdelski M, et al. In situ splitting of the liver in the heart-beating cadaveric organ donor for transplantation in two recipients. Transplantation 1995;59:1081–1083.

[22] Chan KM, Eldeen FZ, Lee CF, Wu TJ, Chou HS, Wu TH, et al. "Left at right" adult liver transplantation: the feasibility of heterotopic implantation of left liver graft. Am J Transplant 2012;12:1511–1518.

[23] Yersiz H, Renz JF, Farmer DG, Hisatake GM, McDiarmid SV, Busuttil RW. One hundred in situ split-liver transplantations: a single-center experience. Ann Surg 2003;238:496–505; discussion 506–497.

[24] Renz JF, Emond JC, Yersiz H, Ascher NL, Busuttil RW. Split-liver transplantation in the United States: outcomes of a national survey. Ann Surg 2004;239:172–181.

[25] Vulchev A, Roberts JP, Stock PG. Ethical issues in split versus whole liver transplantation. Am J Transplant 2004;4:1737–1740.

Chapter 8

Pediatric Liver Transplantation

Julio Cesar Wiederkehr,
Barbara de Aguiar Wiederkehr and
Henrique de Aguiar Wiederkehr

Additional information is available at the end of the chapter

http://dx.doi.org/10.5772/63477

Abstract

Liver transplantation (LT) has become standard management of pediatric liver diseases that lead to acute liver failure or can progress to end-stage liver disease (ESLD). Indications for LT in pediatric patients can be classified into cholestatic disorders, metabolic liver diseases causing liver cirrhosis, metabolic liver diseases without liver cirrhosis, acute liver failure, acute and chronic hepatitis, and liver tumors. The most common indication of PLT is biliary atresia. Generally, the patient is a child with biliary atresia with several prior surgical procedures, extremely malnourished, with stigmata of fat-soluble vitamin deficiency, bleeding diathesis, uncontrolled portal hypertension and massive ascites. Before the technique of liver splitting, pediatric patients were dependent on donors with similar age or size. Partial liver grafts can be obtained either by splitting a cadaveric donor organ or by living-donor liver donation. Living donor liver recipients have a shorter waiting time. The majority of centers employ a regime of' triple therapy with prednisolone, mycophenolate and tacrolimus. LT in the pediatric setting is technically challenging due to the reduced size of the vasculature and biliary tree. Strategies for identification and mitigation of risk factors, prevention of technical complications, and protocols for early detection of vascular complications may reduce mortality, morbidity.

Keywords: organ transplant, liver transplant, pediatric liver disease

1. Introduction

The first successful transplant was performed by Starzl in 1967, on a 1-year-old child with hepatoma [13–15]. The patient survived for over 12 months dying from recurrence of the liver tumor. Throughout the next 15 years, liver transplants (LTs) were performed rarely in a very few centers, with survival rates of only 20–30%. However, the quality of life in pediatric liver transplant (PLT) patients was so good as to support these forerunners to persevere in their efforts and to continue to refine and improve techniques and postoperative care [5].

By March 1980, the liver trials with cyclosporine began in Denver. Twelve patients entered the study between March and September 1980; 11 patients lived for 1 year or longer [2,16]. In 1983, a National Consensus Conference on Liver Transplantation was held in the United States, which became a landmark in the liver transplantation history. This event concluded that liver transplant had advanced from an experimental stage to that of a procedure with a widespread application for patients dying of liver failure. The number of transplants performed both in the United States and elsewhere has grown since then. The number of liver transplant (LT) continues to grow to date as an increasing number of indications for liver replacement are identified [5].

Liver transplantation is the treatment of choice for pediatric liver diseases causing acute liver failure or progressing to end-stage liver disease (ESLD). These include congenital hepatitis, hepatocellular carcinoma, biliary atresia, Wilson's disease (WD), progressive familial intrahepatic cholestasis, and other metabolic syndromes involving injury to the liver [17]. Pediatric acute liver failure (PALF) is a complex, rapidly progressive clinical syndrome that is the final common pathway for many disparate conditions, some known and others yet to be identified. PALF accounts for 10–15% of pediatric liver transplants performed in the United States annually [18–20].

The foremost factor limiting expansion of orthotopic liver transplant (OLT) is donor availability. In small children, scarcity of size-appropriate grafts imposes a significant barrier to PLT. At present, waiting list mortality rate for children less than 6 years of age is four times greater than for children of ages 11–17 years [21]. Living-donor liver transplantation (LDLT) has been developed to address the disparity between the number candidates for transplant and the reduced number of available organs for LT [22].

2. Indications

Various diseases that are indications for LT in pediatric patients can be classified into cholestatic disorders, metabolic liver diseases causing liver cirrhosis, metabolic liver diseases without liver cirrhosis, acute liver failure, acute and chronic hepatitis, and liver tumors. The most common indication of PLT is biliary atresia, approximately 40% of the pediatric candidates [1]. The indications are listed in **Table 1**.

2.1. Biliary atresia

Biliary atresia (BA) is a disease of unknown etiology in which there is obstruction or destruction of the biliary tree [6]. It occurs in approximately 1 of every 15,000 live births [24]. Early diagnosis and palliative surgery—Kasai portoenterostomy are the corner stone for the treatment of BA. In this procedure, the biliary tree is excised to expose biliary channels, and a

Roux-n-Y loop is fashioned for drainage. The procedure is only successful if there is restoration of biliary flow under 6 month of age and is conditional to the age when the operation is performed, the skill of the surgeon, and the degree of fibrosis at operation [25]. BA is the main indication for PLT worldwide and accounts for 76% transplants in children younger than 2 years; 80% of children who have a successful operation do not require transplantation before adolescence [6,23,25].

Chronic liver failure	**Acute liver failure**
Neonatal liver disease	Fulminant hepatitis
Biliary atresia	Autoimmune hepatitis
Idiopathic neonatal hepatitis	Halothane exposure
	Acetaminophen poisoning
	Viral hepatitis
Cholestatic liver disease	Metabolic liver disease
Alagille's syndrome	Fatty acid oxidation defects
Familial intrahepatic cholestasis (FIC)	Neonatal hemochromatosis
Nonsyndromic biliary hypoplasia	Tyrosinemia type I
	Wilson's disease
Inherited metabolic liver disease	
Alfa1 antitrypsin deficiency	
Cystic fibrosis	
Glycogen storage disease type IV	
Tyrosinemia type I	
Wilson's disease	
Chronic hepatitis	**Inborn errors of metabolism**
Autoimmune	Crigler-Najjar type I
Idiopathic	Familial hypercholesterolemia
Postviral (hepatitis B, C, other)	Primary oxalosis
	Organic acidemia
	Urea cycle defects
Other	**Liver tumors**
Cryptogenic cirrhosis	Benign tumors
Fibropolycystic liver disease ± Caroli syndrome	Unresectable malignant tumors

Table 1. Indications for LT in pediatric patients [23].

In several cases, the child needs LT in the first year of life due to the aggressive evolution of the disease leads to cirrhosis accompanied with severe malnutrition. Consequently, technical difficulties related to the limited dimensions of the anatomic structures are faced [26]. Hypoplasia, with or without portal vein thrombosis are relatively frequent in the course of BA. These features are related to a higher incidence of portal vein complications [27]. Previous portoenterostomy procedures cause intra-abdominal adhesions increasing the morbidity due to intraoperative bleeding and eventual bowel perforation. Previous reports have indicated that BA patients display lower survivals than children undergoing LT for other hepatic diseases [26,28,29].

Infants with suspected BA should be evaluated as rapidly as possible because the success of the surgical intervention (hepatoportoenterostomy, the Kasai procedure) diminishes progressively with older age at surgery [30]. The evaluation process involves a series of serologic, laboratory, urine, and imaging tests. The order of diagnostic tests is prioritized based on testing for treatable diseases first, such as biliary obstruction, infections, and some metabolic diseases.

Evaluation of biliary anatomy begins with an ultrasound. The main utility of the ultrasound is to exclude other anatomic causes of cholestasis (i.e., choledochal cyst). In infants with BA, the gallbladder is usually either absent or irregular in shape. When a detailed ultrasonographic protocol is used, additional features can be identified to support the diagnosis of biliary atresia, including abnormal gallbladder size and shape, the "triangular cord" sign, gallbladder contractility, and absence of the common bile duct [31–34]. The triangular cord sign is a triangular echogenic density seen just above the porta hepatis on US scan. Its presence is highly suggestive of biliary atresia [35]. Patency of the extrahepatic biliary tree can be further assessed by hepatobiliary scintigraphy.

The liver biopsy is important for mainly two reasons: to identify histologic changes consistent with obstruction that warrant surgical exploration and to differentiate BA from other causes of intrahepatic cholestasis, which would not need surgical exploration. Biopsy findings that indicate another etiology include bile duct paucity (Alagille syndrome), periodic acid-Schiff (PAS) positive diastase resistant granules (consistent with alpha-one antitrypsin deficiency), or giant cell hepatitis without proliferation of ducts. Characteristic histologic features of BA include expanded portal tracts with bile duct proliferation, portal tract edema, fibrosis and inflammation, and canalicular and bile duct bile plugs. The earliest histological changes associated with BA may be relatively nonspecific, and biopsies done too early may result in a false negative [36].

Histologic findings alone cannot help to distinguish BA from other causes of obstruction, such as choledochal cyst or external compression. Therefore, any evidence of obstruction mandates imaging exploration and a definitive cholangiogram. The intraoperative cholangiogram is the gold standard in the diagnosis of BA. It is essential that patency be investigated both proximally into the liver and distally into the bowel to determine whether BA is present. If the intraoperative cholangiogram demonstrates biliary obstruction (i.e., if the contrast does not fill the biliary tree or reach the intestine), the surgeon should perform a hepatoportoenterostomy (Kasai HPE) at that time [37].

An increase in the number of long-term survivors of biliary atresia has been observed. Nevertheless, the disease is still one of the most challenging problems in the field of pediatric surgery because of progressive fibrosis, portal hypertension, and liver cirrhosis [17]. Kasai portoenterostomy (KPE) may play a role in gaining time for liver transplantation [17,38]. Shinkai et al. [39] showed improvement of post-KPE survival rate with almost 90% for 5 years and nearly 80% for 10 years in patients who were operated on in the 1980s. Still, despite early success with portoenterostomy, a few long-term survivals will present manifestations of portal hypertension, such as esophageal and/or gastric varices, and hypersplenism. Cholangitis and/or hepatic failure caused by progressive ongoing cirrhosis may also occur in patients with long follow-up after KPE. The main cause of comorbidity among long-term survivals of biliary atresia is portal hypertension. Despite the improvement in the long-term survival rate after KPE in biliary atresia, two-thirds of patients who survived over 10 years suffer from various complications including portal hypertension, cholangitis, intrahepatic cyst, and intestinal obstruction in spite of successful KPE. Approximately one-third of these patients will not present any problem. Meticulous follow-up is required since some manifestations of on-going liver cirrhosis will present and therefore planning for liver transplantation is necessary [40].

2.2. Inherited metabolic liver disease

2.2.1. Acute liver failure in inherited metabolic liver disease patients

Metabolic diseases account for at least 10% of acute liver failure cases in North America and Europe [19,41]. While some conditions, such as mitochondrial disease, may present at any age, many metabolic conditions presenting as liver failure segregate within age groups. Metabolic conditions affecting infants in the first few months of life include galactosemia, tyrosinemia, Niemann-Pick type C, mitochondrial hepatopathies, and urea cycle defects [42]. In older infants and young children up to 5 years of age presenting with acute liver failure, metabolic diseases are sometimes identified [18], such as mitochondrial hepatopathies, hereditary fructose intolerance (HFI), argininosuccinate synthetase deficiency (citrullinemia type 1), and ornithine transcarbamylase deficiency. In older children and adolescents, Wilson's disease and mitochondrial disease (fatty acid oxidation defects) may cause acute liver failure [43].

2.2.2. Alpha 1 antitrypsin deficiency

Alpha 1 antitrypsin (AAT) deficiency is the most common form of inherited metabolic liver disease in childhood in Europe. Although 50–70% of children develop persistent liver disease progressing to cirrhosis, only 20–30% require transplantation in childhood or adolescence [44,45].

The presentation of alpha 1 antitrypsin deficiency can include neonatal cholestasis. The frequency of AAT deficiency in infants with neonatal cholestasis ranges from 1 to 10% in different series [46,47]. AAT is an antiprotease and the natural inhibitor of the serine proteases released by activated neutrophils [48]. The "deficiency" state is actually an accumulation of abnormal protein within the endoplasmic reticulum resulting in liver injury in a subset of patients by unclear mechanism [49].

2.2.3. Alagille's syndrome

This autosomal dominant condition has an incidence of 1 case per 100,000 live births. It is a multisystem disorder with cardiac, facial, renal, ocular, and skeletal abnormalities. The condition is caused by mutations in the Jagged 1 gene (JAG1), which encodes a ligand of Notch

1 [50]. The main clinical issues are cholestasis, malnutrition, and cardiac or renal disease [6]. Cholestatic liver disease is of variable severity and may stabilize by school age. It is managed conservatively, with treatment for pruritus and malabsorption as needed. Portoenterostomy (Kasai procedure) is not beneficial and is not recommended [51]. End-stage liver disease develops in approximately 20% of affected children and is amenable to liver transplantation [43,52].

2.2.4. *Tyrosinemia type I*

Tyrosinemia type I, also known as Hepatorenal tyrosinemia [43], is an autosomal recessive disorder caused by a defect of fumaryl acetoacetase (FAA). There is a lifetime risk of developing hepatocellular carcinoma (HCC) [53]. Clinical features are heterogeneous, even within the same family. Young infants present with cholestasis and coagulopathy, which is often disproportionate to the apparent degree of liver disease. Older infants and children may present with chronic liver disease, with or without cholestasis, and painful crises, mimicking porphyria [44]. Management is with a phenylalanine and tyrosine-restricted diet and nitisone, which prevents the formation of toxic metabolites and allows normal growth and development [55]. The long-term outcome has significantly improved with nitisone therapy and transplantation is now only indicated in those adolescents who do not respond to nitisone, or develop HCC [6,54]. Affected individuals have increased urinary excretion of succinylacetone and markedly elevated blood tyrosine concentration [44].

2.2.5. *Cystic fibrosis*

Cystic fibrosis (CF) occurs in 1 in every 3000 live births worldwide [55].

The gene defect is an abnormality in the cystic fibrosis transmembrane conductance regulator (CFTR) located on chromosome 7q31. It is a multiorgan disease mainly affecting the lungs and pancreas [6]. The cystic fibrosis transmembrane conductance regulator is located on the apical surface of the biliary epithelium, explaining some of the biliary tract disease seen in patients with cystic fibrosis [56]. Neonatal cholestasis is an uncommon presentation of cystic fibrosis, occurring in fewer than 5% of patients with CF. In affected infants, jaundice and hepatomegaly slowly resolve. Infants with CF are more likely to present with meconium ileus or steatorrhea with failure to thrive [43]. Cystic fibrosis-associated liver disease (CFLD) occurs in 27–35% of patients and usually presents before the age of 18 years [60]. Cirrhosis and portal hypertension occurs in 5–10% of patients during the first decade of life and present with complications in adolescence or early adult life [57]. The indications for LT include malnutrition unresponsive to nutritional support, intractable portal hypertension, and hepatic dysfunction. It is essential that transplantation be carried out before pulmonary disease becomes irreversible [58].

2.2.6. *Wilson's disease*

Wilson's disease is the most common metabolic condition associated with PALF in children over 5 years of age [18]. It is an autosomal recessive disorder with an incidence of 1 case per 30,000 live births. The defective gene is on chromosome 13 and encodes a copper transporting

P-type adenosinetriphosphatase (ATPase) (ATP7B) [59]. Clinical features in adolescence include hepatic dysfunction (40%) fulminant hepatitis, chronic hepatitis or cirrhosis, and psychiatric symptoms (35%). Neurologic symptoms may be nonspecific, but deteriorating school performance, abnormal behavior, lack of coordination, and dysarthria are common. Renal tubular abnormalities, renal calculi, and hemolytic anemia are associated features [60,61].

The presence of a Coombs-negative hemolytic anemia, marked hyperbilirubinemia, low serum ceruloplasmin, and a normal or subnormal low serum alkaline phosphatase should prompt consideration of WD, but confirming the diagnosis remains a challenge [62]. LT is indicated for those with advanced liver disease (Wilson's score > 6), fulminant liver failure, or progressive hepatic disease despite therapy [60,61].

2.2.7. *Other inborn errors of metabolism*

LT is indicated for those metabolic disorders secondary to hepatic enzyme deficiencies that lead to severe extrahepatic disease such as kernicterus in Crigler-Najjar type I and systemic oxalosis in primary oxaluria. Selection and timing of transplantation depends on the quality of life on medical management and the mortality and morbidity of the primary disease compared with the risks of transplantation [23]. Crigler-Najjar type I is an autosomal recessive condition caused by a deficiency of bilirubin uridine diphosphate glucuronosyltransferase (UDPGT) [63]. Most children require transplantation in early childhood, but those with milder forms may manage with phototherapy into adolescence. Primary hyperoxaluria is a defect of glyoxylate metabolism characterized by the overproduction of oxalate, which is deposited as calcium oxalate in various organs including the kidney [64]. Ideally, liver replacement should be prior to the development of irreversible renal failure. If this is not possible, liver and kidney replacement may be required simultaneously [65]. Children with milder phenotypes will not require intervention until adolescence [6].

2.3. Liver tumors

2.3.1. *Hepatoblastoma*

The most common primary liver tumor in children is hepatoblastoma (HB), accounting for two-thirds of all malignant liver neoplasms in the pediatric population [66]. Neoadjuvant chemotherapy and surgical resection followed by adjuvant chemotherapy is the treatment of choice for patients with HB. When HB shows to be unresectable or unresponsive to chemotherapy, combination of chemotherapy and liver transplantation is an attractive alternative [67]. The United States Surveillance, Epidemiology, and End Results (SEER) from 2002 to 2008 showed an incidence in HB of 10.5 cases/million in children under 1 year of age and 5.2 cases/million in children 1–4 years of age [68]. Histologically, HB cells resemble embryonic liver cells and the incidence is highest at birth suggesting that the process is initiated during gestation [69].

Liver transplantation has resulted in long-term disease-free survival in up to 80% of children with large solitary, and especially multifocal, hepatoblastomas invading all four sectors of the liver [70]. While "extreme" resection of tumors without liver transplant will avoid the need for long-term immunosuppressive therapy, hazardous attempts at partial hepatectomy in children with major venous involvement or with extensive multifocal tumors should be discouraged [71–75]. Only in centers that have a facility for liver transplant extensive hepatic surgery in children should be carried out. In these centers, surgical expertise, as well as willingness to embark on more radical surgery with a transplant "safety net" is likely to be greater [75]. In a review of the United Network for Organ Sharing database in the United States concerning liver transplantation in 135 children transplanted for unresectable or recurrent HB (1987–2004), the 1-, 5-, and 10-year survival was 79, 69, and 66%, respectively [76]. The latest European Liver Transplant Registry (ELTR) report, including 129 patients transplanted for HB, has shown a 1- and 5-year survival of 100 and 74%, respectively [77,78].

The only absolute contraindication for liver transplantation is the persistence of viable extrahepatic tumor deposit after chemotherapy, not amenable to surgical resection. When macroscopic venous invasion occurs (portal vein, hepatic veins, and vena cava), liver resection can be carried on if complete resection of the invaded venous structures is feasible. "En-bloc" and reconstruction should be performed whenever there is evidence or suspicion of invasion of the retrohepatic vena cava. Patients with lung metastases at presentation should not be excluded from liver transplantation if the metastases clear completely after chemotherapy and/ or surgical resection. Liver transplant can only be performed after complete eradication of metastatic lesions, by chemotherapy and surgical resection, of any suspicious remnant after chemotherapy [79]. Rescue liver transplantation, after an incomplete partial hepatectomy or when intrahepatic relapse occurs, may be a relative contraindication because of the disappointing results observed in the SIOPEL-l study and in the reported world experience [77].

2.3.2. Hepatocellular carcinoma

Unlike the adult population, the frequency of I ICC in the pediatric population is low; therefore, the experience in the application of liver transplantation in the pediatric population for HCC is limited [80–83]. Experience with liver transplantation in children with unresectable HCC is somewhat limited but results have significantly improved over the recent years. The Milan criteria—no more than three tumors, each not more than 3 cm in size, or a single tumor, not more than 5 cm in diameter, and no evidence of extrahepatic disease or vascular invasion is commonly used to determine which patients benefit the most with LT [84]. Recently, it has been suggested that the present cut-off for tumor size might be expanded to 6.5 cm or 7 cm, in an otherwise normal liver [89, 90]. Data suggesting that Milan criteria can appropriately identify children with a low-risk tumor recurrence of after transplantation is not yet available. The Milan criteria are derivative from experience treating adult patients with cirrhosis, whereas HCC in children usually is not associated with cirrhosis. The role of OLT in noncirrhotic liver is unknown due to lack of prospective trial in children. Furthermore, there are differences in biology of HCC in adults and in children [85]. The different molecular findings include mutation of c-met gene in children; lower levels of glycin D1 (regulatory protein of G1 phase cycle) expression in children; and higher incidence of loss of heterozygosity on chromosomal arm, 13q, in children [85]. In patients whose disease is confined to the liver, the use of liver transplantation is indicated.

2.4. Acute Liver Failure

Viral hepatitis A and B are the most common causes of acute liver failure in the developing world [86,87]. However, in the United Kingdom and United States, indeterminate hepatitis is the most common cause and has the worst prognosis for spontaneous recovery [18]. The main indications for LT for acute liver failure in adolescence are drug induced, infectious hepatitis, or metabolic disease (e.g., Wilson's disease) [18,88]. Many different drugs cause acute liver failure, including antibiotics, antituberculosis therapy, antiepileptic therapy, and acetaminophen poisoning [89]. Adolescents have a lower incidence of liver failure with acetaminophen overdose than adults, possibly because of the effect of hepatic maturation and glutathione production [90]. Transplantation is more likely to be required if the overdose was taken with another drug (e.g., lysergic acid diethylamide [LSD], ecstasy) or with alcohol [91]. Persistent coagulopathy (INR > 4), metabolic acidosis (pH < 7.3), an elevated creatinine (>300 mmol/l), and rapid progression to hepatic coma grade III are indicatives for liver transplant. Cerebral edema may persist despite evidence of hepatic regeneration and recovery and influence postoperative recovery.

Once the diagnosis of liver disease is made, the most important assessment is to determine the severity of the liver disease and its projected outcome. Patients with evidence of end-stage liver disease, including variceal hemorrhage, intractable ascites, hepatorenal syndrome, recurrent infection, and portosystemic encephalopathy, are candidates for immediate listing for transplantation. Selected patients with well-compensated Child's A cirrhosis and isolated variceal bleeding benefit from surgical portosystemic shunting. The success of transplantation in patients with sequel of end-stage liver disease has also heralded an increasing willingness to apply transplantation in patients with life-disabling complications of liver disease consequent to severe metabolic consequences of chronic liver disease [92].

Thus, the indications for PLT are significantly different to indications in adult LT recipients. In the past, PLT was only performed in curative intent. Nowadays, if life expectancy and/or quality of life can be significantly improved, PLT is also performed. Children diagnosed with metabolic liver diseases not resulting in liver cirrhosis, the indication for LT has to be cautiously evaluated. LT should be performed when the disease can either be cured or if extrahepatic manifestations can be significantly improved [1].

3. Contraindications for transplantation

The few contraindications include severe systemic sepsis—particularly fungal sepsis, at the time of operation; malignant hepatic tumors with extrahepatic spread; severe extrahepatic disease that is not reversible following LT (e.g., severe cardiopulmonary disease for which corrective surgery is not possible), or severe structural brain damage [23].

4. Preoperative management

When transplantation was still perceived as experimental, potential candidates were referred to very late in their course of end-stage liver disease. Generally, the patient was a child with biliary atresia with several prior surgical procedures, who was extremely malnourished, with stigmata of fat-soluble vitamin deficiency, bleeding diathesis, uncontrolled portal hypertension, and massive ascites. One could not imagine a poorer candidate for major surgery. Unfortunately, this is still reality in many centers [2].

Correct preparation before transplantation requires a multidisciplinary approach. The use of new milk formulas specially developed for cholestatic children, parenteral nutrition, may be necessary to correct the nutrition deficit [93]. Gastrointestinal bleeding from esophageal varices should be prevented with sclerotherapy [93], variceal banding [94], and transjugular intrahepatic portosystemic shunt in older children [95]. The remarkable enhancement in the outcomes of liver transplantation, including children, has encouraged an earlier referral, allowing a more elective approach toward liver transplantation [2].

Immunizations should be administered to solid organ transplant candidates as early as possible in the transplant evaluation in order to optimize immune responses and provide immunity to pathogens against which there is only a live vaccine (measles, mumps, rubella, varicella, and zoster). Standard age-appropriate vaccines, as well as vaccines indicated for immunocompromised hosts (e.g., pneumococcal vaccines in adults), should be administered 2–6 months following transplantation, once maintenance immunosuppression levels have been attained. Inactivated vaccines are generally considered to be safe following solid organ transplantation [96].

Live vaccines (measles, mumps, rubella, varicella, zoster, and intranasal influenza vaccine) are not recommended in the majority of solid organ transplant recipients. An exception is varicella-nonimmune pediatric renal or liver transplant recipients who are receiving minimal or no immunosuppression and who have had no recent allograft rejection; such individuals may receive the varicella vaccine [96].

The measles, mumps, and rubella vaccine is considered safe in household contacts of solid organ transplant recipients. We suggest administering the varicella vaccine to nonimmune household contacts. The zoster vaccine should be administered to household contacts when indicated. Vaccinees who develop a rash should avoid contact with transplant recipients for the duration of the rash [1].

In biliary atresia patients, which is the most frequent indication, a sequential strategy with a single attempt at surgical correction, Roux-en-Y portoenterostomy as described by Kasai [97], followed by liver transplantation, when it fails, is consensus by pediatric surgeons [104]. At present, most infants who do not achieve remission following portoenterostomy are referred to and transplanted under the age of 1 year. Malatack et al. [98] proposed a score to choose the timing of transplantation for children with chronic liver failure. Though such a score can be beneficial, it is suggested that liver transplantation should be performed as soon as an appropriate donor is found, even for children in stable condition, at least when the indication is straightforward at any age of the child.

Due to better understanding of the pathophysiology and/or increased of clinical experience, many contraindications accepted in the past are not presently valid. An example is hepatopulmonary syndrome, which can associate with any type of chronic liver disease. Room air PaO_2 level lower than 60 mmHg has been described to be associated with prohibitive mortality after liver transplant [99]. Differently, regardless of the severity of the syndrome, others have shown complete reversion of hepatopulmonary syndrome after LT [107].

4.1. Psychological preparation

A skilled multidisciplinary team, including a psychologist, is essential for counseling and preparation of the patient and his/hers family. Young people need to be involved in the decision making wherever possible, and previous experience of illness, knowledge about their condition and treatment, previous/current adherence to prescribed medical regimens, and self-management behaviors need to be explored. Parents and appropriate relatives must be fully informed of the necessity for LT in their child and of the risks, complications, and the long-term implications of the operation. Particularly, careful counseling is necessary for parents and children being considered for transplantation because of extrahepatic disease due to an inborn error of metabolism. As these young people are not dying from liver disease, they may find it difficult to accept the risks and complications and the necessity for compliance with long-term immunosuppression [6].

4.2. Psychosocial evaluation of live organ donors

Adequate psychosocial evaluation includes assessment of the motivation for donating, decision making and informed consent process, donor-recipient relationship, adequacy of both financial and social support, behavioral and psychological health, and substance use history. A complete assessment of a potential living donor should also address obstacles such as impression management and explicit deception. It should also include ethical aspects, such as the right to donate, donor autonomy, freedom from coercion, and "reasonable" risks to donors. The Transplantation Society Ethics Committee emphasizes that is essential when considering living organ donation, that the well-being of donors, including survival, quality of life, and psychological and social well-being, outweighs the risks to the donor-recipient pair, which include death and medical, psychological, and social morbidities [100]. Like to the psychosocial evaluation of the recipient, the attention should be on the interaction of risk versus protective factors for each donor [109]. Although recent research identifies the needs for standard criteria [101], live organ donor evaluations should be viewed within both individual and contextual frameworks [22].

5. Surgical techniques

Liver transplantation has gained from the knowledge of anesthesiologists handling babies with serious conditions. The pediatric anesthesiologist is an essential member of the team. As in any long operation, exact correction of blood loss, continual monitoring of electrolytes and blood gases, correct identification and treatment of bleeding diathesis, and maintenance of body temperature and diuresis are fundamental. Alongside a correct comprehension of all the surgical techniques, good tactics and technical expertise, proper attention by the surgeon to hemostasis is essential. Although limitation of graft ischemia time is important, the patient will be better off at the end of surgery if the operative field is dry and the small bowel has been preserved from damage during the tedious dissection of tight adhesions, rather than been rushed through surgery by a hurried surgeon [2].

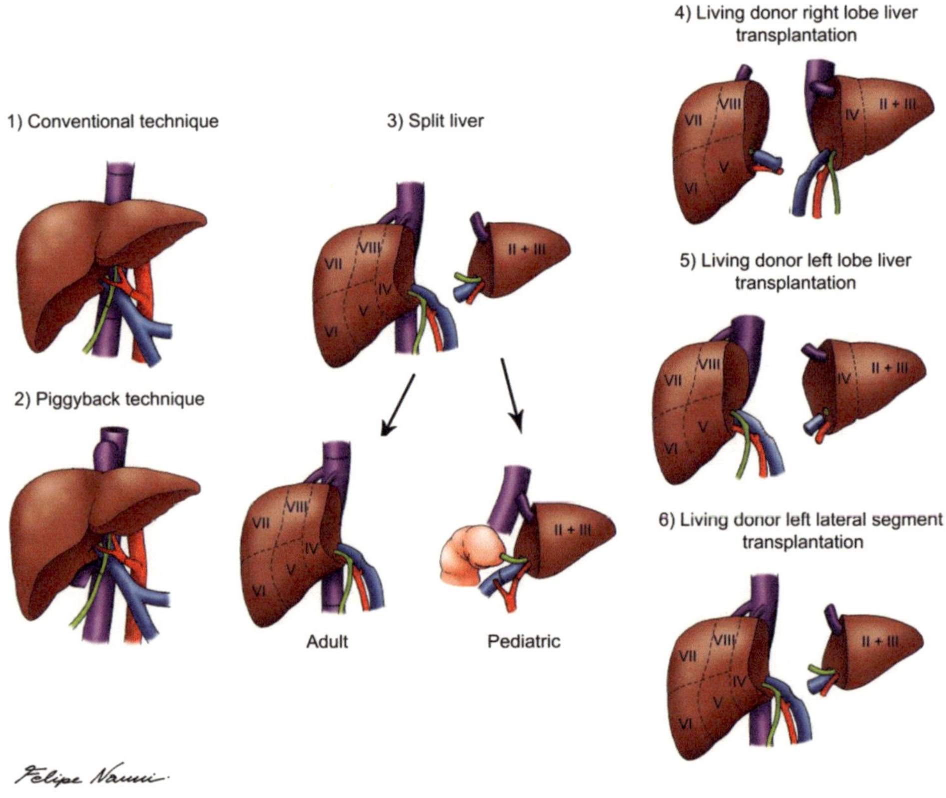

Figure 1. Examples of surgical techniques for orthotopic liver transplantation.

Prior the development of the technique of liver splitting, PLT was dependent on donors with similar age or size. In the early 1980s, Christoph Broelsch and Henri Bismuth were the first applying the technique of reduced-size LT in children [102,103]. Rudolf Pichlmayr performed the first split LT offering one cadaveric liver to two recipients in 1988 [104]. However, pediatric deceased donors as well as organs suitable for split LT remain rare. The numbers of PLTs performed significantly exceed the number of available pediatric organ donors [1,105].

LT in children is comparable to adult LT (piggy back or conventional technique) when full size grafts are transplanted. Partial liver grafts can be obtained either by splitting a cadaveric donor organ or by living-donor liver donation. When liver-splitting technique is used, the anatomical determination of the eight liver segments first described by Couinaud [106,107] in 1957 is essential. **Figure 1** depicts the surgical options for OLT.

The splitting procedure can be performed as anatomical splitting, dividing the liver at Cantlie's line, and splitting along the falciform ligament [117]. When the left lateral segment divided, the technique is much easier to perform than the true right/left lobe split procedure. Additionally, the left lateral segment is preferentially used in PLT. It is the smallest part of the liver when compared to the extended right, the anatomical left, or the right liver lobe.

In small infants, even the left lateral segment of the liver often is too large and techniques to cut down left lateral lobes may be used to prevent graft-size mismatching and the so-called "large-for-size" syndrome [108]. Not rarely, primary closure of the abdominal wall after PLT is not feasible and should not be enforced in order to avoid increase in intra-abdominal pressure. Excessive increase in intra-abdominal pressure may compromise graft perfusion. In such occasions, abdominal wall closure is performed in stages during the first week post-transplant or accomplished by using mesh grafts. This allows for a continuous recovery of the graft from reperfusion injury and edema [109].

5.1. Auxiliary transplantation

Auxiliary partial orthotopic LT (APOLT) is an alternative technique for LT in patients with acute liver failure or in children with metabolic liver diseases without primary hepatocellular dysfunction or cirrhosis. In this technique, a partial graft is implanted without entirely removing the native liver. Gubernatis et al. reported the first successful case in a patient with acute liver failure. After her recovery, the native liver has regenerated and immunosuppressive treatment could be withdrawn [110,111].

In patients with metabolic diseases, APOLT may provide sufficient liver mass to correct the hepatic metabolic function. If the graft fails, the patient's native liver is still present to secure general liver function [112]. When APOLT is performed in acute fulminant liver failure, the immunosuppressive therapy can be stopped if the native liver recuperates, resulting in an atrophy of the transplanted liver [113].

5.2. Living-donor liver donation

After successful implementation of split-liver LT in PLT, this technique leads to the first living-donor liver transplant (LDLT). In 1989, the first series of LDLT in pediatric recipients was performed in Chicago [114], after the pioneer work of Raia et al. [115] in Brazil. As of today, LDLT is an established procedure and the main form of LT due to scarcity of deceased donor organs in most East-Asian countries [116]. In western countries and especially in the UNOS area, use of living-donor organs for LT is less frequent and within UNOS constantly <5% of LT over the last years [117]. Within the European Transplant Network, rates of LDLT in PLT are steadily increasing.

Retrospective analyses have shown favorable or equal results as compared to PLT after deceased donor liver transplant (DDLT) [118–126]. When performing LDLT the scenery include an optimal healthy donor, minimal ischemic time, elective surgery, and timing of transplantation according to the recipients' need. This is particularly pertinent for pediatric patients. During a waiting time for PLT, the underlying disease can complicate and psycho-social long-term morbidity may develop pediatric patient. It has been shown that long-term outcome after PLT significantly correlates with the severity of morbidity at PLT. In a early publication, significant independent predictors of survival after OLT in children with end-stage liver disease were bilirubin (p=0.0024), lower weight (p=0.034), and albumin (p=0.039). Post-transplantation survival rates was statistically significant difference at 1 year (57% vs. 90.5%) and 4 years (49% vs. 90.5%) after OLT(p=0.0001), when one or more of these risk factors - bilirubin >340 μmol/L, lower weight <–2.2 and albumin < 33 g/L, were presente [127]. LDLT offers the possibility and advantage of optimal timing of the transplant procedure before severe morbidity develops.

Living-donor livers recipients have a shorter waiting time when compared to recipients of organs from deceased donors. This reflects in a reduction of waiting list mortality. Nevertheless, live donors are not deprived of risk. Also to considerer is the fact that LDLT is surgically more challenging than whole organ transplantation. Donor major complications, exceeding Clavien's classification grade II, were described in up to 44% after right-lobe LDLT with a mortality risk up to 0.8% [128–130]. Donors of right liver lobe experience operating procedures with longer duration, have significant longer hospital stay and require more blood transfusions [131,132]. For PLT, in most cases, the left lateral segment donation is sufficient. The complication rates after full left lobe or left lateral lobectomy are significantly lower than right lobe donation [133–135]. In order to decrease morbidity and mortality after liver donation, a thorough evaluation of the potential donor is essential to detect and exclude potential increased medical risk factors for the otherwise healthy donor.

5.3. Living related donor liver transplantation in children

5.3.1. Surgical technique

The donor procedure is performed first, except when recipient's diagnosis is malignant liver tumor. The recipient surgery usually starts immediately after the quality of the graft is assured to minimize the cold ischemia time. Left lateral hepatectomy is performed without clamping of the portal triad. The vessels were divided after completion of the parenchymal transection. The whole hilum is dissected and the left hepatic artery is identified. Subsequently, dissection is confined to the left branch of the portal vein and to the left hepatic artery. Minimal dissection was performed around the left hepatic duct to avoid damaging its blood supply. At bench surgery, the graft is perfused with preservation solution.

The liver implantation technique consists of the anastomosis of the left hepatic vein to the native inferior vena cava. This anastomosis can be performed by direct suturing of the donor hepatic veins to the recipient hepatic veins; by a triangular anastomosis after creating a wide triangular orifice in the recipient inferior vena cava at the confluence of all of the hepatic veins; or a wide longitudinal anastomosis in the anterior wall of the inferior vena cava. Subsequently, the portal vein is anastomosed to the trunk of the recipient's portal vein in an end-to-end technique [136].

The liver graft is reperfused after conclusion of the portal vein anastomosis. For the reconstruction of the artery, microsurgical techniques are necessary. The graft hepatic artery is anastomosed to one of the stumps of the main branches or to the trunk of the proper hepatic artery of the recipient in end-to-end fashion using 9-0 or 10-0 prolene sutures. The arterial anastomosis should be performed using microsurgery techniques under surgical microscope (magnification, 8×) or surgical loupes (magnification, 6×), depending on the size of the arteries. Biliary reconstruction is achieved by a Roux-en-Y hepaticojejunostomy. Occasionally, an end-to-end duct anastomosis can be performed [136].

6. Post-transplant care

Immediately after the transplant, the patient is usually ventilated in intensive care for 24-48 h. Graft function is assessed with coagulation studies, blood sugar and acid-base balance, and liver function tests. Initially in the post-operative period, high transaminase levels are usually observed that progressively fall during the first few postoperative days. A rapid reduction of jaundice is an indication of a well-functioning graft.

When abnormal liver function tests are detected, a specific protocol of investigations to determine the cause is necessary. In patients with a t-tube, a cholangiogram will demonstrate patency of the biliary tree. In patients without a t-tube, an ultrasound of the liver can exclude biliary obstruction and demonstrate patency of the portal vein and hepatic artery. In the suspicion of a thrombotic event, angiography should be performed to confirm it. The gold standard for diagnosing a rejection episode is needle biopsy. Liver biopsy should be carried out subsequently. Other diagnoses such as preservation injury or viral hepatitis in the graft can also be diagnosed. For confirmation of viral infections, specific antibody tests usually are necessary [5].

7. Immunossupression

As in adult LT, the introduction of calcineurin inhibitors (CNI) in the early 1980s gave way to long-term survival also for pediatric transplant recipients and until today remains the backbone of immunosuppression practices [1,3,137]. The most popular immunosuppression drugs combination comprises low doses of prednisolone, mycophenolate, and tacrolimus. Despite the high effectiveness of these medications in controling the imune response, rejection is a reality in the majority of liver transplant recipients which can be controlled with the intensification of the steroid dose. Higher doses of immunosuppression are usually associated with a lower incidence of rejection. On the other hand, at the same time, a higher infection rate with considerable morbidity and even morality appears. Moreover, each of the agents has specific toxic effects [5]. Observations made by several groups indicate that after liver transplantation in children require more immunosuppression than adults, with a higher incidence of steroid sensitive and steroid-resistant acute rejection episodes [137].

The period of highest risk for immunologic reactions between graft and host usually is in the early post-transplant phase. Consequently, higher dose of immunosuppression is required during this period. Most protocols include induction therapy, usually interleukin-2 receptor antibodies especially in the pediatric transplant population (Basiliximab® and Daclizumab®), in association with corticosteroids and calcineurin inhibitors (cyclosporine A and tacrolimus) as maintenance therapy [138–143]. In the pediatric transplantation community, the use of other mono- or polyclonal antibodies—monoclonal anti-CD3 antibody preparations (OKT3) and rabbit or equine antithymocyte globulin, for induction therapy has not been adopted. These potent agents can cause undesired short—and uncertain long-term effects on the developing organism and immune system [144]. Several reports showed that the lower doses of immunosuppression can be used based on the individual needs, particularly in pediatric cases which can, ***in long-term***, improve the quality of life of these patients minimizing undesired side effects [145–148].

Common side effects of immunosuppressants include diabetes, deficiency of growth, hypertension, nephrotoxicity, hyperlipidemia, neurologic alterations, hypertrichosis, and bone marrow suppression. Ideal levels of immunosuppression are hard to obtain due to great differences between individuals as well as within the same individual over time. Multiple combination protocols, such as mycophenolate-mofetil and mammalian target of rapamycin inhibitors (sirolimus and everolimus), with and without CNIs have been introduced for maintenance therapy also in pediatric solid organ transplant based on increasing data to safety aspects in the use of different immunosuppressant drugs in the adult population [149–156].

It is well established that long-term immunosuppression increases the risk of infectious and malignant complications. Other side effects, such as nephrotoxicity, disturbances of the lipid profile, arterial hypertension, and cardiovascular disease, are also of concern. These side effects can jeopardize both quality of life and life expectancy. Especially in pediatric liver recipients whose survival can be expected to be more than a few decades; consequently prevention of these side effects is a major objective. The reduction of the global immunosuppression in the first months after the procedure, concerning the total amount of steroids and the target blood levels of calcineurin inhibitors, is the main goal. The use of tacrolimus has allowed complete withdrawal of steroids within the first posttransplant year in most patients, which has been proved to be beneficial. New protocols, specifically designed for children to test new immunosuppressive compounds as well as tolerance inducing strategies, have been more easily introduced [2].

Although immunosuppression drugs is still recommended after liver transplantation, several studies have shown that particularly patients who are transplanted in the early years or receive a parental living liver donation could develop an evident degree of immune tolerance concerning the graft. Single center experiences demonstrate that patients who were withdrawn from immunosuppression because of medical reasons (such as renal insufficiency) or due to noncompliance suggest that around 20% of liver transplant patients develop operationally tolerance regarding the graft [157–162]. Another more aggressive approach to induce immune tolerance in solid organ transplantation is to combine solid organ transplantation with hematopoietic stem cell transplantation from the same donor [1,163–165].

Complete freedom from immunosuppression or significant withdrawal of immunosuppression is possible in long-surviving recipients of liver allografts [159,166,167]. The drug weaning protocol established for pediatric liver transplant patients at the University of Pittsburgh includes long-term survivors who are medically compliant and have normal liver function without recent acute rejection episodes within the past 2 years. Drug withdrawal was begun at a mean time of 6 years after liver transplantation. The baseline immunosuppressant of tacrolimus or cyclosporine was weaned at 2-month to 3-month intervals as long as hepatocellular enzyme tests remained stable. Liver injury tests of aspartate aminotransferase (AST), alanine aminotransferase (ALT), gamma glutamyltransferase (GGTP), and bilirubin are monitored weekly after changes in drug dosage. Tacrolimus or cyclosporine levels are not used in monitoring because baseline levels in this patient population are frequently low or undetectable. Liver biopsy is done for sustained alterations in liver tests. Forty percent (17 of 43) of the patients were off immunosuppression, with a mean time from weaning of 1.7 years. No patient or graft loss has occurred. Rejection has occurred in 14% of patients (6 of 43), being mild in two patients and mild to moderate in four patients, prompting switch to tacrolimus from cyclosporine-based immunosuppression. Pediatric patients have the greatest potential benefit from the significant dosage reductions or complete drug withdrawal that can be potentially realized [2].

However, it is not without risk and it must be done with great care because no marker is available to identify the patients who have developed graft acceptance operational tolerance [168]. Three main objectives should be pursued in PLT regarding immunosuppression: (1) reduction and individualization of immunosuppression in order to diminish long-term side effects; (2) maintenance of long-term allograft function; and (3) monitor and induce tolerance through the development of specific protocols, as well as identify operationally tolerant and nontolerant patients [1].

8. Adherence

Nonadherence to the medical regimen is part of the risk-taking spectrum of behavior [77], and approximately 33–50% of adolescents with a chronic illness are nonadherent in some way with their treatment protocol [169]. There is a clear association between medication nonadherence and unfavorable transplant outcome.

Several studies investigate the role of different factors predisposing to medication nonadherence [170]. In a recent study, 75% of post-LT adolescents were nonadherent and reported poorer health perceptions, lower self-esteem, more limitations in social and school activities, and poorer mental health than those who were adherent [171]. Factors such as history of substance abuse, previous psychiatric problems, older age, female gender, and living in a one-parent household have been associated with poorer adherence [172,173].

Nonadherence to medication is associated with increased medical complications and higher rates of rejection and graft loss [174–176]. In addition, other aspects of nonadherence include clinic nonattendance, missing routine blood tests, and inconsistent timing of medications. The desire to be like their friends can result in nonadherence to different aspects of the treatment regimen. The monitoring and management of nonadherence can be challenging, necessitating a nonjudgmental approach, with a focus on individual adherence plans, improved education, behavioral strategies to encourage self-management and self-motivation and a recognition of the role of treatment burden for patients, and their families [6,177].

9. Complication

The main causes of graft loss in the first week include primary nonfunction (PNF), hepatic artery or portal vein thrombosis, systemic sepsis, and multiorgan failure (<10%). Other significant early complications are acute (50%) or chronic rejection (10%), biliary leaks/strictures (5–25%), viral infections (especially cytomegalovirus (CMV) and Epstein Barr virus), and acute kidney injury and fluid imbalance [7–12]. The most frequent complications are listed in **Table 2**.

Complications after liver transplant
Hemorrhage
Primary nonfunction
Hepatic artery thrombosis
Acute rejection
Chronic rejection
Biliary leak/stenosis
Infection
Bacterial
Opportunistic
Viral (e.g., CMV)
Fungal
Pneumocystis
Acute renal failure
Fluid imbalance

Table 2. Complications after liver transplant.

Intraoperative bleeding in PLT is commonly less of a problem than in adults, even though the majority of the children will have had previous surgery on the liver. This can be explained by the fact that portal hypertension as measured by portal vein pressure is less severe in the child than in the adult, possibly consequence of more effective collateral vessel formation [5].

Thrombosis of the hepatic artery is a major concern in PLT with rates varying from 10 to 25%. This ischemia, when occurring in the early posttransplant period, produces either acute graft failure or biliary tree infarction with bile leakage and intra- or extrahepatic abscess formation [5]. Early hepatic artery thrombosis (HAT) is the most common form of vascular complication and is the main cause of graft loss in pediatric living-related liver transplantation (LRLT) [178]. Early diagnosis and treatment can prevent biliary tract and parenchymal damage [179]. Bekker et al reported an incidence for early HAT in pediatric LT of 8.3% compared to 2.9% in adults. [180]. Hepatic artery stenosis and thrombosis can result in allograft ischemia, which is associated with high mortality and morbidity rate. Arterial complications are frequently diagnosed first by Doppler ultrasound followed by CT angiogram or angiography. Doppler ultrasound showed a sensitivity of 100%, a specificity of 99.5%, a PPV of 95% and NPV of 100%, and overall accuracy of 99.5% in early diagnosis of HAS [179]. According to the interval between LT and development of thrombosis, HAT can be divided into early (within 4 weeks) and late. Usually, early HAT may be the result of technical problems and can have dramatic presentation [181]. Due to the fact that early HAT has a higher mortality comparing to late HAT, intervention is required as urgent procedure [182]. Late HAT is usually due to ischemic or immunologic injuries. Patients with late symptomatic HAT can be initially treated with biliary stent placement and/or endovascular interventions [181].

Positive CMV antibody in donor and negative CMV recipients has been shown to be associated with late HAT [183–186]. Some authors also suggest that perioperative hypercoagulable state as the possible underlying cause for hepatic artery thrombosis [180–187]. Although urgent retransplantation is considered the main therapy for early HAT, endovascular interventions, including PTA, intra-arterial thrombolysis (IAT), and stent placement, may be alternative treatments.

Venous complications after PLT include caval/hepatic vein and portal problems. Clinical manifestations of portal vein stenosis (PVS) include ascites, anemia, splenomegaly, and gastrointestinal bleeding [188–191]. Platelet counts may be below normal limit in pediatric patients with PVS due to hypersplenism [192]. The incidence of portal vein complications is usually higher in pediatric recipients than in adults. Smaller portal vein diameter, size disparity between donor's and recipient's portal vein, and short pedicle of the donor's portal vein are risk factors for portal vein complications [193–196].

Clinically hepatic vein obstruction (HVO) is analogous to Budd-Chiari syndrome [197]. HVO is a general term reflecting any obstruction of the hepatic veins caused by either compression and twisting of the anastomosis. It can be caused by graft regeneration or by intimal hyperplasia and fibrosis at the anastomotic sites [198]. Risk factors related to portal vein complications include technical problems, young age, body weight <6 kg, the recipient's portal vein size <5 mm, graft rotation, previous splenectomy, simultaneous thrombectomy for pre-existing PVT, and use of venous conduits for portal vein reconstruction [9,193,199–204]. Cold ischemia time longer than 12 h can also be a impose risk for developing venous problems. Portal vein stenosis is mostly associated with cryopreserved vein for portal conduits. Portal vein hypoplasia is one of the main risk factors for developing vascular complications in pediatric recipients of LT, particularly when biliary atresia is the indication for LT [205,206]. Suzuki et al. [207] reported a portal vein diameter of <3.5 mm to be the single most sensitive and specific predictor of portal vein stenosis.

Endovascular interventions are less invasive treatment for post-LT vascular complications particularly in pediatric patients. In cases of post-LT HVO, percutaneous endovascular treatment with balloon dilation and/or stent placement can be used as a safe treatment with high success rate. Complications, such as ascites, renal failure, lower limb edema, and splenomegaly, can be resolved after endovascular interventions [208]. Simultaneous obstruction of HV and IVC can also be treated with endovascular interventions. However, isolated HV stenosis is better treated with balloon-expandable stent treatment than with balloon dilation [209].

Although balloon dilation is an effective and relatively safe procedure for treatment of portal vein stenosis, 28–50% of these patients may develop recurrent PVS [210–213]. Previous reports suggest stent placement and repeated balloon dilation as solutions for this problem [212,213]. Sanada et al. [202] showed combined anticoagulant therapy using LMW heparin, warfarin, and aspirin can significantly lower the risk of recurrent PVS [214].

9.1. Biliary complications

The presentation of biliary complications is quite variable. The diagnosis biliary leakages (BL) usually are straightforward and presents early in the posttransplant period. Biliary stenosis (BS) has a more indolent progression and usually is diagnosed later. BS demands a high index of suspicion because in the initial phases the clinical picture can be confused with rejection, infection and primary disease recurrence [215].

Early complications, occurring within 30 days of the transplant, usually are consequence of technical problems. These include handling and harvesting of the graft, preservation injuries, surgical technique of biliary reconstruction, or even vascular insufficiency [216]. Late complications, occurring after 90 days posttransplant, are classified into anastomotic (AS) and nonanastomotic strictures (NAS). NAS are associated to the use of ABO-incompatible grafts, preservation injury, opportunistic infections, recurrent hepatitis, ductopenic rejection, recurrent primary sclerosing cholangitis (PSC), stones or casts, posttransplant lymphoproliferative disorder or other tumors [216].

Long cold ischemia time, hepatic artery thrombosis (HAT), CMV infection, and chronic rejection constitute risk factors for biliary anastomotic complications (leaks and strictures). Also, tissue hypoxia at level of the anastomosis, secondary to hepatopulmonary syndrome, can increase the frequency of biliary complications after liver transplantation [217]. Multiple bile ducts, requiring reconstruction or more than one biliary anastomosis is an independent risk factor for the development of biliary complications with a higher incidence of biliary complications when compared with a single duct (21% versus 9%, respectively) [218].

Treatment strategies are based on the type and severity of the complication and the biliary reconstruction technique applied, duct-to-duct anastomosis or hepaticojejunostomy. Nonoperative management is the first-line approach, and success can be achieved in 70–90% of all BS cases [219–222]. A novel magnetic compression anastomosis has been recently described. Transmural compression with two magnets causes gradual ischemic necrosis, thus creating a new anastomosis between the dilated duct and small intestine or bile duct. This technique has been applied in only few cases, and further experience is necessary before it has broader indications [215,223,224].

The majority of patients will experience at least one episode of acute rejection. However, usually it is treated increasing the steroid. Small bile ducts destruction shown on biopsy is typical finding of chronic rejection. This type of rejection is not reversible by increasing immunosuppression. Repeated biopsy with histological confirmation is necessary to establish this diagnosis. When chronic rejection occurs, the only treatment is retransplantation [5].

Immunosuppressed patients have a higher risk for infection complications. Common bacterial infections, usually in the respiratory and biliary tracts, opportunistic infections are a potential problem. The commonest of these are cytomegalovirus and fungal infections. Donor and recipient CMV status matching of both graft and blood products can minimize CMV infections [5].

When CMV-negative patient receives a CMV-positive graft, prophylactic treatment with acyclovir has been shown to be effective in minimizing the severity of any resulting CMV infection. Fungal infections are not rare after liver transplant, since the majority of children with chronic liver disease are heavily colonized with candida. Limited use of broad-spectrum antibiotics and oral antibiotic prophylaxis may reduce the incidence and severity of fungal sepsis. Pneumocystis infection is an additional risk in these patients. Any of these infections is associated with a high mortality. Prophylaxis with oral cotrimoxazole is nearly always effective for these risks [5].

Another rare complication of LDLT in pediatrics is the graft rotation. Previous studies showed that the graft rotation can lead to venous outflow obstruction and suggested stabilization of the graft to avoid this complication [225,226]. Several surgical factors might have an important role in preventing vascular thrombosis, especially in the transplantation of live donor or split liver allografts. Adequate inflow in the donor vessels is also important to reduce vascular complications. The use of interposition grafts (arteries or veins) is stimulate in the case of small-caliber vessels or a fibrotic and small portal vein, common observed in children with biliary atresia [224].

Oversized grafts are prone to compression after abdominal wall closure, which may compromise the flow in the afferent hepatic vessels increasing the risk for thrombosis. Delayed abdominal wall closure is recommended in these situations, avoiding tight wound closure, and consequently avoiding augmented intra-abdominal pressure. Administration of antiplatelet agents early in posttransplant, such as aspirin, has been advocated to prevent HAT [227, 228].

10. Conclusion

In conclusion, LT in the pediatric setting is technically challenging due to the reduced size of the vasculature and biliary tree. Discrepancies in portal vein and hepatic arterial diameter between the donor and recipient are expected. Despite technical evolution of pediatric liver transplantation, vascular complications are still a significant cause of allograft loss, reflecting in increase of postoperative morbidity and mortality. Arterial complications are more common, occur early in the postoperative period, and are associated with high rates of graft loss and patient mortality. On the other hand, venous complications are less frequent usually occurring in the late postoperative period with no significant effect on graft loss or mortality rates. Important strategies for reduction of mortality, morbidity, and the need for retransplantation include detection and mitigation of risk factors, avoidance of technical complications, and protocols for prompt detection of vascular complications.

Author details

Julio Cesar Wiederkehr[1,2*], Barbara de Aguiar Wiederkehr[2,3] and
Henrique de Aguiar Wiederkehr[3,4]

*Address all correspondence to: julio.wieder@gmail.com

1 Professor of Surgery, Federal University of Parana, Chief, Division of Liver Transplantation Hospital Pequeno Principe, Curitiba, Brazil

2 Resident in Gastrointestinal Surgery, Evangelic University Hospital of Curitiba, Curitiba, Brazil

3 Resident in Gastrointestinal Surgery, Evangelic University Hospital of Curitiba, Curitiba, Brazil

4 Resident in General Surgery Evangelic University Hospital of Curitiba, Curitiba, Brazil

References

[1] Hackl C. Current developments in pediatric liver transplantation. World J Hepatol. 2015;7(11):1509.

[2] Otte JB. History of pediatric liver transplantation. Where are we coming from? Where do we stand? Pediatric Transplant. 2002;6(5):378–387. http://doi.org/10.1034/j.1399-3046.2002.01082.x.

[3] Starzl TE, Iwatsuki S, Klintmalm G, Schröter GP, Weil R, Koep LJ, Porter KA. Liver transplantation, 1980, with particular reference to cyclosporin-A. Transplant Proc. 1981;13:281–285 [PMID: 7022839].

[4] Starzl TE, Todo S, Tzakis AG, Gordon RD, Makowka L, Stieber A, Podesta L, Yanaga K, Concepcion W, Iwatsuki S. Liver transplantation: an unfinished product. Transplant Proc. 1989;21:2197–2200 [PMID: 2469232].

[5] Buckels JA. Paediatric liver transplantation: review of current experience. J Inherited Metab Dis. 1991;14(4):596–603.

[6] Kelly D. The adolescent liver transplant patient pediatric liver transplantation. Adolescent Adherence. Clin Liver Dis 2014;18:613–632.

[7] Duffy JP, Kao K, Ko CY, et al. Long-term patient outcome and quality of life after liver transplantation: analysis of 20-year survivors. Ann Surg. 2010;252(4):652–661.

[8] Kamath BM, Olthoff KM. Liver transplantation in children: update 2010. Pediatr Clin North Am. 2010;57(2):401–414.

[9] Duffy JP, Hong JC, Farmer DG, et al. Vascular complications of orthotopic liver transplantation: experience in more than 4,200 patients. J Am Coll Surg. 2009;208(5): 896–903 [discussion: 903–905].

[10] Anderson CD, Turmelle YP, Darcy M, et al. Biliary strictures in pediatric liver transplant recipients – early diagnosis and treatment results in excellent graft outcomes. Pediatr Transplant. 2010;14(3):358–363.

[11] Martin SR, Atkison P, Anand R, et al. Studies of pediatric liver transplantation 2002: patient and graft survival and rejection in pediatric recipients of a first liver transplant in the United States and Canada. Pediatr Transplant 2004;8(3):273–283.

[12] Heffron TG, Pillen T, Smallwood G, et al. Incidence, impact, and treatment of portal and hepatic venous complications following pediatric liver transplantation: a single-center 12-year experience. Pediatr Transplant. 2010;14(6):722–729.

[13] Reyes J, Mazariegos GV. Pediatric transplantation. Surg Clin N Am. 1999;79(1):163–189.

[14] Starzl TE, et al. Orthotopic homotransplantation of the human liver. Ann Surg. 1968;1680:392415.

[15] Starzl TE, Marchioro TL, Von Kaulla K, et al. Homotransplantation of the liver in humans. Surg Gynecol Obstet. 1963;117659.

[16] Starzl TE, Klintmalm GB, Porter KA, et al. Liver transplantation with use of cyclosporin A and prednisone. N Engl J Med. 1981:305:266–269.

[17] Alpert O, Sharma V, Cama S, Spencer S, Huang H. Liver transplant and quality of life in the pediatric population. Curr Opin Organ Transplant. 2015;20(2):216–221.

[18] Squires RH Jr, Shneider BL, Bucuvalas J, et al. Acute liver failure in children: the first 348 patients in the pediatric acute liver failure study group. J Pediatr. 2006;148:652.

[19] Squires RH Jr. Acute liver failure in children. Semin Liver Dis. 2008;28:153.

[20] Squires RH, Alonso EM. Acute liver failure in children. In: Suchy FJ, Sokol RJ, Balistreri WF (Eds.), Liver Disease in Children, 4th ed. Cambridge University Press, New York, 2012.

[21] OPTN/SRTR 2011 annual data report: liver. Accessed at http://srtr.transplant.hrsa.gov/annual_reports/2011.

[22] Kruper A, Zanowski SC. Parental live liver donation. Curr Opin Organ Transplant. 2015;20(2):140–145.

[23] Kelly DA. Current results and evolving indications for liver transplantation in children. J Pediatr Gastroenterol Nutr. 1998;27:214–221.

[24] McKiernan PJ, Baker AJ, Kelly DA. The frequency and outcome of biliary atresia in the UK and Ireland. Lancet 2000;355:25.

[25] Hartley JL, Davenport M, Kelly DA. Biliary atresia. Lancet. 2009;374(9702):1704–1713.

[26] Tannuri ACA, Gibelli NEM, Ricardi LRS, Silva MM, Santos MM, Pinho-Apezzato ML, et al. Orthotopic liver transplantation in biliary atresia: a single-center experience. Transplant Proc. 2011;43(1):181–183.

[27] Takahashi Y, Nishimoto Y, Matsuura T, et al. Surgical complications after living donor liver transplantation in patients with biliary atresia: a relatively high incidence of portal vein complications. Pediatr Surg Int. 2009;25:745.

[28] Starzl TE, Esquivel V, Gordon R, et al. Pediatric liver transplantation. Transplant Proc 1987;19:3230.

[29] Millis JM, Brems JJ, Hiatt JR, et al. Orthotopic liver transplantation for biliary atresia. Arch Surg. 1988;123:1237.

[30] Serinet MO, Wildhaber BE, Broué P, et al. Impact of age at Kasai operation on its results in late childhood and adolescence: a rational basis for biliary atresia screening. Pediatrics. 2009 May;123(5):1280-1286. doi:10.1542/peds.2008-1949.

[31] Humphrey TM, Stringer MD. Biliary atresia: US diagnosis. Radiology. 2007 Sep;244(3): 845–851.

[32] Lee MS, Kim MJ, Lee MJ, et al. Biliary atresia: color Doppler US findings in neonates and infants. Radiology. 2009 Jul;252(1):282–289. doi:10.1148/radiol.2522080923.

[33] Takamizawa S1, Zaima A, Muraji T, et al. Can biliary atresia be diagnosed by ultrasonography alone? J Pediatr Surg. 2007 Dec;42(12):2093–2096.

[34] Mittal V, Saxena AK, Sodhi KS, et al. Role of abdominal sonography in the preoperative diagnosis of extrahepatic biliary atresia in infants younger than 90 days. AJR Am J Roentgenol. 2011 Apr;196(4):W438–W445. doi:10.2214/AJR.10.5180.

[35] Park WH, Choi SO, Lee HJ, et al. A new diagnostic approach to biliary atresia with emphasis on the ultrasonographic triangular cord sign: comparison of ultrasonography, hepatobiliary scintigraphy, and liver needle biopsy in the evaluation of infantile cholestasis. J Pediatr Surg. 1997 Nov;32(11):1555–1559.

[36] Azar G, Beneck D, Lane B, et al. Atypical morphologic presentation of biliary atresia and value of serial liver biopsies. J Pediatr Gastroenterol Nutr 2002;34:212.

[37] UPTODATE found at http://www.uptodate.com/contents/biliary-atresia?source=search_result&search=Histologic+findings+alone+cannot+help+to+distinguish+BA&selectedTitle=1%7E150 in Feb/2016.

[38] Leonhardt J, Kuebler JF, Leute PJ, Turowski C, Becker T, Pfister ED, et al. Biliary atresia: lessons learned from the voluntary German registry. Eur J Pediatr Surg 2011;2(21)82–87.

[39] Shinkai M, Ohhama Y, Take H, Kitagawa N, Kudo H, Mochizuki K, et al. Long-term outcome of children with biliary atresia who were not transplanted after the Kasai operation: >20-year experience at a children's hospital. J Pediatr Gastroenterol Nutr. 2009;48:443–450.

[40] Jung E, Park WH, Choi SO. Late complications and current status of long-term survivals over 10 years after Kasai portoenterostomy. J Korean Surg Soc. 2011;81(4):271–275. http://doi.org/10.4174/jkss.2011.81.4.271.

[41] Helbling D, Buchaklian A, Wang J, et al. Reduced mitochondrial DNA content and heterozygous nuclear gene mutations in patients with acute liver failure. J Pediatr Gastroenterol Nutr. 2013;57:438.

[42] Sundaram SS, Alonso EM, Narkewicz MR, et al. Characterization and outcomes of young infants with acute liver failure. J Pediatr. 2011;159:813.

[43] UPTODATE. http://www.uptodate.com/contents/acute-liver-failure-in-children-etiology-and-evaluation.

[44] Francavilla R, Castellaneta SP, Hadzic N, et al. Prognosis of alpha-a-antitrypsin deficiency-related liver disease in the era of paediatric liver transplantation. J Hepatol. 2000;32:986–992.

[45] Kayler LK, Rasmussen CS, Dykstra DM, et al. Liver transplantation in children with metabolic disorders in the United States. Am J Transplant 2003;3(3):334–339.

[46] Hoerning A, Raub S, Dechêne A, et al. Diversity of disorders causing neonatal cholestasis — the experience of a tertiary pediatric center in Germany. Front Pediatr. 2014 Jun 23;2:65. doi:10.3389/fped.2014.00065. eCollection 2014.

[47] Fischler B, Papadogiannakis N, Nemeth A. Aetiological factors in neonatal cholestasis. Acta Paediatr. 2001 Jan;90(1):88–92.

[48] Coakley RJ, Taggart C, O'Neill S, McElvaney NG. Alpha1-antitrypsin deficiency: biological answers to clinical questions. Am J Med Sci. 2001 Jan;321(1):33–41.

[49] Perlmutter DH. Alpha-1-antitrypsin deficiency. Semin Liver Dis. 1998;18(3):217–225.

[50] McDaniell R, Warthen DM, Sanchez-Lara PA, et al. NOTCH2 mutations cause Alagille syndrome, a heterogeneous disorder of the notch signaling pathway. Am J Hum Genet. 2006;79(1):169–173.

[51] Kaye AJ1, Rand EB, Munoz PS, et al. Effect of Kasai procedure on hepatic outcome in Alagille syndrome. J Pediatr Gastroenterol Nutr. 2010 Sep;51(3):319–321. doi:10.1097/MPG.0b013e3181df5fd8.

[52] Kamath BM, Yin W, Miller H, et al. Outcomes of liver transplantation for patients with Alagille syndrome: the studies of pediatric liver transplantation experience. Liver Transpl. 2012 Aug;18(8):940–948. doi:10.1002/lt.23437.

[53] Weinberg AG, Mize CE, Worthen HG. The occurrence of hepatoma in the chronic form of hereditary tyrosinemia. J Pediatr 1976;88:434–438.

[54] McKiernan PJ. Nitisinone in the treatment of hereditary tyrosinaemia type 1. Drugs. 2006;66:743–750.

[55] Rowe SM, Miller S, Sorscher EJ. Mechanisms of disease, cystic fibrosis. N Engl J Med. 2005;352:1992–2001.

[56] Colombo C, Battezzati PM, Strazzabosco M, Podda M. Liver and biliary problems in cystic fibrosis. Semin Liver Dis. 1998;18(3):227–235.

[57] Debray D, Lykavieris P, Gauthier F, et al. Outcome of cystic fibrosis-associated liver cirrhosis: management of portal hypertension. J Hepatol. 1999;31:77–83.

[58] Milkiewicz P, Skiba G, Kelly D, et al. Transplantation for cystic fibrosis: outcome following early liver transplantation. J Gastroenterol Hepatol 2002;17:208.

[59] Frydman M, Bonne-Tamir B, Farrer LA, et al. Assignment of the gene for Wilson disease to chromosome 13: linkage to the esterase D locus. Proc Natl Acad Sci USA. 1985;82:1819–1821.

[60] Dhawan A, Taylor RM, Cheeseman P, et al. Wilson's disease in children: 37-year experience and revised King's score for liver transplantation. Liver Transplant 2005;11:441–448.

[61] Rela M, Heaton ND, Vougas V, et al. Orthotopic liver transplantation for hepatic complications of Wilson's disease. Br J Surg. 1993;80:909–911.

[62] UPTODATE. Accessed at http://www.uptodate.com/contents/acute-liver-failure-in-children-etiology-and-evaluation?source=search_result&search=%27Acute+liver

+failure+in+children% 3A+Etiology+and+evaluation%27&selectedTitle=1%7E150 in Jan 2016.

[63] Labrune P, Myara A, Hadchouel M, et al. Genetic heterogeneity of Crigler-Najjar syndrome type I: a study of 14 cases. Hum Genet. 1994;94(6):693–697.

[64] Rezvani I, Auerbach VH. Primaryhyperoxaluria. N Engl J Med. 2013;369(22):2162–2163.

[65] Strobele B, Loveland J, Britz R, et al. Combined paediatric liver-kidney transplantation: analysis of our experience and literature review. S Afr Med J 2013;103(12):925–929.

[66] Ries LAG, Smith MA, Gurney JG, Linet M, Tamra T, Young JL, Bunin GR (Eds.), Cancer Incidence and Survival among Children and Adolescents: United States SEER Program 1975–1995. National Cancer Institute, SEER Program. Bethesda, MD, NIH. Pub. 1999: 99-4649. Available from: URL: http://seer.cancer.gov/archive/publications/childhood/.

[67] Ismail H, Broniszczak D, Kaliciński P, Dembowska-Bagińska B, Perek D, Teisseyre J, Kluge P, Kościesza A, Lembas A, Markiewicz M. Changing treatment and outcome of children with hepatoblastoma: analysis of a single center experience over the last 20 years. J Pediatr Surg. 2012;47: 1331–1339 [PMID: 22813792, doi:10.1016/j.jpedsurg.2011.11.073].

[68] Howlader N, Noone AM, Krapcho M, Neyman N, Aminou R, Waldron W, Altekruse SF, Kosary CL, Ruhl J, Tatalovich Z, Cho H, Mariotto A, Eisner MP, Lewis DR, Chen HS, Feuer EJ, Cronin KA (Eds.), SEER Cancer Statistics Review, 1975–2009 (Vintage 2009 Populations). National Cancer Institute. Based on November 2011 SEER data submission, posted to the SEER web site, April 2012 [Updated August 20, 2012]. Available from: URL: http://seer.cancer.gov/ archive/csr/1975_2009_pops09/.

[69] Litten JB, Tomlinson GE. Liver tumors in children. Oncologist. 2008;13:812–820 [PMID: 18644850 doi: 10.1634/ theoncologist.2008-0011].

[70] Otte JB, De Ville de Goyet J. The contribution of transplantation to the treatment of liver tumors in children. Semin Pediatr Surg. 2015;14:233–238.

[71] Czauderna P, Otte JB, Aronson DC, et al. Guidelines for surgical treatment of hepatoblastoma in the modern era: recommendations from the childhood liver tumour strategy group of the International Society of Paediatric Oncology (SIO-PEL). Eur J Cancer. 2005;41:1031–1036.

[72] Dall'Igna P, Cecchetto G, Toffolutti T, et al. Multifocal hepatoblastoma is there a place for partial hepatectomy? Med Pediatr Oncol. 2003;40:113–116.

[73] Chardot C, Sant Martin C, Gilles A, et al. Living related liver transplantation and vena cava reconstruction after total hepatectomy including the vena cava for hepatoblastoma. Transplantation 2002;73:90–92.

[74] Czauderna P, Mac Kinley G, Perilongo G, et al. Hepatocellular carcinoma in children: results of the first prospective study of the international society of pediatric oncology group. J Clin Oncol. 2002;20:2798–804.

[75] Millar AJW, Hartley P, Khan D, et al. Extended hepatic resection with transplantation back-up for an unresectable tumor. Pediatric Surg Int. 2001;17:378–81.

[76] Austin MT, Leys CM, Feurer ID, et al. Liver transplantation for childhood hepatic malignancy: a review of the United Network for Organ Sharing (UNOS) database. J Pediatr Surg. 2006;41:182–186.

[77] Otte JB. Progress in the surgical treatment of malignant liver tumors in children. Cancer Treat Rev. 2010;36(4):360–371. Elsevier Ltd.

[78] Wiederkehr JC, Coelho IM, Avilla SG, Wiederkehr BA, Wiederkehr HA. Liver tumors in infancy (n.d.).

[79] Hoti E, Adam R. Liver transplantation for primary and metastatic liver cancers. Transplant Int. 2008;21:1107–1117.

[80] Srinivasan P, Mc Call J, Pritchard J, et al. Orthotopic liver transplantation for unresectable hepatoblastoma. Transplantation. 2002;74:652–655.

[81] Tagge EP, Tagge DU, Reyes J, et al. Resection, including transplantation, for hepatoblastoma and hepatocellular carcinoma: impact on survival. J Pediatr Surg. 1992;27:292–296 [discussion 297].

[82] Freeman RB, Jr, Edwards EB. Liver transplant waiting time does not correlate with waiting list mortality: implications for liver allocation policy. Liver Transplant. 2000;6(5):543–552.

[83] Organ Procurement and Transplantation Network-HRSA. Final rule with comment period. Fed Regist. 1998;63:16296–16338.

[84] Mazzaferro V, Regalia E, Doci R, et al.. Liver transplantation for the treatment of small hepatocellular carcinoma in patients with cirrhosis. New Engl J Med. 1996;334:693–699.

[85] Terracciano L, Tornillo L. Cytogenetic alteration in liver cell tumors as detected by comparative genomic hybridization. Pathologica. 2003;95:71–82.

[86] Bravo LC, Gregorio GV, Shafi F, et al. Etiology, incidence and outcomes of acute hepatic failure in 0–18 year old Filipino children. Southeast Asian J Trop Med Public Health. 2012;43(3):764–772.

[87] Baris Z, Saltik Temızel IN, Uslu N, et al. Acute liver failure in children: 20-year experience. Turk J Gastroenterol. 2012;23(2):127–134.

[88] Lee WS, McKiernan P, Kelly DA. Etiology, outcome and prognostic indicators of childhood fulminant hepatic failure in the United Kingdom. J Pediatr Gastroenterol Nutr. 2005;40:575–581.

[89] Murray KF, Hadzic N, Wirth S, et al. Drug-related hepatotoxicity and acute liver failure. J Pediatr Gastroenterol Nutr. 2008;47:395–405.

[90] Lauterberg BH, Vaishnar Y, Stillwell WB, et al. The effects of age and glutathione depletion on hepatic glutathione turnover in vivo determined by acetaminophen probe analysis. J Pharmacol Exp Ther. 1980;213:54–58.

[91] Mahadevan SB, McKiernan PJ, Davies P, et al. Paracetamol induced hepatotoxicity. Arch Dis Child 2006;91(7):598–603.

[92] Yao FY, Ferrell L, Bass NM, et al. Liver transplantation for hepatocellular carcinoma: expansion of the tumor size limits does not adversely impact survival. Hepatology. 2001;33:1394–1403.

[93] Sokal EM, Van Hoorebeeck N, Van Obbergh L, et al. Upper gastro-intestinal tract bleeding in cirrhotic children candidates for liver transplantation. Eur J Pediatr. 1992:151:326–328.

[94] Hall RJ, Lilly JR, Stiegmann GV Endoscopic esophageal varix ligation: technique and preliminary results in children. J Pediatr Surg. 1988:23:1222–1223.

[95] Berger H, Bugnon F, Goffette P, et al. Percutaneous transjugular intrahepatic stent shunt for treatment of intractable varicose bleeding in paediatric patients. Eur J Pediatr. 1994:153:721–725.

[96] UPTODATE. Accessed at http://www.uptodate.com/contents/immunizations-in-solid-organ-transplant-candidates-and-recipients in Jan 2016.

[97] Kasai M, Kimura S, Asakura Y, et al. Surgical treatment of biliary atresia. J Pediatr Surg. 1968:3:665–675.

[98] Malatack JJ, Schaid DJ, Urbach AH, et al. Choosing a pediatric recipient for orthotopic liver transplantation. J Pediatr. 1987:111:479–489.

[99] Hobeika J, Houssin D, Bernard O, et al. Orthotopic liver transplantation in children with chronic liver disease and severe hypoxemia. Transplantation 1994;57:224–228.

[100] Ventura K. Ethical considerations in live liver donation to children. Prog Transplant 2010; 20:186–190.

[101] Duerinckx N, Timmerman L, Van Gogh J, et al. Predonation psychosocial & evaluation of living kidney and liver donor candidates: a systematic literature review. Transplant Int. 2014;27:2–18.

[102] Broelsch CE, Emond JC, Thistlethwaite JR, Whitington PF, Zucker AR, Baker AL, Aran PF, Rouch DA, Lichtor JL. Liver transplantation, including the concept of reduced-size liver transplants in children. Ann Surg. 1988;208:410–420 [PMID: 3052326].

[103] Broelsch CE, Emond JC, Thistlethwaite JR, Rouch DA, Whitington PF, Lichtor JL. Liver transplantation with reduced-size donor organs. Transplantation. 1988;45:519–524 [PMID: 3279573].

[104] Pichlmayr R, Ringe B, Gubernatis G, Hauss J, Bunzendahl H. Transplantation of a donor liver to 2 recipients (splitting transplantation)—a new method in the further development of segmental liver transplantation. Langenbecks Arch Chir. 1988;373:127–130 [PMID: 3287073].

[105] Eurotransplant International Foundation. EAR 2013. Available from: http://www.eurotransplant.org/cms/index.php?page=annual_reports.

[106] Couinaud C. Liver lobes and segments: notes on the anatomical architecture and surgery of the liver. Presse Med. 1954;62:709–712 [PMID: 13177441].

[107] Couinaud C. Liver anatomy: portal (and suprahepatic) or biliary segmentation. Dig Surg. 1999; 16:459–467 [PMID: 10805544].

[108] Kanazawa H, Sakamoto S, Fukuda A, Uchida H, Hamano I, Shigeta T, Kobayashi M, Karaki C, Tanaka H, Kasahara M. Living-donor liver transplantation with hyperreduced left lateral segment grafts: a single-center experience. Transplantation. 2013;95:750–754 [PMID: 23503505, doi: 10.1097/TP.0b013e31827a93b4].

[109] Caso Maestro O, Abradelo de Usera M, Justo Alonso I, Calvo Pulido J, Manrique Municio A, Cambra Molero F, García Sesma A, Loinaz Segurola C, Moreno González E, Jiménez Romero C. Porcine acellular dermal matrix for delayed abdominal wall closure after pediatric liver transplantation. Pediatr Transplant. 2014;18:594–598 [PMID: 25039398, doi:10.1111/petr.12319].

[110] Gubernatis G, Pichlmayr R, Kemnitz J, Gratz K. Auxiliary partial orthotopic liver transplantation (APOLT) for fulminant hepatic failure: first successful case report. World J Surg. 1991; 15:660–665; discussion 665–666 [PMID: 1949867].

[111] Melter M, Grothues D, Knoppke B. Pädiatrische Lebertrans- plantation. Monatsschr Kinderheilkd. 2012;160:343–357 [doi:10.1007/s00112-011-2561-9].

[112] Faraj W, Dar F, Bartlett A, Melendez HV, Marangoni G, Mukherji D, Vergani GM, Dhawan A, Heaton N, Rela M. Auxiliary liver transplantation for acute liver failure in children. Ann Surg. 2010; 251: 351–356 [PMID: 20054274, doi:10.1097/SLA.0b013e3181b dfef6].

[113] Shanmugam NP, Dhawan A. Selection criteria for liver trans- plantation in paediatric acute liver failure: the saga continues. Pediatr Transplant. 2011;15:5–6 [PMID: 21241436, doi:10.1111/j.1399-3046.2010.01457.x].

[114] Broelsch CE, Emond JC, Whitington PF, Thistlethwaite JR, Baker AL, Lichtor JL. Application of reduced-size liver transplants as split grafts, auxiliary orthotopic grafts, and living related segmental transplants. Ann Surg. 1990;212:368–375; discussion 375–377 [PMID: 2396888].

[115] Raia S, et al. Liver transplantation from live donors. Lancet. 334(8661):497.

[116] Lee SG, Moon DB. Living donor liver transplantation for hepatocellular carcinoma. Recent Results Cancer Res. 2013;190:165–179 [PMID: 22941020, doi: 10.1007/978-3-642-16037-0_11].

[117] Organ Procurement and Transplantation Network. [Accessed 2014 Dec 1]. Available from: URL: http://optn.transplant.hrsa.gov/ converge/latestdata/rptData.asp.

[118] Bhangui P, Vibert E, Majno P, Salloum C, Andreani P, Zocrato J, Ichai P, Saliba F, Adam R, Castaing D, Azoulay D. Intention-to-treat analysis of liver transplantation for hepatocellular carcinoma: living versus deceased donor transplantation. Hepatology. 2011;53:1570–1579 [PMID: 21520172, doi:10.1002/hep.24231].

[119] Gondolesi GE, Roayaie S, Muñoz L, Kim-Schluger L, Schiano T, Fishbein TM, Emre S, Miller CM, Schwartz ME. Adult living donor liver transplantation for patients with hepatocellular carcinoma: extending UNOS priority criteria. Ann Surg. 2004;239:142–149 [PMID: 14745320, doi: 10.1097/01.sla.0000109022.32391.eb].

[120] Grant RC, Sandhu L, Dixon PR, Greig PD, Grant DR, McGilvray ID. Living vs. deceased donor liver transplantation for hepatocellular carcinoma: a systematic review and meta-analysis. Clin Transplant. 2013;27:140–147 [PMID: 23157398, doi:10.1111/ctr.12031].

[121] Kaihara S, Kiuchi T, Ueda M, Oike F, Fujimoto Y, Ogawa K, Kozaki K, Tanaka K. Living-donor liver transplantation for hepatocellular carcinoma. Transplantation. 2003;75:S37–S40 [PMID: 12589138, doi:10.1097/01.TP.0000047029.02806.16].

[122] Sandhu L, Sandroussi C, Guba M, Selzner M, Ghanekar A, Cattral MS, McGilvray ID, Levy G, Greig PD, Renner EL, Grant DR. Living donor liver transplantation versus deceased donor liver transplantation for hepatocellular carcinoma: comparable survival and recurrence. Liver Transplant. 2012;18:315–322 [PMID: 22140013, doi: 10.1002/lt.22477].

[123] Todo S, Furukawa H. Japanese Study Group on Organ Transplantation. Living donor liver transplantation for adult patients with hepatocellular carcinoma: experience in Japan. Ann Surg. 2004; 240:451–459; discussion 459–461 [PMID: 15319716].

[124] Saidi RF, Jabbour N, Li Y, Shah SA, Bozorgzadeh A. Is left lobe adult-to-adult living donor liver transplantation ready for widespread use? The US experience (1998–2010). HPB (Oxford) 2012;14:455–460 [PMID: 22672547, doi:10.1111/j.1477-2574.2 012.00475.x].

[125] Saidi RF, Markmann JF, Jabbour N, Li Y, Shah SA, Cosimi AB, Bozorgzadeh A. The faltering solid organ donor pool in the United States (2001–2010). World J Surg. 2012;36(12):2909–2913 [PMID: 22933050, doi: 10.1007/s00268-012-1748-0].

[126] Muzaale AD, Dagher NN, Montgomery RA, Taranto SE, McBride MA, Segev DL. Estimates of early death, acute liver failure, and long-term mortality among live liver

donors. Gastroenterology. 2012;142:273–280 [PMID: 22108193, doi:10.1053/j. gastro. 2011.11.015].

[127] Rodeck B, Melter M, Kardorff R, Hoyer PF, Ringe B, Burdelski M, Oldhafer KJ, Pichlmayr R, Brodehl J. Liver transplantation in children with chronic end stage liver disease: factors influencing survival after transplantation. Transplantation. 1996;62:1071–1076 [PMID: 8900304].

[128] Roll GR, Roberts JP. Left versus right lobe liver donation. Am J Transplant. 2014;14:251–252 [PMID: 24304562, doi:10.1111/ ajt.12556].

[129] Roll GR, Parekh JR, Parker WF, Siegler M, Pomfret EA, Ascher NL, Roberts JP. Left hepatectomy versus right hepatectomy for living donor liver transplantation: shifting the risk from the donor to the recipient. Liver Transplant. 2013;19:472–481 [PMID: 23447523, doi:10.1002/lt.23608].

[130] Ghobrial RM, Freise CE, Trotter JF, Tong L, Ojo AO, Fair JH, Fisher RA, Emond JC, Koffron AJ, Pruett TL, Olthoff KM. Donor morbidity after living donation for liver transplantation. Gastroenterology. 2008;135:468–476 [PMID: 18505689, doi:10.1053/ j.gastro.2008.04.018].

[131] Kousoulas L, Becker T, Richter N, Emmanouilidis N, Schrem H, Barg-Hock H, Klempnauer J, Lehner F. Living donor liver transplantation: effect of the type of liver graft donation on donor mortality and morbidity. Transplant Int. 2011;24:251–258 [PMID: 21062368, doi:10.1111/j.1432-2277.2010.01183.x].

[132] Kousoulas L, Emmanouilidis N, Klempnauer J, Lehner F. Living-donor liver transplantation: impact on donor's health-related quality of life. Transplant Proc. 2011;43:3584–3587 [PMID: 22172809, doi:10.1016/j.transproceed.2011.10.038].

[133] Lo CM. Complications and long-term outcome of living liver donors: a survey of 1,508 cases in five Asian centers. Transplantation. 2003;75:S12–S15 [PMID: 12589131].

[134] Morioka D, Egawa H, Kasahara M, Ito T, Haga H, Takada Y, Shimada H, Tanaka K. Outcomes of adult-to-adult living donor liver transplantation: a single institution's experience with 335 consecutive cases. Ann Surg. 2007;245:315–325 [PMID: 17245187, doi:10.1097/01.sla.0000236600.24667.a4].

[135] Umeshita K, Fujiwara K, Kiyosawa K, Makuuchi M, Satomi S, Sugimachi K, Tanaka K, Monden M; Japanese Liver Transplantation Society. Operative morbidity of living liver donors in Japan. Lancet. 2003;362:687–690 [PMID: 12957090, doi:10.1016/ S0140-6736(03)14230-4].

[136] Tannuri ACA, Gibelli NEM, Ricardi LRS, Santos MM, Maksoud-Filho JG, Pinho-Apezzato ML et al. Living related donor liver transplantation in children. Transplant Proc. 2011;43(1):161–164. http://doi.org/10.1016/j.transproceed.2010.11.013.

[137] Mcdiarmid SV. Special considerations for pediatric immunosuppression after liver transplantation. In: Busuttil RW, Klintmalm GB (Eds.), Transplantation of the Liver. Philadelphia, London: W.B. Saunders Co., 1996. pp. 250–261.

[138] Ganschow R, Grabhorn E, Burdelski M. Basiliximab in paediatric liver-transplant recipients. Lancet 2001;357:388 [PMID: 11211016, doi:10.1016/S0140-6736(00)03654-0].

[139] Ganschow R, Grabhorn E, Schulz A, Von Hugo A, Rogiers X, Burdelski M. Long-term results of basiliximab induction immunosuppression in pediatric liver transplant recipients. Pediatr Transplant. 2005;9:741–745 [PMID: 16269045, doi:10.1111/ j. 1399-3046.2005.00371.x].

[140] Grabhorn E, Schulz A, Helmke K, Hinrichs B, Rogiers X, Broering DC, Burdelski M, Ganschow R. Short- and long-term results of liver transplantation in infants aged less than 6 months. Transplantation. 2004;78:235–241 [PMID: 15280684].

[141] Heffron TG, Pillen T, Smallwood GA, Welch D, Oakley B, Romero R. Pediatric liver transplantation with daclizumab induction. Transplantation. 2003;75:2040–2043 [PMID: 12829908, doi:10.1097/01.TP.0000065740.69296.DA].

[142] Schuller S, Wiederkehr JC, Coelho-Lemos IM, Avilla SG, Schultz C. Daclizumab induction therapy associated with tacrolimus-MMF has better outcome compared with tacrolimus-MMF alone in pediatric living donor liver transplantation. Transplant Proc. 2005;37:1151–1152 [PMID: 15848653, doi:10.1016/j.transproceed.200 5.01.023].

[143] Strassburg CP, Manns MP. Partial liver transplantation and living donation from the viewpoint of internal medicine. Der Internist 2002;43:1551–1558.

[144] Di Filippo S. Anti-IL-2 receptor antibody vs. polyclonal anti-lymphocyte antibody as induction therapy in pediatric transplantation. Pediatr Transplant. 2005;9:373–380 [PMID: 15910396, doi:10.1111/j.1399-3046.2005.00303.x].

[145] Dell-Olio D, Kelly DA. Calcineurin inhibitor minimization in pediatric liver allograft recipients. Pediatr Transplant. 2009;13:670–681 [PMID: 19413716, doi:10.1111/j. 1399-3046.2009.01184. x].

[146] Tönshoff B, Höcker B. Treatment strategies in pediatric solid organ transplant recipients with calcineurin inhibitor-induced nephrotoxicity. Pediatr Transplant. 2006;10:721–729 [PMID: 16911497, doi:10.1111/j.1399-3046.2006.00577.x].

[147] Tredger JM, Brown NW, Dhawan A. Immunosuppression in pediatric solid organ transplantation: opportunities, risks, and management. Pediatr Transplant. 2006;10:879–892 [PMID: 17096754, doi:10.1111/j.1399-3046.2006.00604.x].

[148] Turmelle YP, Nadler ML, Anderson CD, Doyle MB, Lowell JA, Shepherd RW. Towards minimizing immunosuppression in pediatric liver transplant recipients. Pediatr Transplant. 2009;13:553–559 [PMID: 19067920, doi:10.1111/j.1399-3046.2008.01061. x].

[149] Evans HM, McKiernan PJ, Kelly DA. Mycophenolate mofetil for renal dysfunction after pediatric liver transplantation. Transplantation. 2005;79:1575–1580 [PMID: 15940048].

[150] Ferraris JR, Duca P, Prigoshin N, Tambutti ML, Boldrini G, Cardoni RL, D'Agostino D. Mycophenolate mofetil and reduced doses of cyclosporine in pediatric liver transplantation with chronic renal dysfunction: changes in the immune responses. Pediatr Transplant. 2004;8:454–459 [PMID: 15367280, doi:10.1111/ j.1399-3046.2004.00172.x].

[151] Filler G, Gellermann J, Zimmering M, Mai I. Effect of adding Mycophenolate mofetil in paediatric renal transplant recipients with chronical cyclosporine nephrotoxicity. Transplant Int 2000; 13:201–206 [PMID: 10935703].

[152] Hoyer PF, Ettenger R, Kovarik JM, Webb NJ, Lemire J, Mentser M, Mahan J, Loirat C, Niaudet P, VanDamme-Lombaerts R, Offner G, Wehr S, Moeller V, Mayer H. Everolimus in pediatric de nova renal transplant patients. Transplantation. 2003;75:2082–2085 [PMID: 12829916, doi:10.1097/01.TP.0000070139.63068.54].

[153] Jiménez-Rivera C, Avitzur Y, Fecteau AH, Jones N, Grant D, Ng VL. Sirolimus for pediatric liver transplant recipients with post- transplant lymphoproliferative disease and hepatoblastoma. Pediatr Transplant. 2004;8:243–248 [PMID: 15176961, doi:10.1111/ j.1399-3046.2004.00156.x].

[154] Scheenstra R, Torringa ML, Waalkens HJ, Middelveld EH, Peeters PM, Slooff MJ, Gouw AS, Verkade HJ, Bijleveld CM. Cyclosporine A withdrawal during follow-up after pediatric liver transplantation. Liver Transplant. 2006;12:240–246 [PMID: 16447209, doi:10.1002/lt.20591].

[155] Sindhi R, Ganjoo J, McGhee W, Mazariegos G, Reyes J. Preliminary immunosuppression withdrawal strategies with sirolimus in children with liver transplants. Transplant Proc. 2002;34:1972–1973 [PMID: 12176651].

[156] Vester U, Kranz B, Wehr S, Boger R, Hoyer PF; RAD B 351 Study Group. Everolimus (Certican) in combination with neoral in pediatric renal transplant recipients: interim analysis after 3 months. Transplant Proc. 2002;34:2209–2210 [PMID: 12270366].

[157] Feng S, Ekong UD, Lobritto SJ, Demetris AJ, Roberts JP, Rosenthal P, Alonso EM, Philogene MC, Ikle D, Poole KM, Bridges ND, Turka LA, Tchao NK. Complete immunosuppression withdrawal and subsequent allograft function among pediatric recipients of parental living donor liver transplants. JAMA. 2012;307:283–293 [PMID: 22253395, doi: 10.1001/jama.2011.2014].

[158] Koshiba T, Li Y, Takemura M, Wu Y, Sakaguchi S, Minato N, Wood KJ, Haga H, Ueda M, Uemoto S. Clinical, immunological, and pathological aspects of operational tolerance after pediatric living-donor liver transplantation. Transplant Immunol. 2007;17:94–97 [PMID: 17306739, doi:10.1016/j.trim.2006.10.004].

[159] Mazariegos GV, Reyes J, Marino IR, Demetris AJ, Flynn B, Irish W, McMichael J, Fung JJ, Starzl TE. Weaning of immunosuppression in liver transplant recipients. Transplantation. 1997;63:243–249 [PMID: 9020325].

[160] Mazariegos GV, Sindhi R, Thomson AW, Marcos A. Clinical tolerance following liver transplantation: long term results and future prospects. Transplant Immunol. 2007;17:114–119 [PMID: 17306742, doi:10.1016/j.trim.2006.09.033].

[161] Starzl TE, Demetris AJ, Trucco M, Ricordi C, Murase N, Thomson AW. The role of cell migration and chimerism in organ transplant acceptance and tolerance induction. Transplant Sci. 1993;3:47–50 [PMID: 21572595].

[162] Takatsuki M, Uemoto S, Inomata Y, Egawa H, Kiuchi T, Fujita S, Hayashi M, Kanematsu T, Tanaka K. Weaning of immunosuppression in living donor liver transplant recipients. Transplantation. 2001;72:449–454 [PMID: 11502975].

[163] Donckier V, Troisi R, Le Moine A, Toungouz M, Ricciardi S, Colle I, Van Vlierberghe H, Craciun L, Libin M, Praet M, Noens L, Stordeur P, Andrien M, Lambermont M, Gelin M, Bourgeois N, Adler M, de Hemptinne B, Goldman M. Early immunosuppression withdrawal after living donor liver transplantation and donor stem cell infusion. Liver Transplant. 2006;12:1523–1528 [PMID: 17004249, doi:10.1002/lt.20872].

[164] Kawai T, Cosimi AB, Spitzer TR, Tolkoff-Rubin N, Suthanthiran M, Saidman SL, Shaffer J, Preffer FI, Ding R, Sharma V, Fishman JA, Dey B, Ko DS, Hertl M, Goes NB, Wong W, Williams WW, Colvin RB, Sykes M, Sachs DH. HLA-mismatched renal transplantation without maintenance immunosuppression. N Engl J Med. 2008;358:353–361 [PMID: 18216355, doi:10.1056/ NEJMoa071074].

[165] Scandling JD, Busque S, Dejbakhsh-Jones S, Benike C, Millan MT, Shizuru JA, Hoppe RT, Lowsky R, Engleman EG, Strober S. Tolerance and chimerism after renal and hematopoietic-cell transplantation. N Engl J Med. 2008;358:362–368 [PMID: 18216356, doi:10.1056/NEJMoa074191].

[166] Starzl TE, et al. Cell migration and clmerism after whole-organ transplantation: the basis of graft acceptance. Hepatology. 1993;171127–171152.

[167] Ramos HC, Reyes J, Abu-Elmagd K, et al. Weaning of immunosuppression in long-term liver transplant recipients. Transplantation. 1995;59:212–217

[168] Wong T, Nouri-Aria K T, Devlin J, et al. Tolerance and latent cellular rejection in long-term liver transplant recipients. Hepatology. 1998:28:443–449.

[169] Smith BA, Shuchman M. Problem of nonadherence in chronically ill adolescents: strategies for assessment and intervention. Curr Opin Pediatr. 2005;17:613–618.

[170] Hind JM, Kelly DA. Pediatric liver transplantation: review of the literature 2007–2008. Pediatric Transplant. 2009;13(1):14–24. http://doi.org/10.1111/j.1399-3046.2009.01238.x.

[171] Fredericks EM, Magee JC, Opipari-Arrigan L, et al. Adherence and health-related quality of life in adolescent liver transplant recipients. Pediatr Transplant. 2008;12:289–299.

[172] Berquist RK, Berquist WE, Esquivel CO, et al. Non-adherence to post-transplant care: prevalence, risk factors and outcomes in adolescent liver transplant recipients. Pediatr Transplant. 2008;12:194–200.

[173] Lurie S, Shemesh E, Sheiner PA, et al. Non-adherence in pediatric liver transplant recipients–an assessment of risk factors and natural history. Pediatr Transplant. 2000;4:200–206.

[174] Dew MA, Dabbs AD, Myaskovsky L, et al. Meta-analysis of medical regimen adherence outcomes in pediatric solid organ transplantation. Transplantation. 2009;88:736–746.

[175] Burra P. The adolescent and liver transplantation. J Hepatol. 2012;56:714–722.

[176] Stuber ML, Shemesh E, Seacord D, et al. Evaluating non-adherence to immunosuppressant medications in pediatric liver transplant recipients. Pediatr Transplant. 2008;12:284–288.

[177] O'Grady JG, Asderakis A, Bradley R, et al. Multidisciplinary insights into optimizing adherence after solid organ transplantation. Transplantation. 2010;89:627–632.

[178] Maksoud-Filho JG, Tannuri U, Gibelli NEM, et al. Intimal dissection of the hepatic artery after thrombectomy as a cause of graft loss in pediatric living-related liver transplantation. Pediatr Transplant. 2008:12:91–94.

[179] Uller W, Knoppke B, Schreyer Ag, et al. Interventional radiological treatment of perihepatic vascular stenosis or occlusion in pediatric patients after liver transplantation. Cardiovasc Intervent Radiol. 2013:36:1562–1571.

[180] Bekker J, Ploem S, De Jong K P. Early hepatic artery thrombosis after liver transplantation: a systematic review of the incidence, outcome and risk factors. Am J Transplant. 2009:9:746–757.

[181] Porrett P M, Hsu J, Shaked A. Late surgical complications following liver transplantation. Liver Transplant. 2009:15(Suppl 2):S12–S18.

[182] Oh C K, Pelletier S J, Sawyer R G, et al. Uni- and multi-variate analysis of risk factors for early and late hepatic artery thrombosis after liver transplantation. Transplantation. 2001:71:767–772.

[183] Silva MA, Jambulingam PS, Gunson BK, et al. Hepatic artery thrombosis following orthotopic liver transplantation: a 10-year experience from a single centre in the United Kingdom. Liver Transplant. 2006:12:146–151.

[184] Gunsar F, Rolando N, Pastacaldi S, et al. Late hepatic artery thrombosis after orthotopic liver transplantation. Liver Transplant. 2003:9:605–611.

[185] Valente JF, Alonso MH, Weber FL, Hanto DW. Late hepatic artery thrombosis in liver allograft recipients is associated with intrahepatic biliary necrosis. Transplantation. 1996:61:61–65.

[186] Tzakis AG, Gordon RD, Shaw BW Jr, Iwatsuki S, Starzl TE. Clinical presentation of hepatic artery thrombosis after liver transplantation in the cyclosporine era. Transplantation. 1985:40:667–671.

[187] Singhal A, Stokes K, Sebastian A, et al. Endovascular treatment of hepatic artery thrombosis follow- ing liver transplantation. Transplant Int. 2010:23:245–256.

[188] Hasegawa T, Sasaki T, Kimura T, et al. Successful percutaneous transluminal angioplasty for hepatic artery stenosis in an infant undergoing living-related liver transplantation. Pediatr Transplant. 2002:6:244–248.

[189] Maruzzelli L, Miraglia R, Caruso S, et al. Percutaneous endovascular treatment of hepatic artery stenosis in adult and pediatric patients after liver transplantation. Cardiovasc Intervent Radiol. 2010: 33:1111–1119.

[190] Wakiya T, Sanada Y, Mizuta K, et al. Endovascular interventions for hepatic artery complications immediately after pediatric liver transplantation. Transplant Int. 2011:24:984–990.

[191] Wakiya T, Sanada Y, Mizuta K, et al. Interventional radiology for hepatic artery complications soon after living donor liver transplantation in a neonate. Pediatr Transplant. 2012:16:E81–E85.

[192] Carnevale FC, De Tarso Machado A, Moreira AM, et al. Long-term results of the percutaneous transhepatic venoplasty of portal vein stenoses after pediatric liver transplantation. Pediatr Transplant. 2011:15:476–481.

[193] Umehara M, Narumi S, Sugai M, et al. Hepatic venous out-flow obstruction in living donor liver transplantation: Balloon angioplasty or stent placement? Transplant Proc. 2012:44:769–771.

[194] Shibasaki S, Taniguchi M, Shimamura T, et al. Risk factors for portal vein complications in pediatric living donor liver transplantation. Clin Transplant. 2010:24:550–556.

[195] Kawano Y, Mizuta K, Sugawara Y, et al. Diagnosis and treatment of pediatric patients with late-onset portal vein stenosis after living donor liver transplantation. Transplant Int. 2009:22:1151–1158.

[196] Kawano Y, Akimaru K, Taniai N, et al. Successful transjugular balloon dilatation of the hepatic vein stenosis causing hypoalbuminemia after pediatric living-donor liver transplantation. Hepatogastroenterology. 2007:54:1821–1824.

[197] Carnevale FC, Borges MV, Pinto RA, Oliva JL, Andrade WDE C, Maksoud JG. Endovascular treatment of stenosis between hepatic vein and inferior vena cava following liver transplantation in a child: a case report. Pediatr Transplant. 2004:8:576–580.

[198] Carnevale FC, Borges MV, Moreira AM, Cerri GG, Maksoud JG. Endovascular treatment of acute portal vein thrombosis after liver transplantation in a child. Cardiovasc Intervent Radiol. 2006:29:457–461.

[199] Ueda M, Oike F, Kasahara M, et al. Portal vein complications in pediatric living donor liver transplantation using left-side grafts. Am J Transplant. 2008:8:2097–2105.

[200] Azzam A Z, Tanaka K. Management of vascular complications after living donor liver transplantation. Hepatogastroenterology. 2012;59:182–186.

[201] Yilmaz A, Arikan C, Tumgor G, Kilic M, Aydogdu S. Vascular complications in living-related and deceased donation pediatric liver transplantation: Single center's experience from Turkey. Pediatr Transplant. 2007;11:160–164.

[202] Sanada Y, Kawano Y, Mizuta K, et al. Strategy to prevent recurrent portal vein stenosis following interventional radiology in pediatric liver transplantation. Liver Transplant. 2010:16:332–339.

[203] Mitchell A, John PR, Mayer DA, Mirza DF, Buckels JAC, De Ville De Goyet J. Improved technique of portal vein reconstruction in pediatric liver transplant recipients with portal vein hypoplasia. Transplantation. 2002;73:1244–1247.

[204] Millis JM, Seaman DS, Piper JB, et al. Portal vein thrombosis and stenosis in pediatric liver transplantation. Transplantation. 1996;62:748–754.

[205] Orlandini M, Feier FH, Jaeger B, Kieling C, Vieira SG, Zanotelli ML. Frequency of and factors associated with vascular complications after pediatric liver transplantation. J Pediatr. (Rio J.) 2013:90:169–175.

[206] Llad OL, Fabregat J, Castellote J, et al. Management of portal vein thrombosis in liver transplantation: Influence on morbidity and mortality. Clin Transplant. 2007:21:716–721.

[207] Suzuki L, De Oliveira I R S, Widman A, et al. Real-time and Doppler US after pediatric segmental liver transplantation. I. Portal vein stenosis. Pediatr Radiol. 2008:38:403–408.

[208] Uller W, Knoppke B, Schreyer AG, et al. Interventional radiological treatment of perihepatic vascular stenosis or occlusion in pediatric patients after liver transplantation. Cardiovasc Intervent Radiol. 2013;36:1562–1571.

[209] Buell JF, Funaki B, Cronin DC, et al. Long-term venous complications after full-size and segmental pediatric liver transplantation. Ann Surg. 2002:236:658–666.

[210] Shibasaki S, Taniguchi M, Shimamura T, et al. Risk factors for portal vein complications in pediatric living donor liver transplantation. Clin Transplant. 2010:24:550–556.

[211] Kishi Y, Sugawara Y, Matsui Y, Akamatsu N, Makuuchi M. Late onset portal vein thrombosis and its risk factors. Hepatogastroenterology. 2008;55:1008–1009.

[212] Sakamoto S, Nakazawa A, Shigeta T, et al. Devastating outflow obstruction after pediatric split liver transplantation. Pediatr Transplant. 2013:17:E25–E28.

[213] Bertram H, Pfister E-D, Becker T, Schoof S. Transsplenic endovascular therapy of portal vein stenosis and subsequent complete portal vein thrombosis in a 2-year-old child. J Vasc Interv Radiol. 2010:21:1760–1764.

[214] Kamran Hejazi Kenari S, Mirzakhani H, Eslami M, Saidi RF. Current state of the art in management of vascular complications after pediatric liver transplantation. Pediatr Transplant. 2015;19(1):18–26. http://doi.org/10.1111/petr.12407.

[215] Feier FH, da Fonseca EA, Seda-Neto J, Chapchap P. Biliary complications after pediatric liver transplantation: risk factors, diagnosis and management. World J Hepatol. 2015;7(18):2162–2170. http://doi.org/10.4254/wjh.v7.i18.2162.

[216] Ostroff JW. Management of biliary complications in the liver transplant patient. Gastroenterol Hepatol (N Y). 2010;6:264–272 [PMID: 20567581].

[217] Gupta S, Castel H, Rao RV, Picard M, Lilly L, Faughnan ME, Pomier-Layrargues G. Improved survival after liver transplantation in patients with hepatopulmonary syndrome. Am J Transplant. 2010;10:354–363 [PMID: 19775311, doi:10.1111/j. 1600-6143.2 009.02822.x].

[218] Salvalaggio PR, Whitington PF, Alonso EM, Superina RA. Presence of multiple bile ducts in the liver graft increases the incidence of biliary complications in pediatric liver transplantation. Liver Transplant. 2005;11:161–166 [PMID: 15666393, doi:10.1002/ lt. 20288].

[219] Kling K, Lau H, Colombani P. Biliary complications of living related pediatric liver transplant patients. Pediatr Transplant. 2004;8:178–184 [PMID: 15049799, doi: 10.1046/j.1399-3046.2003.001 27.x].

[220] Feier FH, Chapchap P, Pugliese R, da Fonseca EA, Carnevale FC, Moreira AM, Zurstrassen C, Santos AC, Miura IK, Baggio V, Porta A, Guimarães T, Cândido H, Benavides M, Godoy A, Leite KM, Porta G, Kondo M, Seda-Neto J. Diagnosis and management of biliary complications in pediatric living donor liver transplant recipients. Liver Transplant. 2014;20:882–892 [PMID: 24760734, doi:10.1002/lt.23896].

[221] Anderson CD, Turmelle YP, Darcy M, Shepherd RW, Weymann A, Nadler M, Guelker S, Chapman WC, Lowell JA. Biliary strictures in pediatric liver transplant recipients—early diagnosis and treatment results in excellent graft outcomes. Pediatr Transplant. 2010;14:358–363 [PMID: 20003138, doi:10.1111/j.1399-3046.2 009.01246.x].

[222] Miraglia R, Maruzzelli L, Caruso S, Riva S, Spada M, Luca A, Gridelli B. Percutaneous management of biliary strictures after pediatric liver transplantation. Cardiovasc Intervent Radiol. 2008;31:993–998 [PMID: 18574628, doi:10.1007/s00270-008-9378-5].

[223] Marubashi S, Nagano H, Yamanouchi E, Kobayashi S, Eguchi H, Takeda Y, Tanemura M, Maeda N, Tomoda K, Hikita H, Tsutsui S, Doki Y, Mori M. Salvage cystic duct

anastomosis using a magnetic compression technique for incomplete bile duct reconstruction in living donor liver transplantation. Liver Transplant. 2010;16:33–37 [PMID: 20035518, doi:10.1002/lt.21934].

[224] Muraoka N, Uematsu H, Yamanouchi E, Kinoshita K, Takeda T, Ihara N, Matsunami H, Itoh H. Yamanouchi magnetic compression anastomosis for bilioenteric anastomotic stricture after living-donor liver transplantation. J Vasc Interv Radiol. 2005;16:1263–1267 [PMID: 16151070, doi:10.1097/01.RVI.0000173280.56442.9E].

[225] Wakiya T, Sanada Y, Mizuta K, et al. A comparison of open surgery and endovascular intervention for hepatic artery complications after pediatric liver transplantation. Transplant Proc. 2013 45:323–329.

[226] Funaki B, Rosenblum J D, Leef J A, et al. Percutaneous treatment of portal venous stenosis in children and adolescents with segmental hepatic transplants: long-term results. Radiology. 2000;215:147–151.

[227] Hashikura Y, Kawasaki S, Okumura N, et al. Prevention of hepatic artery thrombosis in pediatric liver transplantation. Transplantation. 1995:10:1109–1112.

[228] Shay R, Taber D, Pilch N, et al. Early aspirin therapy may reduce hepatic artery thrombosis in liver transplantation. Transplant Proc. 2013;45:330–334.

Chapter 9

Portopulmonary Hypertension

Emica Shimozono, Cristina A. A. Caruy,
Adilson R. Cardoso, Derli C. M. Servian and
Ilka F. S. F. Boin

Additional information is available at the end of the chapter

http://dx.doi.org/10.5772/63073

Abstract

Portopulmonary hypertension (PPH) is characterized by the development of pulmonary arterial hypertension (PAH) associated with portal hypertension, with or without liver disease. It is defined as a mean pulmonary artery pressure (MPAP) greater than 25 mmHg, pulmonary vascular resistance (PVR) above 240 dynes.s.cm^{-5}, pulmonary artery occlusion pressure (PAOP) normal when less than 15 mmHg or transpulmonary gradient (TPG) > 10 mmHg. In the pulmonary hypertension classification PPH is classified in Group I. Pulmonary arterial hypertension in association with cirrhosis and portal hypertension is underdiagnosed. Epidemiological studies estimated that about 2–6% of patients with portal hypertension develop PPH. Mortality is directly proportional to measured MPAP and PVR. Mean pulmonary artery pressure is an independent predictor of mortality, and many centers consider that values greater than 50 mmHg is an absolute contraindication to liver transplantation (LT). The aim of the review is to explore the current aspects of PPH relative to concept, diagnosis, and treatment.

Keywords: pulmonary hypertension, portal hypertension, portopulmonary hypertension, diagnosis, liver transplantation

1. Introduction

Pulmonary hypertension (PH) is defined as a mean pulmonary artery pressure greater than or equal to 25 mmHg at rest, and above 30 mmHg during exercise, measured by right heart catheterization (RHC) [1].

Pulmonary arterial hypertension (PAH) is a complex clinical entity, classified as Group I from the classification of PH. It may be idiopathic (formally called primary pulmonary hypertension), hereditary, induced by drugs or toxins, or associated with connective tissue diseases, human immunodeficiency virus, portal hypertension, congenital heart disease, schistosomiasis, and others [1–3].

Portal hypertension is a hemodynamic disorder that usually results from chronic liver disease or cirrhosis. Portal blood flow in adults is about 1000–1200 mL/min, creating a normal intraportal pressure of 7 mmHg. In the normal liver, the gradient between the portal vein and hepatic veins or the right atrium usually does not exceed 5 mmHg. Portal hypertension is defined by a gradient greater than 6 mmHg. When pressure gradients reach 10–12 mmHg, portal blood flow is shunted into the systemic circulation, resulting in the development of esophageal varices, ascites, and splenomegaly. Diagnosis can be made by abdominal ultrasonography and endoscopy [4].

Portopulmonary hypertension (PPH) is a form of pulmonary hypertension, associated with portal hypertension, with or without advanced liver disease [5–9].

In liver transplantation (LT) candidates, a large deconstructed pulmonary vasculature can occur. Vasculature alteration may range from hepatopulmonary syndrome (HPS), characterized by pulmonary vascular dilatation to portopulmonary hypertension, with pulmonary vascular resistance elevated, causing severe clinic hypoxemia, right heart failure, and death [5, 10, 11].

Mantz and Craige were the first to describe an association between pulmonary hypertension and portal hypertension in 1951. Those authors reported a case of a 53-year-old patient diagnosed with axial portal vein thrombosis and spontaneous portocaval shunt. Autopsy revealed changes in the pulmonary arterial vascular bed and reduction in portal vein diameter with normal liver parenchyma [12, 13].

Since the 1980s, PPH has gained recognition and importance, following the evolution of liver transplantation. In some cases, LT can be beneficial for the disease [6, 11].

In 1983, the National Institutes of Health Consensus Development Conference concluded that LT should be considered a therapeutic procedure for patients with chronic and end-stage liver disease lack of alternative treatment [14].

PPH was classified as a subtype of primary pulmonary hypertension in 1981 by the National Institute of Health Registry for Characterization of Primary Pulmonary Hypertension [8].

PPH was classified as secondary pulmonary hypertension in 1993, and since then it has become known as portopulmonary hypertension [5, 11, 15].

The Second World Pulmonary Hypertension Symposium was held in Evian (France) in 1998, where pulmonary hypertensive diseases were classified into five groups according to similarities in pathophysiologic mechanisms, clinical presentation, and therapeutic options [2].

At the Third World Pulmonary Hypertension Symposium in 2003 in Venice (Italy) and the Fourth World Symposium in 2008 in Dana Point (California, USA), PPH was categorized into Group I Pulmonary Hypertension [1, 2, 16, 17].

During the Fifth World Pulmonary Hypertension Symposium held in 2013 in Nice, France, the consensus was to maintain the general disposition of previous classification, with some modifications and updates [18], as seen in **Table 1**.

Group I. Pulmonary arterial hypertension
• Idiopathic
• Hereditary: mutation in the bone morphogenetic protein receptor type 2 (BMPR2), activin type I receptor kinase-like gene (ALK-1), endoglin (ENG), mothers against decapentaplegic 9 (SMAD9), caveolin 1 (CAV1), gene encoding potassium channel superfamily K member 3 (KCNK3) or unknown causes
• Drug and toxin induced
• Associated with: connective tissue disease, congenital heart disease, acquired immunodeficiency syndrome,**portal hypertension**, schistosomiasis
1′-Veno-occlusive pulmonary disease and/or pulmonary capillary hemangiomatosis
1″-Persistent pulmonary hypertension of the newborn (PPHN)
Group II. Pulmonary hypertension due to left heart disease
• Systolic dysfunction, diastolic dysfunction, valvular disease, congenital/acquired left heart inflow/outflow tract obstruction and congenital cardiomyopathies
Group III. Pulmonary hypertension due to lung diseases and/or hypoxia Chronic obstructive pulmonary disease, interstitial lung disease, other pulmonary diseases with mixed restrictive and obstructive pattern, sleep disordered breathing, alveolar hypoventilation disorders, chronic exposure to high altitude, developmental lung diseases
Group IV. Chronic thromboembolic disease (CTEPH)
Group V. Pulmonary hypertension with unknown multifactorial mechanisms

Table 1. Classification of pulmonary hypertension—2013 Nice/France [18].

Based on diagnostic criteria, PPH can also be defined as: an increase in mean pulmonary artery pressure (MPAP) > 25 mmHg, increased pulmonary vascular resistance (PVR) > 240 dynes.s.cm^{-5}, and a mean pulmonary artery occlusion pressure (PAOP) normal < 15 mmHg, in patients with portal hypertension and no other causes of pulmonary hypertension. These hemodynamic criteria are consistent with the definitions and classification proposed by the Third World Pulmonary Hypertension Symposium, according to the European Respiratory Society (ERS) Task Force on Pulmonary-Hepatic Vascular Disorders (PHD). Furthermore, a transpulmonary gradient (TPG) > 10 mmHg was finally recommended by the ERS Task Force on PHD [19], as seen in **Table 2**.

1.	Portal hypertension (with and without cirrhosis)
2.	Abnormal pulmonary hemodynamics
a.	MPAP > 25 mmHg
b.	PVR > 240 dynes.s.cm^{-5}
c.	PAOP < 15 mmHg

MPAP, mean pulmonary artery pressure; PVR, pulmonary vascular resistance; PAOP, pulmonary artery occlusion pressure.

Table 2. Diagnostic criteria for portopulmonary hypertension (according to ERS Task Force on PHD) [19].

The addition of transpulmonary gradient,TPG (MPAP-PAOP), was suggested because it can distinguish between excess volume (TPG < 10 mmHg) and vascular abnormalities (TPG > 10 mmHg) [19].

Approximately 30–50% of patients with cirrhosis have a high-flow circulatory state, owing to splanchnic vasodilation and hyperdynamic circulation, and this may cause an increase in MPAP, despite lack of pulmonary vasculature remodeling. The hyperdynamic circulation is characterized by a high cardiac output (CO), a low systemic vascular resistance (SVR), and a low PVR [6, 20]. Therefore, the proposed classification for severity of PPH was based on MPAP [19, 21], as described in **Table 3**.

Severity rate	Mean pulmonary artery pressure (mmHg)
Mild	25 to < 35
Moderate	35 to < 45
Severe	≥ 45

Table 3. Classification of severity of portopulmonary hypertension based on MPAP (mean pulmonary artery pressure) [19].

Mild PPH appears to have no impact on outcomes following LT. However, significant increases in pulmonary artery pressures are associated with high mortality rates. MPAP > 50 mmHg is associated with 100% mortality in patients undergoing LT. Mortality is 35–40% in MPAP ranging from 35 to 50 mmHg and from zero to 17% in MPAP < 35 mmHg [22].

2. Prevalence and survival

The first autopsy studies were carried by McDonnell et al. in 1983. Those authors reported a prevalence of 0.13% in PAH non-cirrhotic patients compared to 0.73% in patients with cirrhosis and portal hypertension. In biopsies of other clinical studies, the prevalence of PAH ranged from 0.61% to 2% in cirrhotic patients [8, 23, 24].

Hemodynamic data from prospective studies revealed that approximately 2–6% of patients with portal hypertension develop PPH [25, 26].

The incidence of PPH in patients undergoing LT ranges from 4 to 6%, while some studies show percentages as high as 8.5–12.5% [13, 25, 27, 28].

In a study involving 362 patients from 1985 to 1993, Castro et al. [27] used the criteria MPAP > 25 mmHg and PVR > 120 dynes.s.cm^{-5} for diagnosis of PPH. Those authors concluded that increased MPAP is common in patients with advanced liver disease (20%), although PPH occurred in only 4% of patients (15 patients).

Ramsay et al. [28] reviewed severe PH in patients with advanced liver disease in a study from Baylor University Medical Center. Those authors evaluated 1205 consecutive LTs, between December 1984 and October 1995. The incidence of PPH was 8.5% (102 patients with MPAP > 25 mmHg, and 6.72% in the mild form, 1.16% in the moderate form, and 0.58% in the severe form), using the same criteria. Mortality was 30% in three years in mild to moderate PPH, 42% in nine months in severe PPH, and 71% at three years post-LT.

In 1990, Robalino et al. [29] found that patients suffering from PAH associated with portal hypertension had a 15-month survival mean and a 50% mortality rate within six months of diagnosis, compared to those with primary pulmonary hypertension who survived two to three years and had a 57% survival rate within two years of diagnosis.

In a retrospective cohort study (data collection from 1997 to 2001 at the University of Pennsylvania, with a 3-year follow-up), Kawut et al. [30] compared survival and hemodynamics in patients with PPH (n=13) and PAH (n=33, pulmonary arterial hypertension was idiopathic, familial or associated with anorexics). Many of those patients were treated with epoprostenol. Those authors concluded that death risk in patients with PPH increased two fold compared to patients with PAH. Estimates of 1-year and 3-year-survival rates were 85% and 38% for patients with PPH, 82% and 72% for patients with PAH respectively. Although PPH patients had a higher cardiac index and lower PVR than PAH, patient outcome was worse, and could be attributed to complications of portal hypertension.

In a retrospective analysis of 154 PPH patients diagnosed from 1984 to 2004 and referred to the French Center for Pulmonary Arterial Hypertension, Le Pavec et al. [31] found a survival rate of 88%, 75%, and 68% at one, three, and five years, respectively. In this study, mortality was related to cirrhosis severity (higher in patients with Child-Turcotte-Pugh class B and C) and to low cardiac index.

In another French study (data obtained from the 2002/2003 National Registry including 17 university hospitals), Humbert et al. [25, 32] evaluated 674 cases diagnosed with PAH, showing that 10.4% of this population had PPH. Among all causes, PPH was the fourth cause of PAH, following idiopathic PAH (39.2%), PAH associated with connective tissue disease (15.3%), and PAH associated with congenital heart disease (11.3%). At diagnosis, 75% of patients were New York Heart Association (NYHA) class II or IV. Diagnosis was made following diagnostic criteria, according to RHC. Survival rate of PAH was 88% within one year.

In a retrospective Mayo Clinic study, Swanson et al. [33] reviewed 74 patients with PPH, between 1994 and 2007. Using current diagnostic criteria, hemodynamic data (averages and ranges) were: MPAP= 49 mmHg (27–86); PVR = 515 dynes.s.cm^{-5} (241–1285); PAOP = 12 mmHg (3-29); TPG = 36 mmHg (14-77). Patients were categorized into three subgroups: (I) 19 patients without therapy for PAH or LT represented the natural history of the disease, (II) 43 patients with therapy for PAH, and (III) 12 patients with therapy for PAH and LT. In subgroup (I), the 5-year survival rate was 14%, and 54% of patients had died within one year of diagnosis. In subgroup (II), the five-year survival rate was 45% and 12% of the patients had died within one year of diagnosis. In subgroup (III), the 5-year survival rate was 67% in nine patients undergoing LT and therapy for PH, and 25% in patients undergoing only LT. The authors concluded that mortality was not related to baseline hemodynamic variables, type of liver disease or severity of liver dysfunction. Medical therapy for PPH should be considered in all patients with PPH. However, its effects and impact on potential LT candidates deserve further study.

In a recent research study carried out by REVEAL (Registry to Evaluate The Early and Long-Term PAH Disease Management), Krowka et al. [34] conducted an observational study of 174 patients with PPH, compared to 1392 patients with idiopathic PAH and 85 patients with familial PAH. Survival in patients with PPH was 67% within two years and 40% within five years, and 85% and 64% in patients with PAH, respectively. The authors concluded that despite better hemodynamics, survival was worse in PPH. A delay in diagnosis, different treatment patterns, late onset of treatment of pulmonary hypertension, and liver-related complications had an impact on survival in PPH patients. However, further controlled studies are needed to elucidate this issue. Those authors concluded that PPH accounted for 7–10% of Group I pulmonary hypertension cases.

Nowadays with the advent of better patient selection for LT and appearance of new drugs, it is hoped that this limited scenary will be changed.

2.1. Pathophysiogenesis

The development of PPH is independent on the cause of portal hypertension and severity of underlying liver disease. It is weakly correlated with the Child-Turcotte-Pugh [35] classification and is associated with mortality beyond that predicted by the MELD score (Model End-Stage Liver Disease) [16, 36].

The pathogenesis mechanisms of PPH remain unclear, and the knowledge on its development comes from PAH because of features similarity. Both disorders are characterized by obstruction of pulmonary arterial blood flow with increased PVR. The lesions detected are: medial hypertrophy, intimal proliferation and fibrosis of muscular pulmonary arteries, thickening of the adventitia, and *in situ* thrombosis. Plexiform lesions are typically found in small muscular arteries, adjacent to a larger parent vessel, and large arterial vasodilatation. Necrosis of muscular arteries cause leakage of plasma proteins into the arterial wall, resulting in necrotizing inflammatory arteritis, a probable precursor of plexiform lesions [8, 19, 37].

All these changes lead to increased pulmonary vascular resistance with vasoconstriction, arterial wall remodeling, and *in situ* microthrombosis, among other angiogenic factors investigated, such as genetic susceptibility, increased production of inflammatory mediators, and neurohormones [19].

It is believed that hyperdynamic circulation with high cardiac output can cause PPH, which are influenced by hepatic dysfunction caused by liver cirrhosis. This condition of increased pulmonary blood flow seen in patients with portal hypertension determines an increase shear stress at the level of vasculature, that may lead to endothelial injury and dysfunction with vasoconstriction and progressive vascular remodeling [25, 38].

Investigators have postulated that high concentrations vasoactive substances secondary to an imbalance between vasoconstrictor and vasodilator factors could reach the pulmonary circulation due to portosystemic shunts or defective hepatic metabolism, and initiate the pulmonary vascular injury present in PPH [19, 25].

The mediator substances envolving in this process may be ET-1A, tromboxane A2, interleukin-1, interleukin-6, angiotensin-1, glucagon, and serotonin. PPH patients showed elevated ET-1 and interleukin levels compared to patients with cirrhosis without PPH [38, 39].

ET-1 is produced by the pulmonary endothelium and liver, and binding ET-1A and ET-1B receptors on smooth muscle cells results in vasoconstriction and mitogenesis [19].

In a prospective multicenter case-control study of 175 patients with liver disease, Kawut et al. [40] identified 34 patients with PPH. Those authors demonstrated that the risk of developing PPH was higher in females and patients suffering from autoimmune hepatitis, and lower in those with hepatitis C virus.

In a recent study, Roberts et al. [41] showed that genetic variation in estrogen signaling and cell growth regulators is associated with PPH.

In another study, the same authors demonstrated that serotonin transporter polymorphism is not associated with PPH [42].

The fact that the presence of a high cardiac output, can result in a degree of pulmonary hypertension with normal or near normal pulmonary vascular resistance, which might have led to erroneous interpretation and overestimation of the incidence of PPH [43].

2.2. Clinical presentation

Patients with PPH usually have symptoms similar to those observed in other forms of PAH [1, 25].

Symptoms produced by the disease may be nonspecific. The most common symptoms are dyspnea, fatigue, and chest pain. Syncope, palpitations, and peripheral edema are less commonly observed. Symptoms arise when mean pulmonary artery pressure exceeds 40 mmHg [5, 44].

Clinical symptoms of liver disease and portal hypertension may be present [25, 45].

A prospective study by Hadengue et al. showed that 60% of patients with PPH were asymptomatic and 40% had exertional dyspnea [11, 35].

Investigating a small number of patients with PPH, Robalino and Moodie found that symptomatic patients had a higher incidence of dyspnea (81%), followed by syncope (26%), chest pain (24%), asthenia (15%), hemoptysis (12%), and orthopnea (12%) [29].

Regarding cardiac auscultation, an increased pulmonic component of the second heart sound (P2) occurred in 82% of cases. A systolic murmur of tricuspid regurgitation was present in 69%, edema in 35%, and signs suggestive of right heart failure in 34% [22, 29].

Differences between hepatopulmonary syndrome and portopulmonary hypertension are described according to Rodriguez-Roisin et al., as seen in **Table 4** [6, 19, 43, 46].

	HPS	PPH
Symptoms	progressive dyspnea	progressive dyspnea, chest pain, syncope
Clinical examination	cyanosis, finger clubbing, spider angiomas	no cyanosis, RV heave, pronounced P2 component
ECG	none	RBBB Rightward axis RV hypertropy
Arterial blood gas	moderate/severe hypoxaemia	no or mild hypoxaemia
Chest radiograph	normal	cardiomegaly hilar enlargement
CEE	always positive, left atrial opacification for > 3-6 cardiac cycles after RA opacification	usually negative
Pulmonary angiography	normal/spongy appearence (type I) elevated PVR Discrete AVC (type II)	large main pulmonary arteries
^{99m}TcMAA	≥6%	<6%
Hemodynamics	normal/ low PVR	elevated PVR/ normal PAOP
OLT indicated	even in severe stages	only in mild/ moderate stages

Abbreviations: RV, right ventricle; P2, hyperphonesis of the pulmonic component of the second heart sound; ECG, electrocardiography; RBBB, right bundle-branch block; CEE, contrast-enhanced echocardiography; RA, right atrium; PVR, pulmonary vascular resistance; AVC, arteriovenous comunication; ^{99m}TcMAA, technetium^{99m} labelled macroaggregated albumin; PAOP, pulmonary artery occlusion pressure; OLT, orthotopic liver transplantation. Rodriguez-Roisin R, Krowka MJ, Herve P, Fallon MB. Pulmonary-hepatic vascular disorders (PHD). Eur Respir J 2004; 24 (5):873 [19].

Table 4. Differences between hepatopulmonary syndrome (HPS) and portopulmonary hypertension (PPH).

2.3. Diagnosis

PPH is usually diagnosed after a diagnosis of portal hypertension is made. The mean interval between diagnoses of both conditions is 28 ± 38 months, according to a prospective study by Hadengue et al. [35]. Those authors reported that 40% of dyspneic patients were overlooked on clinical examination.

According to currently established and recognized diagnostic criteria, the American Association for the Study of Liver Disease (AASLD) has proposed transthoracic echocardiography screening of all LT candidates for noninvasive identification of any form of PH and patient selection for RHC [47].

Transthoracic echocardiography (TTE) provides a number of variables that correlate with right heart hemodynamics, including pulmonary artery pressure. Estimated pulmonary artery pressure (PAP) is based on maximum tricuspid regurgitant jet velocity. The simplified Bernoulli equation describes the relationship between tricuspid regurgitant jet velocity and peak tricuspid regurgitant pressure gradient is equal to 4X (tricuspid regurgitant jet velocity)^2. This equation allows us to estimate systolic pulmonary artery pressure (SPAP), taking into account right atrial pressure (RAP):

SPAP = (tricuspid regurgitant pressure gradient) + estimated RAP (which is equal to 5 or 10 mmHg), or *Equation (1):*

$$SPAP = [4x(tricuspid\ regurgitation\ jet\ velocity)^2 + meanRAP] \quad (1)$$

In patients with severe tricuspid regurgitation, calculation of SPAP may be underestimated, thus the pulmonary hypertension is not precisely defined by Doppler for a threshold value of SPAP obtained [1].

Doppler TTE is a sensitive method for detection of PH, despite its low positive predictive value. Consequently, pulmonary hemodynamics should be measured by RHC in positive cases to substantiate diagnosis [1, 19, 46, 47].

In a recent study, Raevens et al. [48–50] analyzed the accuracy of TTE in the detection of all forms of PPH for different cutoff values of SPAP. In SPAP values of 30 mmHg, those authors found a sensitivity of 100%, a specificity of 54%, a positive predictive value of 10%, and a negative predictive value of 100%. In SPAP values of 38 mmHg, findings were: 100% sensitivity, 82% specificity, 22% positive predictive value, and 100% negative predictive value. In SPAP values of 50 mmHg, 86% sensitivity, 95% specificity, 46% positive predictive value, and 99% negative predictive value were found.

The authors incorporated the presence or absence of right ventricle dilatation, concluding that TTE is a highly sensitive screening test for PPH detection. Currently, in the performance of RHC to confirm or rule out PPH, an SPAP cutoff of 30 mmHg may produce a high number of false-positive tests, resulting in low specificity, and low positive predictive values. An SPAP of 38 mmHg was associated with a lower number of false-positive tests and higher specificity, ensuring a negative predictive value of 100%, safely reducing the number of patients referred to RHC. An SPAP of 50 mmHg is associated with a decreased sensitivity of 86% and a risk of canceling LT at the time of surgery.

Right heart catheterization is the gold standard for diagnostic confirmation of pulmonary arterial hypertension, including PPH. RHC measures pressure, flow, and resistance, provides assessment of severity of hemodynamic impairment, and is useful for vasoreactivity testing of the pulmonary circulation. The following variables are measured systolic, diastolic and mean pulmonary artery pressure, RAP, PAOP, right ventricular pressure (RVP), cardiac output (CO) by thermodilution or by the Fick method, allowing calculation of pulmonary vascular resistance [19, 48]. The PVR is calculed using following formula, *Equation (2):*

$$PVR = \frac{MPAP - PAOP \times 80}{CO} \tag{2}$$

In PPH, the vasoreactivity test should be performed to determine disease severity and identify which patients could benefit from vasodilator therapy. A acute vasodilator testing should be commonly performed using intravenous epoprostenol (IV) or inhaled nitric oxide (NO). The test is considered positive when MPAP decreases by ≥ 10 mmHg to an absolute value of MPAP ≤ 40 mmHg with increased or no change in CO [1, 19].

MPAP may increase in different situations. First, many patients with advanced liver disease present a hyperdynamic, high-flow circulatory state, resulting from splanchnic vasodilation caused by portal hypertension, leading to a marked increase in MPAP and CO. However, PVR remains normal or decreased. Second, elevation of MPAP is due to increased central blood volume due to left ventricular (LV) abnormalities measured by PAOP, which reflects end-diastolic LV volume, resulting in varying effects on PVR. Traspulmonary gradient (TPG = MPAP - PAOP) can distinguish between excess volume (TPG < 10 mmHg) and vascular pulmonary abnormalities (TPG > 10 mmHg) [19]. Third, MPAP is elevated regardless of disease severity, due to increased PVR caused by changes in the pulmonary vascular bed with progressive obliteration to pulmonary arterial blood flow from the right ventricle (RV) to the lungs [19, 36].

Type	MPAP	PAOP	CO	PVR
1. Hyperdynamic circulatory state	↑	N or ↓	↑↑	↓
2. Excess volume	↑	↑↑↑	↑	NA
3.Portopulmonary hypertension	↑↑↑	↓	↑follow by ↓	↑↑↑

MPAP, mean pulmonary artery pressure; PAOP, pulmonary artery occlusion pressure; CO, cardiac output; PVR, pulmonary vascular resistance; N, normal; NA, no alteration.

Table 5. Hemodynamic data obtained by right heart catheterization in advanced liver disease [19].

In all patients with pulmonary hypertension, RHC is essential for diagnostic confirmation and assessment of disease severity [1, 19, 36].

Diagnostic confirmation of cirrhosis by liver biopsy may strengthen the diagnosis of PPH [5, 8].

Pulmonary artery catheterization obtained the following hemodynamic data [19, 36], as observed in **Table 5**.

2.4. Treatment

Specific treatment of PAH are use in PPH and includes different classes of vasodilators, such as prostacyclin analogs, endothelin receptor antagonists, and phosphodiesterase type 5 inhibitors [19, 25, 38].

The goal of therapies is to improve haemodynamics by reducing mean pulmonary artery pressure and pulmonary vascular resistance, to improve the haemodynamic right ventricle, thus creating possibility for patients to become eligible for LT [51, 52].

These drugs are used only after diagnostic confirmation of the disease by RHC, and patients meet diagnostic criteria for PPH, according to the ERS Task Force on PHD [16, 19].

A decrease of > 20% in MPAP and PVR indicates that patients are responsive to vasodilators [11]. Publications and reports of a recent small case series have indicated that use of these drugs before and after LT results in clinical improvement. However, further studies are needed [53–55].

2.4.1. Prostacyclins

Prostacyclin analogs (prostanoids), such as epoprostenol, beraprost, iloprost.

Epoprostenol is administered by continuous intravenous infusion. It is a potent pulmonary and systemic vasodilator, it has antiproliferative effects, and potent inhibitor of platelet aggregation. The drug also reduces MPAP, and probably improves exercise tolerance and hemodynamic parameters, but common adverse effects and complications are attributable to this drug: jaw pain, headache, diarrhea, nausea, and vomiting; others effects are described as infecction in infusion line, ascites, right heart failure, splenomegaly, severe thrombocytopenia, and leukopenia [1, 19, 25, 56].

2.4.2. Endothelin receptor antagonists

Bosentan, ambrisentan, and sitaxentan.

Endothelin are endogenous vasoconstrictors with a major role in the pathogenesis of PAH.

Bosentan is an orally active dual antagonist of endothelin 1A and 1B that reduces PVR, improving exercise capacity, functional class, pulmonary and cardiac hemodynamics, and even prevents clinical deterioration. It can elevate liver enzymes despite limited experience in PPH [1, 19].Bosentan use should be avoided in patients with moderate to severe liver dysfunction and elevated liver enzymes.

Ambrisentan is a selective ET-1A with minimal effect on liver function and sitaxentan was withdrawn from the market due fatal liver injury registration [38].

2.4.3. Phosphodiesterase inhibitors (PDE 5 inhibitors)

Sildenafil, vardenafil, tadalafil.

These drugs block cyclic GMP degradation. Cyclic GMP is a second messenger for nitric oxide, thereby prolonging vasodilator mediation of NO, producing lower MPAP and PVR [1]. These should be use cautiously because it may increase portal hypertension by splanchnic vasodilation [38].

Reichenberger et al. [16, 57] used sildenafil in 14 patients with PPH for 12 months. Of these patients, six received inhaled iloprost or treprostinil. Hemodynamics improved significantly within three months and was maintained at 12 months, when diagnosed by RHC. Other small studies have shown clinical improvement after safe and effective use of this drug.

Yamashita et al. [58] reported cases of two patients with advanced liver disfunction and thrombocytopenia who were successfully treated with a combination of two oral vasodilators, ambrisentan and tadalafil. They concluded that it may be a safe and effective option for selected patients with severe and rapidly progressing PPH.

Retrospective studies involving postoperative liver transplant have stated that PPH was an absolute contraindication to transplantation because of high perioperative mortality. It is currently known that better preoperative evaluation, early initiation of drug, and improved anesthetic and surgical conditions offer new treatment possibilities.

PPH can thus become more common in liver transplantation centers [1, 5, 19, 56, 59].

2.5. Liver transplantation

Liver transplantation is a highly complex procedure, since the organ is responsible for multiple functions in the body. The first unsuccessful attempt at orthotopic LT in humans was carried out in the United States in 1963 by Thomas Earl Starzl and staff. Starzl was named the father of modern transplantation. The first successful case was recorded in 1967. By the end of the 1960s, 33 transplants had been described worldwide. Subsequently, other teams started performing this surgery with a low survival rate [14].

PPH patients have a high mortality rate related to right heart failure. There are few treatment options and LT has become an attractive therapy with a potential for cure. The role of LT in the treatment of PPH has evolved over the past 15 years [16]. Over time, better results will be achieved by advances in the understanding of new immunosuppressive drugs, biologic drug activity, metabolism, surgical technique, evaluation and intraoperative monitoring in anesthesiology and intensive care [14]. The anesthesiologist has an important role in managing these high risk patients [60].

Perioperative mortality risk is 100% in patients with a MPAP above 50 mmHg. However, a patient with MPAP $\leq$ 35 mmHg, observed in intraoperative period, can safely undergo LT. An

MPAP ranging from 35 to 50 mmHg poses a dilemma if these values are associated with PVR > 240 dynes.s.cm^{-5}, mortality rate hovers around 50% [61–63].

Studies have proved successful in practice, with the introduction of pulmonary arterial vasodilators after PPH diagnosis, lower pulmonary artery pressure, and improving right ventricular function obtained for patient referral to LT [16, 19, 64].

Kwo et al. [65] reported that four patients with severe PPH showed a marked reduction in MPAP and PVR after long-term use of epoprostenol, providing better results for LT candidates.

Mair et al. [66] described a poor outcome in a case report. The patient received epoprostenol for eight months before LT. PVR was reduced from 12 units to 3 Wood units, but the patient developed right heart failure unresponsive to conventional inhaled therapy in the LT perioperative period, and died 28 days later.

LT is a special case of right ventricular stress with a sharp 5–10% increase in CO during reperfusion. However, an increase in CO is unpredictable and may reach up to 300%, precipitating right heart failure in a RV that is already under strain [61, 67]. Increased CO probably results from removal of blood flow obstruction through the portal vein in the diseased liver, associated with systemic vasodilatation caused by acid rain, and other metabolites originating from the new graft. There is a significant decrease in myocardial contractility, chronotropy, and systemic vascular resistance [61, 68]. Once this occurs, a patient suffering from pulmonary hypertension is at great risk [61].

2.6. Study justification

We believe that understanding the aspects and nuances of this severe disease may raise awareness about the issue and increase scientific knowledge. Following recommendations proposed by the international scientific community will certainly contribute to solidify work done by a multidisciplinary team to decrease morbidity and mortality in PPH patients undergoing liver transplantation.

2.7. Nomenclature

ALK 1	Activin-like receptor kinase-1
AASLD	American Association for the Study of Liver Disease
BMPR2	Bone morphogenetic protein receptor type 2
CAV1	Caveolin-1
CO	Cardiac output
ENG	Endoglin
ERS	European Respiratory Society
ET-1A	Endothelin-1A

ET-1B	Endothelin-1B
cGPM	Cyclic guanosine monophosphate
HPS	Hepatopulmonary syndrome
IV	Intravenous
KCNK3	Gene encoding potassium channel
LT	Liver transplantation
LV	Left ventricle
MELD	Model end-stage for liver disease
MPAP	Mean pulmonary artery pressure
NO	Nitric oxide
NYHA	New York Heart Association
PAH	Pulmonary arterial hypertension
PAOP	Pulmonary artery occlusion pressure
PAP	Pulmonary artery pression
PDE	Phosphodiesterase
PH	Pulmonary hypertension
PHD	Pulmonary hepatic vascular disorders
PPH	Portopulmonary hypertension
PVR	Pulmonary vascular resistance
RAP	Right atrial pressure
RHC	Right heart catheterization
RV	Right ventricle
SPAP	Systolic pulmonary artery pressure

Author details

Emica Shimozono*, Cristina A. A. Caruy, Adilson R. Cardoso, Derli C. M. Servian and Ilka F. S. F. Boin

*Address all correspondence to: emicashi@hotmail.com

Unit of Liver Transplantation - Clinics Hospital - State University of Campinas (HC - Unicamp), Campinas - São Paulo, Brazil

References

[1] Galiè N, Hoeper MM, Humbert M, Torbicki A, Vachiery JL, Barbara JA et al. ESC Committee for Practice Guidelines. Guidelines for the diagnosis and treatment of pulmonary hypertension: the Task Force for the diagnosis and treatment of pulmonary hypertension of the European Society of Cardiology (ESC) and the European Respiratory Society (ERS), endorsed by the International Society of Heart and Lung Transplantation (ISHLT). Eur Heart J. 2009;30(20): 2493–537. DOI: 10.1093/eurheartj/ehp297

[2] Simonneau G, Galiè N, Rubin LJ, Langleben D, Seeger W, Domenighetti G et al. Clinical classification of pulmonary hypertension. J Am Coll Cardiol. 2004;43:5S–12S. DOI: 10.1016/j.jacc.2004.02.037

[3] Galiè N, Humbert M, Vachiery JL, Gibbs S, Lang I, Torbicki A et al. 2015 ESC/ERS Guidelines for the diagnosis and treatment of pulmonary hypertension of the European Society of Cardiology (ESC) and European Respiratory Society (ERS). Eur Heart J. 2016;37(1):67–119. DOI: 10.1093/eurheartj/ehv317

[4] Kurram B, Guadalupe Garcia-Tsao. Treatment of portal hypertension. World J Gastroenterol. 2012;18(11):1166–1175. DOI: 10.3748/wjg.v18.i11.1166

[5] Garcia E, Moreira JS, Brandão ABM, Zille AI, Fernandes JC. Hipertensão Portopulmonar. J Bras Pneumol. 2005;31(2):157–61. DOI: 10.1590/s1806-37132005000200012

[6] Golbin JM, Krowka MJ. Portopulmonary hypertension. Clin Chest. 2007;28:203–218. DOI: 10.1016/j.ccm.2006.11.004

[7] Krowka MJ. Hepatopulmonary syndrome versus portopulmonary hypertension: distinctions and dilemmas. Hepatology. 1997;25:1282–84. DOI: 10.1002/hep.510250540

[8] Mandell MS, Groves BM. Pulmonary hypertension in chronic liver disease. Clin Chest Med. 1996;17(1):17–33. DOI: 10.1016/S0272-5231(05)70296-3

[9] Naeye RL. Primary pulmonary hypertension with coexisting portal hypertension. A retrospective study of six cases. Circulation. 1960;22: 376–84. DOI: 10.116/01.CIR.22.3.376

[10] Møller S, Henriksen JH, Bendtsen F. Extrahepatic complications to cirrosis and portal hypertension: Haemodynamic and homeostatic aspects. World J Gastroenterol. 2014;20(42):15499–517. DOI: 10.3748/wjg.v20.i42.15499

[11] Hervé P, Lebrec D, Brenot F, Simonneau G, Humbert M, Sitbon O et al. Pulmonary vascular disorders in portal hypertension. Eur Respir J. 1998;11:1153–66. DOI: 10.1183/09031936.98.11051153

[12] Mantz FA, Craige E. Portal axis thrombosis with spontaneous portocaval shunt and resultant cor pulmonale. Arch Pathol Lab Med. 1951;52: 91–97.

[13] Kuo PC, Plotkin JS, Gaine S, Schroeder RA, Rustgi VK, Rubin LJ, Jonhson LB. Portopulmonary hypertension and the liver transplantation candidate. Transplantation. 1999;67(8):1087–93. DOI: 10.1097/00007890-199904270-00001

[14] Mies S. Transplante de Fígado. Rev Ass Med Brasil. 1998;44(2):127–34. DOI: 10.1590/S0104-42301998000200011

[15] Gaine SP, Rubin LJ. Primary pulmonary hypertension. Lancet. 1998; Aug 29; 352(9129): 719–25. DOI: 10.1016/S0140-6736(98)02111-4

[16] Safdar Z, Bartolome S, Sussman N. Portopulmonary hypertension: An update. Liver Transpl. 2012;18(8): 881–91. DOI: 10.1002/lt.23485

[17] Simonneau G, Robbins IM, Beghetti M, Channick RN, Decroix M, Denton CP et al. Updated clinical classification of pulmonary hypertension. J Am Coll Cardiol. 2009;54(1 suppl):S43-S54. DOI: 10.1016/j.jacc.2009.04.012

[18] Simonneau G, Gatzoulis MA, Adatia I, Celermajer D, Denton C, Ghofrani A et al. Update clinical classification of pulmonary hypertension. J Am Coll Cardiol. 2013;62(25 suppl):D34-D41. DOI: 10.1016/j.jacc.2013.10.029

[19] Rodriguez-Roisin R, Krowka MJ, Hervé P, Fallon MB. ERS Task Force Pulmonary-Hepatic Vascular Disorders (PHD) Scientific Committee. Eur Respir J. 2004;24(5):861–880. DOI: 10.1183/09031936.04.00010904

[20] Saleemi S. Portopulmonary hypertension. Ann Thorac Med. 2010;5(1):5–9. DOI: 10.4103/1817-1737.58953

[21] Chemla D, Castelain V, Hervé P, Lecarpentier Y, Brimioulle S. Haemodynamic evaluation of pulmonary hypertension. Eur Respir J. 2002; 20:1314–1331. DOI: 10.1183/09031936.02.00068002

[22] Singh C, Sager JS. Pulmonary complications of cirrhosis. Med Clin N Am. 2009;93:871–83. DOI: 10.1016/j.mcna.2009.03.006

[23] McDonnell PJ, Toye PA, Hutchins GM. Primary pulmonary hypertension and cirrhosis are they related? Am Rev Respir Dis. 1983;127:437–41. DOI: 10.1164/arrd.1983.127.4.437

[24] Taura P, Garcia-Valdecasas JC, Beltran J, Izquierdo E, Navasa M, Sala- Blanch J et al. Moderate primary pulmonary hypertension in patients undergoing liver transplantation. Anesth Analg. 1996;83:675–680. DOI: 10.1097/00000539-199610000-00003

[25] Giusca S, Jinga M, Jurcut C, Jucurt R, Serban M, Ginghina C. Portopulmonary hypertension: From diagnosis to treatment. European Journal of Internal Medicine. 2011;22:441–47. DOI: 10.1016/j.ejim.2011.02.018

[26] Colle IO, Moreau R, Godinho E, Belghiti J, Ettori F, Cohen-Solal A et al. Diagnosis of portopulmonary hypertension in candidates for liver transplantation: a prospective study. Hepatology. 2003;37:401–09. DOI: 10.1053/jhep.2003.50060

[27] Castro M, Krowka MJ, Schroeder DR, Beck KC, Plevak DJ, Rettke SR et al. Frequency and clinical implications of increased pulmonary artery pressures in liver transplant patients. Mayo Clin Proc. 1996;71:543–51. DOI: 10.4065/71.6543

[28] Ramsay MA, Simpson BR, Nguyen AT, Ramsay KJ, East C, Klintmalm GB. Severe pulmonary hypertension in liver transplant candidates. Liver Transpl Surg. 1997;3:494–500. DOI: 10.1002/lt.500030503

[29] Robalino BD, Moodie DS. Association between primary pulmonary hypertension and portal hypertension: Analysis of its pathophysiology and clinical, laboratory and hemodynamic manifestations. J Am Coll Cardiol. 1991;17:492–98. DOI: 10.1016/S0735-1097(10)80121-4

[30] Kawut SM, Taichman DB, Ahya VN, Kaplan S, Archer-Chicko CL, Kimmel SE et al. Hemodynamics and survival of patients with portopulmonary hypertension. Liver Transpl. 2005;11(9):1107–11. DOI: 10.1002/lt.20459

[31] Le Pavec J, Souza R, Hervé P, Lebrec D, Savale L, Tcherakian C et al. Portopulmonary hypertension: survival and prognostic factors. Am J Respir Crit Care Med. 2008;178: 637–43. DOI: 10.1164/rccm.200804-6130C

[32] Humbert M, Sitbon O, Chaouat A, Bertocchi M, Habib G, Gressin V et al. Pulmonary artery
hypertension in France: results from a national registry. Am J Rev Respir Crit Care Med. 2006;173:1023–1030. DOI: 10.1164/rccm.200510-166680C

[33] Swanson KL, Wiesner RH, Nyberg SL, Rosen CB, Krowka MJ. Survival in portopulmonary hypertension: Mayo Clinic experience categorized by treatment groups. Am J Transpl. 2008;8:2445–53. DOI: 10.1111/j.1600-6143.2008.02384.x

[34] Krowka MJ, Miller DP, Barst RJ, Taichman D, Dweik RA, Badesch DB et al. Portopulmonary hypertension: a report from the US-based REVEAL Registry. Chest. 2012;141:906–15. DOI: 10.1378/chest.11-0160

[35] Hadengue A, Benhayoun MK, Lebrec D, Benhamou JP. Pulmonary hypertension complicating portal hypertension: prevalence and relation to splanchnic hemodynamics. Gastroenterology. 1991;100(2):520- 28. PMID: 1985048

[36] Krowka MJ, Swanson KL, Frantz RP, MacGoon MD, Wiesner RH. Portopulmonary hypertension: Results from a 10 year screening algorithm. Hepatology. 2006;44(6): 1502–10. DOI: 10.1002/hep.21431

[37] Nayak RP, Li D, Matuschak GM. Portopulmonary hypertension. Current Gastroenterol Rep. 2009;11(1):56–63. DOI: 10.1007/s11894-009-0009-3

[38] Raevens S, Geerts A, Van Steenkiste C, Verheist X, Van Vlierberghe H, Colle I. Hepatopulmonary syndrome and portopulmonary hypertension: recent knowledge in pathogenesis and overview of clinical assessment. Liver International. 2015;35(6):1646–60. DOI: 10.1111/liv.12791

[39] Pellicelli AM, Barbaro G, Puoti C, Guarascio P, Lusi EA, Bellis Let al. Plasma cytokines and portopulmonary hypertension in patients with cirrhosis waiting for orthotopic liver transplantation. Angiology. 2010;61:802–6. DOI: 10.1177/0003319710369101

[40] Kawut SM, Krowka MJ, Trotter JF, Roberts KE, Benza RL, Badesch DB et al. Clinical risk factors for portopulmonary hypertension. Hepatology. 2008;48:196–203. DOI: 10.1002/hep.22275

[41] Roberts KE, Fallon MB, Krowka MJ, Brown RS, Trotter JF, Peter I et al. Genetic risk factors for portopulmonary in patients with advanced liver disease. Am J Resp Crit Care Med. 2009;179:835–42. DOI: 10.1164/rccm.200809-14720C

[42] Roberts KE, Fallon MB, Krowka MJ, Benza RL, Knowles JA, Badesch DB et al. Serotonin transporter polymorphisms in patients with portopulmonary hypertension. Chest. 2009;135:1470–75. DOI: 10.1378/chest.08-1909

[43] Hoeper MM, Kowka MJ, Strassburg CP. Portopulmonary hypertension and hepatopulmonary syndrome. Lancet. 2004;363:1461–68. DOI: 10.1016/S0140-6736(04)16107-2

[44] Hopps E, Valenti A, Caimi G. Portopulmonary hypertension. Clin Inves Med. 2011;34(3):E111–118. PMID: 216311986

[45] Minemura M, Tajiri K, Shimizu Y. Systemic abnormalities in liver disease. World J Gastroenterol. 2009; june 28;15(24):2960–2974. DOI: 10.3748/wjg.15.2960

[46] Krowka MJ, Mandell MS, Ramsay MAE, Kawut SM, Fallon MB, Manzarbeitia C et al. Hepatopulmonary syndrome and portopulmonary hypertension: a report of multicenter liver transplant database. Liver Transpl. 2004;10(2):174–82. DOI: 10.1002/lt.20016

[47] Murray KF, Carithers RL Jr. AASLD practice guidelines: evaluation of the patient for liver transplantation. Hepatology. 2005;41(6):1407–32. DOI: 10.1002/hep.20704

[48] Krowka MJ. Portopulmonary hypertension: diagnostic advances and caveats. Liver Transpl. 2003;9:1336–37. DOI: 10.1002/lt.500091215

[49] Raevens S, Colle I, Reyntjens K, Geerts A, Berrevoet F, Rogiers X et al. Echocardiography for the detection of portopulmonary hypertension in liver transplant candidates: an analysis of cutoff values. Liver Transp. 2013; 19(6):602–10. DOI: 10.1002/lt.23649

[50] Porres-Aguilar M, Duarte-Rojo A, Krowka MJ. Transthoracic Echocardiography screening for the detection of portopulmonary hypertension: a work in progress. Liver Transpl. 2013;19:573–74. DOI: 10.1002/lt.23663

[51] Porres-Aguilar M, Mukherjee D. Portopulmonary hypertension: An update. Respirology. 2015;20(2):235–42. DOI: 10.1111/resp.12455

[52] Medarov BI, Chopra A, Judson MA. Clinical aspects of portopulmonary hypertension. Respir Med. 2014;108(7):943–54. DOI: 10.1016/j.rmed.2014.04.004

[53] Krowka MJ, Frantz RP, MacGoon MD, Severson C, Plevak DJ, Wiesner RH. Improvement in pulmonary hemodynamics during intravenous epoprostenol (prostacyclin): a

study of 15 patients with moderate to severe portopulmonary hypertension. Hepatology. 1999;30:641–648. DOI: 10.1002/hep.510300307

[54] Kett DH, Acosta RC, Campos MA, Rodriguez MJ, Quartin AA, Schein RMH. Recurrent portopulmonary hypertension after liver transplantation: management with epoprostenol and resolution after retransplantation. Liver Transpl. 2001;7:645–648. DOI: 10.1053/jlts.2001.25358

[55] Minder S, Fischler M, Muelhaupt B, Zalunardo MP, Jenni R, Clavien PA et al. Intravenous iloprost bridging to liver transplantation in portopulmonary hypertension. Eur Resp J. 2004;24:703–707. DOI: 10.1183/09031936.04.00133203

[56] Savalle L, O'Callaghan DS, Magnier R, Le Pavec J, Hervé P, Jais Z et al. Current management approaches to portopulmonary hypertension. Int J Clin Pract Suppl. 2011;65(169):11–8. DOI: 10.1111/j.1742.2010.02600.x

[57] Reichenberger F, Voswinckel R, Steveling E, Enke B, Kreckel A, Olschewski H et al. Sildenafil treatment for portopulmonary hypertension. Eur Resp J. 2006;28:563–567. DOI: 10.1183/09031936.06.00030206

[58] Yamashita Y, Tsujino I, Sato T, Yamada A, Watanabe T, Ohira H et al. Hemodynamic effects of ambrisentan-tadalafil combination therapy on progressive portopulmonary hypertension. World J Hepatol. 2014;6(11):825–9. DOI: 10.4254/wjh.v6.i11.825

[59] Raevens S, De Pauw M, Reyntjens K, Geerts A, Verhelst X, Berrevoet F et al. Oral vasodilator therapy in patients with moderate to severe portopulmoary hypertension as a bridge to liver transplantation. Eur J Gastroenterol Hepatol. 2013;25(4):495–502. DOI: 10.197/MEG.0b013e32835c504b

[60] Aldenkortt F, Aldenkortt M, Caviezel L, Walber JL, Weber A, Schiffer E. Portopulmonary hypertension and hepatopulmonary syndrome. World J Gastroenterol. 2014;20(25):8072–81. DOI: 10.3748/wjg.v20.i25.8072

[61] Ramsay MA. Perioperative mortality in patients with portopulmonary hypertension undergoing liver transplantation. Liver Transp. 2000;6 (4):451–2. DOI: 10.1053/jlts.2000.8859

[62] Mancuso L, Scordato F, Pieri M, Valerio E, Mancuso A. Management of portopulmonary hypertension: news perspectives. World J Gastroenterol. 2015;19(45):8252–7. DOI: 10.3748/wjg.v19.i45.8252

[63] Machicao VI, Balakrishnan M, Fallon MB. Pulmonary complication in chronic liver disease. Hepatology. 2014;59(4):1627–37. DOI: 10.1002/hep.26745

[64] Cartin-Ceba R, Krowka MJ. Portopulmonary hypertension. Clin Liver Dis. 2014;18(2): 421–38. DOI: 10.1016/j.cld.2014.01.004

[65] Kuo PC, Jonhson LB, Plotkin JS, Howell CD, Bartlett ST, Rubin LJ. Continuous intravenous infusion of epoprostenol for the treatment of portopulmonary hypertension. Transplantation. 1997;63:604–6. DOI: 10.1097/00007890-199702270-00020

[66] Mair P, Kaehler CH, Pomaroli A, Schwarz B, Vogel W, Margreiter R. Orthotopic liver transplantation in a patient with severe portopulmonary hypertension. Acta Anaesthesiol Scand. 2001;45(4):513–18. DOI: 10.1034/j.1399-6576.2001.045004513.x

[67] Khaderi S, Khan R, Safdar Z, Stribling R, Vierling JM, Goss A, Sussman NL. Long-term follow-up of portopulmonary hypertension patients after liver transplantation. Liver Transpl. 2014;20(6):724–7. DOI: 10.1002/lt.23870

[68] Rudnick MR, De Marchi L, Plotkin JS. Hemodynamic monitoring during transplantation: A state of the art review. World J Hepatol. 2015;7(10):1302–11. DOI: 10.4254/wjh.v7.i10.1302

Section 4

Heart and Lung Transplantation

Chapter 10

Ex-Vivo Lung Perfusion: From Bench to Bedside

Nader Aboelnazar, Sayed Himmat,
Darren Freed and Jayan Nagendran

Additional information is available at the end of the chapter

http://dx.doi.org/10.5772/62449

Abstract

Lung transplantation is an established treatment option for eligible patients with end-stage lung disease. Nonetheless, there exists an imbalance between donor lungs considered suitable for transplantation and the ever-growing number of patients dying on the waiting list. This chapter reflects the potential alternative, normothermic ex-vivo lung perfusion (EVLP), which has emerged to address this issue and how it can expand the currently limited donor pool. Normothermic ex-vivo lung perfusion (EVLP), as a novel preservation technique, is capable of assessing, evaluating, and improving lung function prior to lung transplantation. Here, we (1) contrast the various available commercial EVLP available and used around the world; (2) outline the University of Alberta novel EVLP circuit; (3) discuss the limitations present between clinical and laboratory applications; and (4) present what we are currently working on at the laboratory to further improve the assessment techniques used on EVLP.

Keywords: donor lung preservation, donor lung repair, ex-vivo lung perfusion, lung transplantation, lung health index

1. Lung transplantation

1.1. History

Human lung transplantation (LTx) has been widely accepted as a modality of treatment for advanced stage lung disease [1]. The annual report from the Registry of the International Society for Heart and Lung Transplantation (ISHLT) states more than 45,000 LTx cases performed worldwide since the 1990s. In 2012, ISHLT reported that in that year it had the second highest annual activity, following the highest activity level in 2011, in LTx performed. "The number of adult primary lung transplants in 2012 was 40-fold higher than the number of pediatric primary lung transplants" [1]. The agency for healthcare policy and research in the United States mentioned that "lung transplantation has evolved as a clinical procedure achieving a favourable risk–benefit ratio and acceptable 1- and 2-year survival rates" [1].

In the 1940s and the 1950s, a rise in animal experimentation verified feasibility of LTx procedure [2–4]. However, it was not until 1963 when the first human lung transplantation was performed. The recipient of that first lung transplantation received a left lung, which was donated from a cardiocirculatory death donor (DCD); however, the recipient survived for only 18 days [5]. From 1963 to 1980, almost 44 lung transplantations were attempted worldwide; due to rejections and problems with anastomotic bronchial and tracheal healing, the survival rates were only several days [6, 7].

The introduction of cyclosporine A in the 1980s, a powerful immunosuppressant, generated a renewed interest in organ transplantation, including LTx. In 1983, Dr. Cooper from Toronto performed the first successful human single lung transplantation, while Dr. Patterson performed the first double lung transplantation in 1988 [6, 7]. Despite the relatively short history of thoracic transplantation, there has been significant improvement in post-transplantation mortality rate from only weeks to several months and years. This success can be attributed to the advent of the heart–lung machine, improved preservation solutions, immunosuppression regimes, and specialized patient care by transplant clinics.

1.2. Indications

Lung transplantation is considered for patients with end-stage lung disease. Referral for transplantation is urgent when the lung disease begins to limit basic daily activities and poses a high risk of death in the short term.

According to ISHLT, the most common primary indication for adult lung transplants between January 1995 and June 2013 was chronic obstructive pulmonary disease (COPD, 33%) not associated with α_1-antitrypsin deficiency (A1ATD), followed by interstitial lung disease (ILD, 24%), including idiopathic pulmonary fibrosis (IPF), cystic fibrosis (CF, 16%) associated with bronchiectasis, and 6% of COPD associated with A1ATD [8, 9]. For the 45,711 lung transplants that occurred from 1990 to 2012, recipients with COPD not associated with A1ATD, ILD, and CF contributed to the greatest amount of growth in the number of LTx [8, 9].

1.3. Criteria

The appropriate timing for patients to be referred for lung transplantation is when they are believed to have less than 50% of a survival chance in 24–36 month period. An additional consideration is the patient's quality of life. The following are the guidelines for referral for LTx, based on the underlying lung disease [10] (**Table 1**).

Criteria for referral in patients with COPD and alpha1-antitrypsin deficiency emphysema are as follows: • BODE index > 5 • Postbronchodilator FEV_1 < 25% predicted • Resting hypoxemia (i.e., PaO_2 < 55–60 mm Hg) • Hypercapnia ($PaCO_2$ > 50 mm Hg) • Secondary pulmonary hypertension • Clinical course marked by rapid rate of decline in FEV_1 or life-threatening exacerbations FEV_1, forced expiratory volume in 1 s; PaO_2, partial pressure of arterial oxygen; $PaCO_2$, partial pressure of arterial carbon dioxide	The BODE index, a multidimensional 10-point scale, can be used to assess the need for transplantation in patients with COPD. It consists of the following [46]: • B—Body mass index • O—Degree of airflow obstruction • D—Degree of dyspnea, as measured by the modified Medical Research Council dyspnea scale • E—Exercise capacity (E), which is measured with a 6 min walk test
Criteria for referral in patients with cystic fibrosis are as follows: • Postbronchodilator FEV_1 < 30% predicted • Resting hypoxemia, i.e., PaO_2 < 55 mm Hg • Hypercapnia ($PaCO_2$ > 50 mm Hg) • Clinical course—Increasing frequency and severity of exacerbations (ICU stays) • Development of pulmonary hypertension	
Criteria for referral in patients with idiopathic pulmonary fibrosis are as follows: • DLCO < 39%, predicted • A 10% or greater decrement in forced vital capacity (FVC) during 6 months' follow-up • FVC < 60–65%, predicted • Decrease in oxygen saturations <88% during 6 min walk test DLCO, diffusion capacity of carbon monoxide; FVC, forced vital capacity.	

Table 1. Guideline criteria for referral to lung transplantation, based on underlying lung diseases [10].

1.4. The burden

The Canadian Organ Replacement Registry (CORR) has reported that in the past decade, the annual number of lung transplants has gradually increased over the years [11]; meanwhile, the waiting list increases at a much faster rate. Therefore, a staggering increase in the morbidity rate and a high waiting list mortality rate have been reported [11]. With the advancements of medical knowledge and specialized patient care over the years, lung disease patients with other ailments can now have their nonrelated lung conditions managed appropriately and live longer till they require a lung transplant.

Currently, more than 80% of donor lungs are potentially injured and therefore not considered suitable for transplantation [12]. At the University of Alberta, we report that from 2007 to 2011 there have been a total of 681 lungs offered, and only 183 lungs deemed acceptable for LTx. This equates to approximately a 27% utilization rate over the past 5 years. With the University of Alberta/Mazankowski Alberta Heart Institute acting as a catchment for over 6 million Canadians, this institute performs the majority of thoracic transplantations for several provinces in Canada. Unfortunately, with such a low lung utilization rate, there are more than 24 deaths/year for patients waiting for a suitable donor lung. Having said that, various strategies need to be implemented to increase the utilization rate of the current standard lung donor pool.

During recent years, transplant centers worldwide have started to include the use of lungs from extended/marginal criteria donors, living lobar donors, as well as tapping into the unused pool of donors after circulatory death (DCD) [13, 14]. Normothermic ex-vivo lung perfusion (EVLP) emerged as a new and promising platform, with the clinical potential to increase the number of transplantable lungs and improve the early and late outcome post-transplantation. EVLP has the potential to assess, evaluate, and recondition lungs, and eventually expand the limited donor pool. Currently, EVLP is limited to only 4–6 h of a reconditioning window [13]. This narrows therapeutic interventions that can be applied during this short perfusion time. The need for an extended clinical EVLP protocol (≥12 h) is critical to achieve its full potential. Gene therapy and stem cell therapy are promising therapeutic examples. However, their respective delivery techniques using EVLP are yet to be optimized.

2. Normothermic ex-vivo lung perfusion

2.1. Lung preservation

Since the late 1980s, conventional donor lung preservation has been focused around the use of cold static preservation (CSP): placing them on ice for transportation to a recipient site. CSP supports the slowing down of cell metabolism, thus, reducing the demand for oxygen and other substrates [15]. Low metabolic state decreases enzymatic activity related to ischemia and hypoxia, thereby protecting the graft from their deleterious effects. However, the associated decrease in function of vital enzymes such as Na^+/K^+ ATPase causes an ionic imbalance, leading to edema and a rise in intracellular calcium, which causes cellular injury [16]. With the lungs inflated during CSP, studies have shown significant generation of reactive oxygen species, leading to more damage of the donated lungs [17, 18].

Over the years, there has been a predominant effort to optimize retrograde and antegrade flushing solutions, with the compositions representing mostly extracellular characteristics [19]. Further studies reported better results utilizing flush solutions, with temperatures at 10°C, whereas others supported the routine use of solutions in the 4–8°C range [20]. This was achieved after flushing the lungs with the respective flush solution and storing them on ice for the duration of the transport of the donor lungs to the recipient site. Cold preservation was thought to benefit the lungs more than other organs, given the ability to store them inflated with oxygen, allowing for efficient aerobic metabolism and maintaining their gas-exchange surface [21].

2.2. Definition and history

Physiological normothermic ex-vivo lung perfusion is a novel method that maintains the organ in a more physiological protective condition, outside the body, during preservation. EVLP will help increase the utilization of donor lungs by allowing trained professionals to accurately evaluate and assess the functionality of lungs (which otherwise would be unutilized) during the transport period. While the lungs are on EVLP, they will be maintained under normothermic physiological conditions to help alleviate the deleterious ischemia reperfusion injury that is observed with CSP, furthermore, permitting the treatment/reconditioning of the lungs prior to transplantation. Currently, with CSP, lungs have no way to be truly assessed for injury that occurs during the transport period which can range from 6 to 8 h. Thus, transplanting lungs that have suboptimal functions can result in poor postlung transplantation outcome and increase the severity of primary graft dysfunction/failure.

Ex-vivo perfusion of organs began with the work of Carrel and Lindbergh in 1935 [22]. They have documented 26 perfusions of whole organs: ovary, thyroid, kidney, and heart. Organs that were perfused were functional for several days with active cellular proliferation. Since the advent of the work of Carrel and Lindbergh on ex-vivo perfusion, ex-vivo systems were limited to the study of organ physiology, including lungs [23]. It was not until 2001 that Stig Steen first described the use of EVLP in clinical lung transplantation. Using a proprietary lung-perfusion solution (STEEN Solution™), put together in Dr. Stig Steen and his team's lab, the group was able to reassess uncontrolled donation after cardiocirculatory death (DCD) lungs [24, 25]. Until then, the majority of donor lungs were from brain-dead donors (BDD). With the help of EVLP, the successful reconditioning of these DCD lungs (an unutilized donor pool) resulted in a cascade of research to revisit the possibility of utilizing donor lungs from the DCD pool.

It was not until further modifications of the EVLP system and perfusion technique by the University of Toronto group, which allowed perfusion of pig lungs on EVLP from only 4 to 6 h [25] to a prolonged 12-hour ex-vivo perfusion, without damaging the organ [26]. The group went on to determine the impact of prolonged EVLP using injured ischemic donor pig lungs. To mimic the clinical scenario, where lungs undergo a period of cold ischemia during transportation, pig lungs were preserved under CSP for 12 h and subsequently divided into two groups: cold static preservation (the current gold standard) and normothermic EVLP for a further 12 h of perfusion (total 24 h of preservation) [27].

It became evident that unlike CSP, normothermic EVLP demonstrated noticeable improvement with regard to overall lung function: less edema formation post-transplantation, better alveolar–epithelial cell tight junction integrity, enhanced metabolic function, and improved oxygenation [25].

2.3. The circuit

As described in more detail in reference [14], in general, most EVLP platforms utilized around the world (used experimentally or clinically) consist of the same components. The circuit consists of a perfusion circuit with tubing, a reservoir, a pump, membrane gas exchanger, a leukocyte depletion filter, and an ICU-type ventilator [14] (**Figure 1**). The system is then primed with their respective perfusate and additives, and then warmed to 32–34°C. Once this temperature is achieved, careful institutional specific lung ventilation commences, allowing the lungs to continue to reach a perfusate temperature of normothermia (37°C).

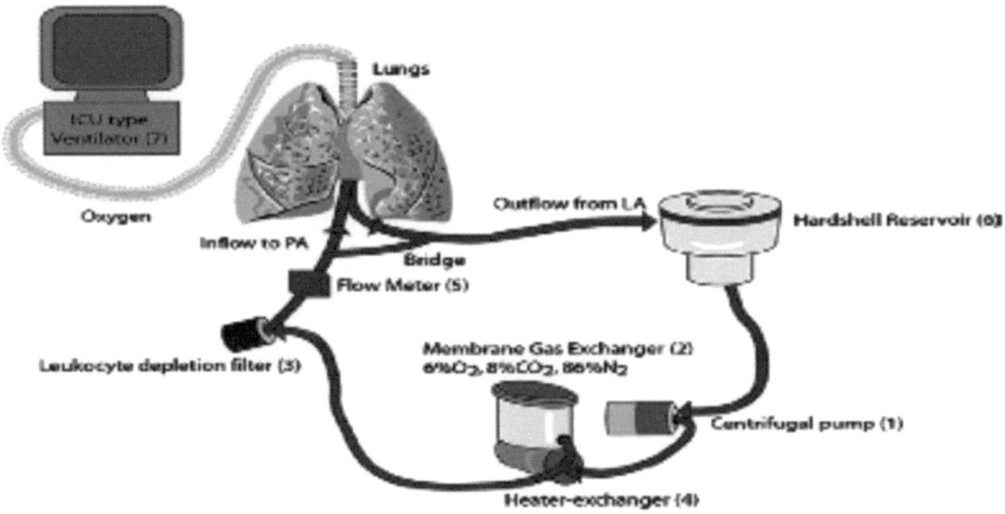

Figure 1. Schematic of the standard ex-vivo lung perfusion circuit [26].

The lungs are placed in a specially designed organ chamber. A pump, roller or centrifugal, circulates the perfusate from the reservoir through a gas-exchange membrane and a leukocyte filter, before entering the lungs via the pulmonary artery. Before entering the leukocyte filter, the gas-exchange membrane is connected to a heat exchanger and a special gas tank: the heat exchanger warms up/maintains the perfusate at normothermic temperatures, while the special gas tank consists of a low oxygen mixture to deoxygenate the perfusate before returning to the lungs (6% O_2, 8% CO_2, and 86% N_2) [14]. The outflow perfusate returns to the reservoir either through a left atrial (LA) cannula or via an open atrium, where it is then recirculated. Catheters or pressure transducers are used to continuously monitor and measure pulmonary artery pressures (PAP) and left atrial pressures (LAP), if it is a closed left atrial system. A temperature probe monitors the circuit temperature throughout the perfusion, and flow probes measure PA and LA perfusate flow (if the circuit has a closed left atrium). Finally, lungs are ventilated with a standard intensive care unit (ICU) ventilator [14].

2.4. EVLP protocols

Reference [14] outlines an in-depth review on the currently utilized EVLP platforms and their protocols. As of today, there currently exist three different EVLP protocols utilized around the world: (1) Toronto protocol, (2) Lund protocol, and (3) Organ Care System™ (OCS) protocol (TransMedics, Andover, MA). These protocols vary in composition of their respective perfusate, in perfusion and ventilation settings, and in the equipment used for their circuits [14] (**Table 2**). In general, after cold pulmonary flush and retrieval using an extracellular fluid (ECF)-type solution (low-potassium dextran solution, known as Perfadex®), the donor lungs will be instrumented in the donor hospital or recipient hospital (after experiencing a period of cold ischemia during transport) and placed on the EVLP platform for either immediate or delayed normothermic perfusion, respectively. Interestingly, reference [28] investigated the best timing for EVLP: at the donor hospital immediately after cold pulmonary flush or at the recipient hospital after transport and a period of cold storage (delayed EVLP) [14, 28]. It was further found that lower levels of inflammatory markers on bronchoalveolar lavage were present, and less histological lung injury and superior post-transplant oxygenation were seen in the group of delayed EVLP (4 h of cold storage followed by 4 h of EVLP) [14, 28].

Parameter	Toronto	Lund	OCS
Perfusion			
Target flow	40% CO	100 % CO	2.0–2.5 1/min
PAP	Flow dictated	≤20 mm Hg	≤20 mm Hg
LA	Closed	Open	Open
Perfusate	Steen™ Solution	Steen™ Solution + RBC's hct 14%	OCS™ solution+ RBC's hct 15–25 %
Ventilation			
Start temp (°C)	32	32	34
Tidal volume	7 ml/kg bw	5–7 ml/kg bw	6 ml/kg bw
RR (bpm)	7	20	10
PEEP	5 cm H_2O	5 cm H_2O	5–7 cm H_2O
FiO_2 (%)	21	50	12

All parameters are listed for perfusion in steady state (preservation); values may vary during monitoring of the graft. bw, body weight donor; bpm, breaths per minute; CO, cardiac output; FiO_2, inspired fraction of oxygen; hct, hematocrit; LA, left atrium; PAP, pulmonary artery pressure; RBCs, red blood cells; RR, respiratory rate; PEEP, positive end-expiratory pressure; Temp, temperature.

Table 2. Comparison among the three different protocols currently used for EVLP [14].

2.4.1. Toronto protocol

The Toronto group uses an acellular perfusate, STEEN Solution™ (XVIVO Perfusion, Goteborg, Sweden), which was originally described by Stig Steen and coworkers from the Lund

University [25]. This proprietary solution is an extracellular solution, with the addition of human albumin, which maintains optimal colloid pressure, and dextran-40, which protects the endothelium from complement- and cell-mediated injuries and inhibits coagulation and platelet aggregation [14, 25]. Once the LA cannula is filled with STEEN Solution™ (XVIVO Perfusion, Goteborg, Sweden), perfusion commences at 10% of the calculated cardiac output flow, and is incrementally increased till the final 40% cardiac output flow for the remainder of the perfusion run, by 50 min from the start of perfusion [12–15]. Ventilation is initiated once the perfusate temperature reaches 32°C at an immediate 7 ml/kg tidal volume, positive end-expiratory pressure (PEEP) of 5 cm H_2O, respiratory rate (RR) of 7 breaths/min, and with an inspired fraction of oxygen (FiO_2) of 21% [12–15] (**Table 2**). Unlike the other two protocols, the Toronto method elects to have a closed left atrium and has the height of the reservoir adjusted manually to maintain a positive LA pressure between 3 and 5 mm Hg [12–15]. Finally, the Toronto group carefully monitors and maintains the mean pulmonary arterial pressure (PAP) to stay below 15–20 mm Hg, which is flow-dictated. This is believed to avoid development of hydrostatic pulmonary edema [14, 15].

2.4.2. Lund protocol

The Lund group utilizes a cellular perfusate, STEEN Solution™ (XVIVO Perfusion, Goteborg, Sweden), mixed with packed red blood cells (pRBCs) to obtain a hematocrit of 14% [14, 25] (**Table 2**). In the Lund technique, ventilation begins at a tidal volume of 3 ml/kg at 32°C and gradually increases by 1 l/min, for each degree, until it reaches 5–7 ml/kg at 37°C [14]. Other parameters that differ from the Toronto protocol are the open LA system at 100% cardiac output flow, respiratory rate (RR) of 20 breaths/min, and a FiO_2 of 50% [14, 25, 29] (**Table 2**).

2.4.3. OCS (transMedics) protocol

The OCS™ protocol is based on a cellular perfusate like the Lund protocol; however, in this protocol, the perfusate is composed of an OCS™ Solution® (TransMedics) or Perfadex® (XVIVO Perfusion AB, Goteborg, Sweden) and pRBCs to achieve a hematocrit between 15 and 25% [14, 30]. Both of these solutions are low-potassium dextran-40 based solutions, without the addition of human albumin (unlike STEEN Solution™) [14]. Perfusion flow is set to 2–2.5 l/min, PAP maintained less than 20 mm Hg, with an open LA system, initiating ventilation at 34°C and 6 ml/kg, a RR of 10 breaths/min, PEEP of 5–7 cm H_2O, and an FiO_2 of 12% [14, 15, 30]. The variations among these protocols have been summarized in **Table 2**.

2.5. EVLP application

2.5.1. Commercial application of EVLP

There are several commercially available EVLP platforms, under different stages of development. Today, there exist four EVLP platforms used commercially that differ in their technology and perfusion protocol, and in the concept for clinical use.

Equipment	OCS™ Lung	Vivoline® LS1	Lung Assist®	XPS™
Pump type	Piston	Roller	Centrifugal	Centrifugal
Flow	Pulsatile	Continuous	Continuous	Continuous
Ventilator	Yes	No	No	Yes
Monitor	Yes	Yes	No	Yes
Gas cylinder	Yes	No	Yes	Yes
Gas analyzer	Portable	No	No	In-line
Real time	No	No	No	Yes
X-Ray				
Portability	Yes	No	Yes	No

OCS™ Lung (Transmedics); source: www.transmedics.com. Vivoline® LS1 (Vivoline Medical); source: www.vivoline.se. Lung Assist® (Organ Assist), source: www.organ-assist.nl. XPS™ (XVIVO Perfusion AB); source: www.xvivoperfusion.co.

Table 3. Comparison between commercially available devices for EVLP [14].

1. OCS™ Lung (TransMedics) is a portable device that uses a cellular-based perfusate, piston pump (creating a pulsatile-type flow), LA open system, with all the required equipment on board: batteries, gas cylinders for preservation and monitoring, and a ventilator for use during transport of organs from donor to recipient hospital [14]. Whether there is any benefit for pulsatile versus nonpulsatile flows has been a topic of controversy over the years; however, some document that the presence of a pulsatile-type flow may be beneficial for recruitment of the pulmonary vasculature, while being perfused under physiological conditions [14, 31].

   OCS™ Lung (TransMedics) was included in an international INSPIRE trial used to compare normothermic preservation versus cold static preservation, ending its trial in January 2014 [14, 30, 32, 33]. The University of Alberta Hospital being one of the centers involved in this trial, we demonstrated the feasibility of prolonged EVLP using the OCS system. Our results revealed how complications, postoperatively, in regards to primary graft dysfunction (an acute lung injury that can occur in the first 72 h after transplantation), were resolved after 30 days. Moreover, the patient/recipient demonstrated excellent pulmonary function at 1 year post-transplantation, despite getting reconditioned extended criteria lungs that otherwise would have been discarded [33].

2. Vivoline® LS1 (Vivoline Medical, Lund, Sweden) is a nonportable device that uses the Lund technique, requires the availability of an external ventilator and gas cylinder, and has an internal roller pump to create a continuous flow (nonpulsatile). It was utilized in the United Kingdom under the "Donor Ex-Vivo Lung Perfusion in United Kingdom" (DEVELOP-UK) trial to assess reconditioned extended criteria lungs versus standard-criteria lungs; the trial ended in October 2015 [34].

3. Lung Assist® (Organ Assist, Groningen, the Netherlands) is deemed "a less robust device with its individual components fixed on a frame designed for EVLP, and for in situ evaluation of lungs from uncontrolled DCD at the donor site, prior to explanting the organs from the body" [14, 35].

4. XPS™ (XVIVO Perfusion AB) utilizes the Toronto protocol and only differs by the addition of various in-line monitors to streamline organ assessment [32]. It contains a centrifugal pump that delivers a continuous flow (nonpulsatile); it is a fully integrated device, and unlike the other commercially available devices, it offers X-ray possibilities during EVLP [14]. XPS™ (XVIVO Perfusion AB) has been involved in the FDA NOVEL lung trial: "Normothermic Ex-Vivo Lung Perfusion as an Assessment of Extended/Marginal Donor Lungs," since May 2011–May 2014 to compare the reconditioned extended criteria lungs versus standard-criteria lungs in the United States [14, 36]. A summary of the various commercially available devices and their technological differences is described in **Table 3**.

Figure 2 provides a visual representation of the four commercially available devices previously mentioned.

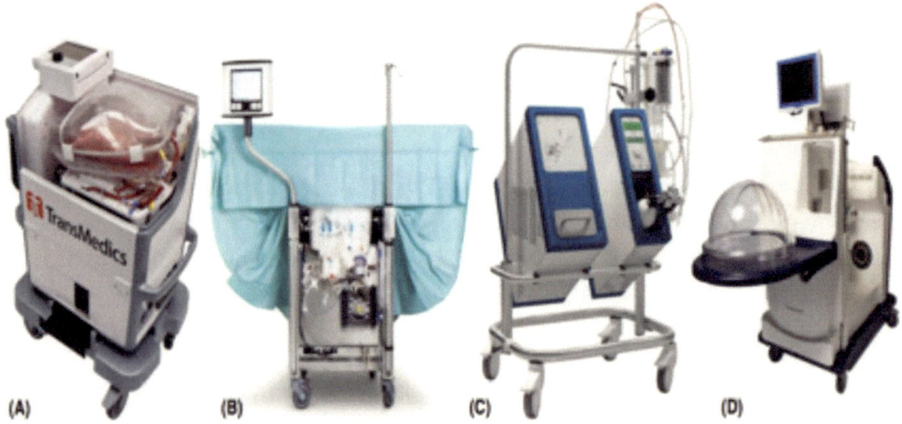

Figure 2. Commercially available ex-vivo lung perfusion devices. (**A**) OCS™ Lung (TransMedics); source: www.transmedics.com. (**B**) Vivoline LS1 (Vivoline Medical); source: www.vivoline.se. (**C**) Lung Assist (Organ Assist); source: www.organ-assist.nl. (**D**) XPS™ (XVIVO Perfusion AB); source: www.xvivoperfusion.com [37].

2.5.2. Potential applications of EVLP

As described in more detail in reference [38], there are a few applications that can benefit from the platform of EVLP:

Transplantation

- Extended donor lung preservation
- Functional assessment prior to transplantation

http://dx.doi.org/10.5772/62449

- Biological assessment before implantation
- Enabling organ's natural recovery processes
- Active repair of injured lungs using various therapies
- Active molecular treatments for organ preparation
- Xenotransplantation studies

Regenerative medicine

- Bioreactive for lung de-cellularization and regeneration
- Stem cell and gene therapy for lung injury

Respiratory medicine

- Study of acute lung injury
- Functional studies for endobronchial interventions for chronic obstructive pulmonary disease
- Study of lung physiology

Cancer

- Study of chemotherapeutic agents to evaluate lung toxicity and antitumor activity
- Lung cancer treatments

2.6. EVLP and lung transplantation

The first clinical use of EVLP was in 2001 by Stig Steen [39]. Steen evaluated lungs from DCD donors and six extended criteria donor lungs for 60 min on EVLP before transplantation. It was observed that the mean time in the intensive care unit (ICU) was longer for the perfused lungs with EVLP compared to the standard criteria lungs. However, the 30-day survival rate post lung transplantation from the perfused groups with EVLP was 100% [39–41].

Human ex-vivo lung perfusion (HELP) trial in 2011 was the first prospective clinical trial done at Toronto General Hospital. Of the 23 lungs from high-risk brain death (BDD) and cardiac death donors (DCD) that underwent 4 h of EVLP, 20 were considered suitable and later transplanted [12, 26, 38, 42]. The criteria to terminate perfusion and discard lungs included pulmonary vascular resistance (PVR), dynamic compliance (C_{dyn}), and peak inspiratory pressure (PIP) decline by more than 15%, and also a change in partial pressure of oxygen/fraction of inspired oxygen ratio ($\Delta PaO_2/FiO_2$ or P/F ratio) of less than 350 mm Hg. Again, there were no significant differences in primary graft dysfunction (PGD) trends, extubation time, ICU/hospital stay, and 30-day mortality rate, compared to the standard criteria lungs [12].

In Europe, Zych et al. [43], from Hartfield, evaluated 13 sets of rejected lungs, of which 6 improved during EVLP and were later implanted: no difference in ICU stay and in 3 and 6 months survival compared to the standard criteria lungs [43]. From Vienna, Aigner et al. [44] perfused and reassessed 13 sets of lungs, of which 9 showed improvement after EVLP.

Currently, FDA mandated multicenter clinical trial (the NOVEL lung trial) to approve the clinical use of EVLP for assessment of extended/marginal donor lungs. Eight centers using a nonrandomized, controlled, clinical study in the United States were involved in the trial using inclusion/exclusion criteria for perfusion on EVLP, described in the HELP trial [29, 38] (**Table 4**). The trial began in May 2011 and ended in May 2014; first report of 30 patients who received EVLP lungs were comparable to 31 control groups of non-EVLP transplants. The 2014 updates described 76 EVLPs yielding 42 transplants [45]. No significant difference was present between transplanted lungs after EVLP reconditioning and the 42 non-EVLP perfused controls in regards to the 1-year survival rates.

Inclusion	Exclusion
Best $PaO_2/FiO_2 < 300$ mm Hg	Pneumonia
Pulmonary edema	Severe mechanical trauma
Bilateral infiltrates	Contusion more than one lobe
Chest radiograph	Gross gastric acid aspiration
Transplant team evaluation (poor lung deflation/inflation)	
Blood transfusion (>10 units)	
Donation after cardiac death	
(PaO_2/FiO_2) ratio—partial pressure of arterial oxygen/fraction of inspired oxygen	

Table 4. Inclusion and exclusion criteria for the HELP trial [29].

The end of the trial compared data from 84 recipients regarding their 30-day post-transplant mortality as the primary endpoint between standard donor lungs (42 cases) and extended criteria donor lungs (42 cases) after EVLP reconditioning (Using Toronto protocol and XPS™ device) [14]. The secondary endpoints included PGD, days before extubation, need for extracorporeal membrane oxygenation (ECMO) after transplant, ICU stay, and 1-year survival [29].

The Gothenburg group published a study where 11 EVLPs were done over the course of 18 months period. Eight double and three single post-EVLP transplants were done. Despite the reported 100% survival of the EVLP cohort, ICU stay and ventilation time were longer in perfused lungs compared to that in controls [45].

2.7. University of Alberta experience with EVLP

The University of Alberta Hospital Transplant Program is the most geographically isolated lung transplantation program in the world. Due to this geographical isolation and the large catchment area served to Canadians, compounded by the shortage of suitable donor lungs, we began experimenting with EVLP on a large porcine model in 2014. Our laboratory effort thus far has primarily focused on one of the most prevailing questions in literature regarding EVLP: which perfusate, acellular or cellular-based, is more optimal for perfusing the lungs and how can we overcome the current limitation we observe clinically to extend EVLP from merely 4–6 h to >12 h safely?

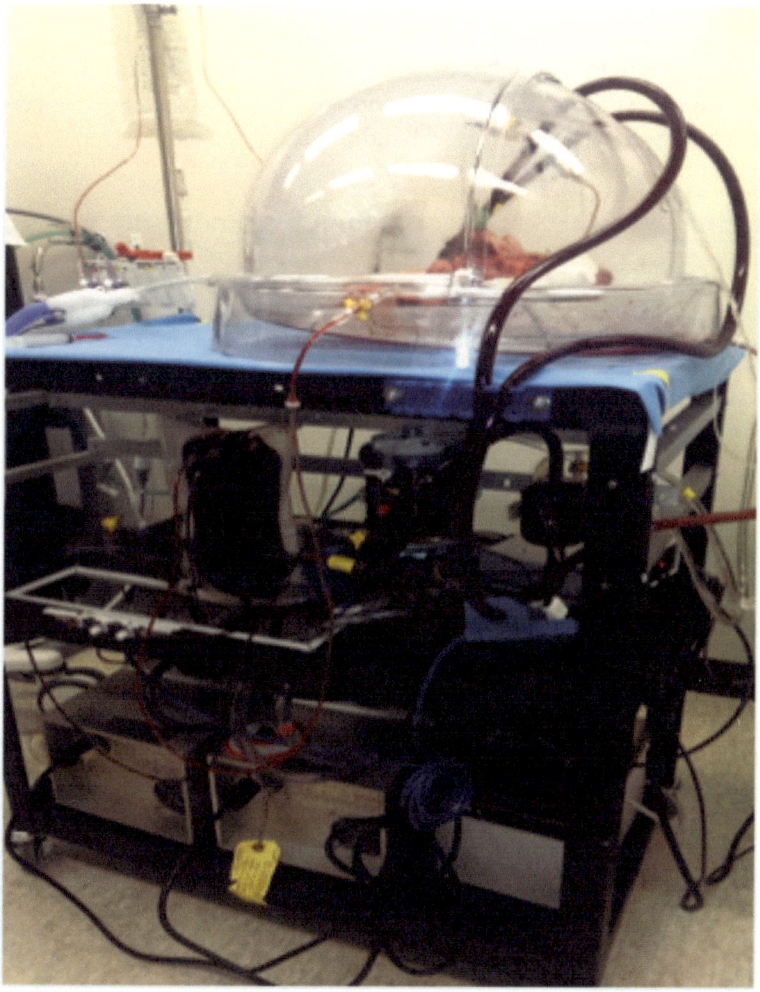

Figure 3. The fully automated and mobile EVLP circuit at the U of A.

We began with constructing a circuit that should help us relieve our main issue here at the University of Alberta—geographical isolation. As seen in **Figure 3**, our circuit contains all the universal components that are present in the commercially available circuits discussed earlier and illustrated in **Figure 1**: centrifugal pumps, a reservoir, tubing, deoxygenator/heat exchanger, a leukocyte filter, pressure/flow probes, and an ICU-type ventilator. However, our's is the only laboratory in the world that currently uses a circuit that is fully automated and does not require constant monitoring and/or manual manipulation throughout the perfusion.

Unlike the EVLP circuit utilized at the University of Alberta, the Toronto group using the XPS™ (XVIVO Perfusion AB) and the OCS™ Lung (TransMedics) are not fully automated. Our circuit is capable of controlling and manipulating the flow, pulmonary arterial (PA) and left atrial (LA) pressures, in real time without the need for manual alterations. Our software-driven microcontroller (**Figure 4**) receives PA/LA pressures and flow in real time, while adjusting the centrifugal pumps' RPMs accordingly to maintain desired constant PA flow/pressure control (user-selectable) and constant LA pressure. This is unlike that in the OCS™ Lung (TransMedics), where the desired flow would need to be manually changed by an attendee, or that in the XPS™ (XVIVO Perfusion AB), where the LA pressures are manually altered by the use of gravity (adjusting the height of the reservoir).

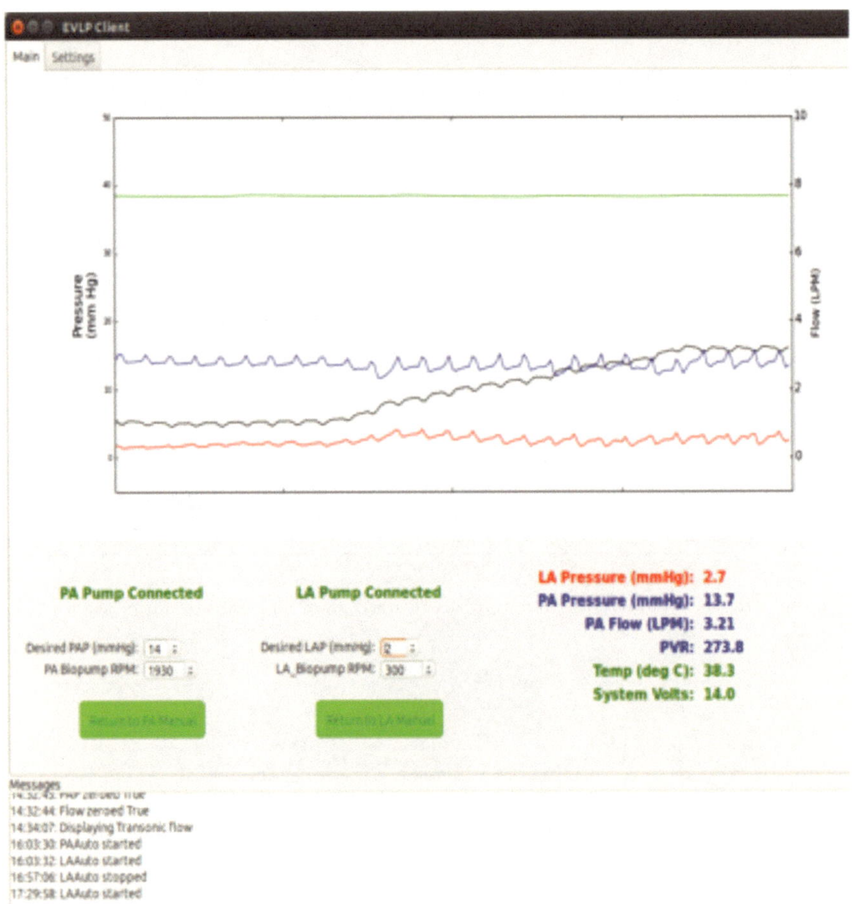

Figure 4. Microcontroller interface for the EVLP circuit parameters.

The current design of our circuit provides us with the freedom of portability, with full automation, to decrease the amount of cold ischemia the lungs experience when performing our porcine experiments. That being said, so far our lab has been capable to demonstrate a reproducible technique to successfully perfuse these large porcine lungs up to 12 h. With preliminary unpublished data demonstrating that an acellular based perfusate results in 50% more edema formation after 12 h of perfusion, compared to perfusing with either cellular based perfusate – whole blood or packed red blood cells (pRBCs) ($p < 0.01$). Here, edema formation corresponds with the deteriorating lung vasculature and integrity. We believe that despite the lungs showing stable physiological parameters during EVLP, especially with acceptable lung oxygenation (*P*/*F* ratios) of >300 mm Hg, lung oxygenation is not a sensitive parameter of lung health, even though it has been a widely accepted modality for evaluating lung integrity. Our data confirms what others have shown, that the focus when assessing lung integrity/health after EVLP should be with the trends of compliance over the duration of EVLP than oxygenation of the perfusate (*P*/*F* ratios) [27, 47–49]. Moreover, we believe that the blunting we observe in lung vasculature tone throughout the duration of the perfusion (with serial hypoxic challenges) can be another more sensitive physiological index of lung health. The decrease in magnitude in hypoxic pulmonary vasoconstriction (HPV) response likely correlates with the diminishing lung quality during EVLP, as supported by an ongoing cytokine profile that accumulates over time.

3. Conclusion

Lung transplantation has shown over the years to be a life-saving therapy for patients that are suffering from end-stage lung disease. However, despite the improvements in techniques, lung donor grafts have the lowest graft acceptance rate of any solid organ [50]. With only 15–25% of lungs from multiorgan brain death donors (BDD) currently deemed suitable for clinical transplantation, the rest acquire too much injury during brain death, ICU-related complications, or the onset of a prolonged cold ischemic time, rendering the donor lungs unusable. Therefore, as observed at the University of Alberta, the mortality rate on the waiting list continues to grow as clinicians must remain conservative in their donor selection to avoid post-transplantation primary graft dysfunction (PGD). The advent of normothermic ex-vivo lung perfusion (EVLP), as a novel donor preservation and reconditioning technique, has demonstrated over the years results that are positive if not different between lungs deemed unsuitable (marginal/extended) and standard (unperfused) criteria lungs, after lung transplantation [12, 41].

Normothermic ex-vivo lung perfusion (EVLP) has the capability, as a platform, for real-time functional assessment, evaluation, and reconditioning through administration of targeted therapies, prior to lung transplantation—a capability that clinicians were unable to perform, prior to the establishment of this platform, in 2001. Moreover, EVLP has permitted us to re-explore other donor pools: marginal lungs, extended criteria lungs, and cardiocirculatory death (DCD) lungs. As more research goes into developing the technology and improving the current evaluative/assessment techniques, simplifying EVLP will help more centers around the world to utilize its beneficial attributes and save lives: by expanding the currently limited donor pool. Our transplant program at the University of Alberta serves as a massive catchment area for the majority of thoracic transplantation, spanning 6 million km^2 for more than 7 million

Canadians. Being the most geographically isolated transplantation program in the world, our continuous research to further develop our program one of a kind fully automated circuit and to make it truly portable is imperative. We can save 24 human lives per year, if EVLP is used just twice a month to recondition lungs that otherwise would be discarded because they incurred too much damage or came from an unusable donor pool.

There is still much to investigate with EVLP and to refine. As we continue to seek out EVLP techniques that will allow us to safely extend the limited clinical perfusion of human lungs from merely 4–6 h to >12 h, it will open up more avenues for therapeutic interventions such as cell and gene therapies. Normothermic ex-vivo lung perfusion is the future, and it will help usher in a new era in medicine and lung transplantation, sooner than we think.

Acknowledgements

The authors acknowledge all the hardwork of their lab colleagues (Dr. Sanaz Hatami and Dr. Christopher White) and the summer students. Furthermore, The University of Alberta Faculty of Medicine and Dentistry, Department of Surgery, Experimental Surgery; finally, the continuous support from their funders, in no specific order:

1. Canada Foundation for Innovation
2. University Hospital Foundation
3. Canadian National Transplant Research Program
4. Canadian Institute for Health & Research

Abbreviations

1. LTx – Lung Transplantation
2. ISHLT – International Society for Heart and Lung Transplantation
3. DCD – Cardiocirculatory Death Donor
4. BDD – Brain-Dead Donor
5. COPD – Chronic Obstructive Pulmonary Disease
6. A1ATD – α_1-antitrypsin deficiency
7. ILD – Interstitial Lung Disease
8. IPF – Idiopathic Pulmonary Fibrosis
9. CF – Cystic Fibrosis
10. PaO_2 – Partial Pressure of Arterial Oxygen

http://dx.doi.org/10.5772/62449

11. $PaCO_2$ – Partial Pressure of Arterial Carbon Dioxide
12. CORR – Canadian Organ Replacement Registry
13. CSP – Cold Static Preservation
14. LA – Left Atrial/Atrium
15. PA – Pulmonary Arterial
16. PAP – Pulmonary Arterial Pressure
17. LAP – Left Arterial Pressure
18. ICU – Intensive Care Unit
19. ECF – Extracellular Fluid
20. PEEP – Positive End-Expiratory Pressure
21. RR – Respiratory Rate
22. FiO_2 – Inspired Fraction of Oxygen
23. pRBCs – Packed Red Blood Cells
24. PVR – Pulmonary Vascular Resistance
25. C_{dyn} – Dynamic Compliance
26. PIP – Peak Inspiratory Pressure
27. P/F or PaO_2/FiO_2 – Partial Pressure of Oxygen/Fraction of Inspired Oxygen
28. ECMO – Extracorporeal Membrane
29. HPV – Hypoxic Pulmonary Vasoconstriction

Author details

Nader Aboelnazar[1], Sayed Himmat[1], Darren Freed[1,2,3,4] and Jayan Nagendran[1,2,3,4*]

*Address all correspondence to: jayan@ualberta.ca

1 Department of Experimental Surgery, University of Alberta, Edmonton, Alberta, Canada

2 Mazankowski Alberta Heart Institute, Edmonton, Alberta, Canada

3 Alberta Transplant Institute, Edmonton, Alberta, Canada

4 Canadian National Transplant Research Program, Edmonton, Alberta, Canada

References

[1] Yusen RD, Christie JD, Edwards LB, *et al.* (2014). The registry of the international society for heart and lung transplantation: thirty-first adult lung and heart–lung transplant report—2014; focus theme: retransplantation. *J Heart Lung Transplant* 2014;33:1009–1024. DOI: http://dx.doi.org/10.1016/j.healun.2014.08.004

[2] William EA. Experimental Transplantation of Vital Organs. BY V. P. DEMIKHOV. Authorized translation from the Russian by Basil Haigh, M.A., M.B., B.Chir. Cloth. Pp. 285, Consultants Bureau, 227 W. 17th St., New York City. 1962. *Anesthesiology* 1963;24:408. http://anesthesiology.pubs.asahq.org/article.aspx?articleid=1967289

[3] Cooper DKC. Transplantation of the heart and both lungs: I. Historical review. *Thorax* 1969;24:383–390. PMCID: PMC472000 - http://www.ncbi.nlm.nih.gov/pmc/articles/PMC472000/

[4] Konstantinov IE. At the cutting edge of the impossible: a tribute to Vladimir P. Demikhov. *Texas Heart Inst J* 2009;36:453–458. http://www.ncbi.nlm.nih.gov/pmc/articles/PMC2763473/#r3-20

[5] Hardy JD, Eraslan S, Dalton ML Jr. Autotransplantation and homotransplantation of the lung: further studies. *J Thorac Cardiovasc Surg* 1963;46:606–615. PMID:14087734 - http://europepmc.org/abstract/med/14087734

[6] Toronto Lung Transplant Group. Unilateral Lung transplantation for pulmonary fibrosis. *N Engl J Med* 1986;314:1140–1145. DOI: 10.1056/NEJM198605013141802

[7] Patterson GA, Cooper JD, Goldman B, *et al.* Technique of successful clinical double-lung transplantation. *Ann Thoracic Surg* 1988;45:626–633. PMID: 3288141 - http://www-ncbi-nlm-nih-gov.login.ezproxy.library.ualberta.ca/pubmed/?term=5.%09Patterson+GA%2C+C.+J.+%281988%29.+Technique+of+successful+clinical+double-lung+transplantation.+Ann+Thoracic+Surg%2C+626-33.

[8] Travis WD, Costabel U, Hansell DM, *et al.* An official American Thoracic Society/European Respiratory Society statement: update of the international multidisciplinary classification of the idiopathic interstitial pneumonias. *Am J Respir Crit Care Med* 2013;188:733–748. DOI: 10.1164/rccm.201308-1483ST

[9] Simonneau G, Gatzoulis MA, Adatia I, *et al*. Updated clinical classification of pulmonary hypertension. *J Am Coll Cardiol* 2013;62:D34–D41. DOI: 10.1016/j.jacc.2013.10.029

[10] Orens JB, Estenne M, Arcasoy S, *et al*. International Guidelines for the Selection of Lung Transplant Candidates: 2006 Update-A Consensus Report From the Pulmonary Scientific Council of the International Society for Heart and Lung Transplantation. *J Heart Lung Transplant* 2006;25:745–755. DOI: http://dx.doi.org/10.1016/j.healun.2006.03.011

[11] Canadian Organ Replacement Register Annual Report: Treatment of End-Stage Organ Failure in Canada 2003–2012. Ottawa, ON: Canadian Institute for Health Information.

[Internet]. 2014. Available from: https://secure.cihi.ca/free_products/2014_CORR_Annual_Report_EN.pdf [Accessed: 2016-01-05]

[12] Cypel M, Yeung JC, Liu M, *et al.* Normothermic ex vivo lung perfusion in clinical lung transplantation. *N Engl J Med* 2011;364:1431–1440. DOI: 10.1056/NEJMoa1014597

[13] Yeung JC, Cypel M, Waddell TK, *et al.* Update on donor assessment, resuscitation, and acceptance criteria, including novel techniques–nonheart-beating donorlung retrieval and exvivo donor lung perfusion. *Thorac Surg Clin* 2009;19:261–274. DOI: 10.1016/j.thorsurg.2009.02.006

[14] Raemdonck VD, Neyrinck A, Cypel, M. and Keshavjee, S. Ex-vivo lung perfusion. *Transplant Int* 2015;28:643–656. DOI: 10.1111/tri.12317

[15] Machuca TN, Cypel M, Keshavjee S. Advanves in lung preservation. *Surg Clin N Am* 2013;93:1373–1394. DOI: 10.1016/j.suc.2013.08.001

[16] Boutilier RG. Mechanisms of cell survival in hypoxia and hypothermia. *J Exp Biol* 2001;204:3171–3181. http://jeb.biologists.org/content/204/18/3171.long

[17] Zhao G, al-Mehdi AB, Fisher AB. Anoxia-reoxygenation versus ischemia in isolated rat lungs. *Am J Physiol Lung Cell Mol Physiol* 1997;273:L1112–L1117. http://ajplung.physiology.org/content/273/6/L1112?ij-key=64301b235cc7cc4994e5267adae8a6528099c962&keytype2=tf_ipsecsha

[18] Hochachka PW. Defense strategies against hypoxia and hypothermia. *Science* 1986;231:234–241. DOI: 10.1126/science.2417316

[19] Keshavjee SH, Yamazaki F, Cardoso PF, *et al.* A method for safe twelve hour pulmonary preservation. *J Thoracic Cardiovasc Surg* 1989;98:529–534. http://www.ncbi.nlm.nih.gov/pubmed/2477644

[20] Date H, Lima O, Matsumura A, *et al.* In a Canine model,lung preservation at ten degrees C is superior to that at 4 degrees. A comparison of two preservation temperatures on lung functionand on adenosine triphosphate level measured by phosphorus 31-nuclear magnetic resonance. *J Thoracic Cardiovasc Surg* 1992;103:773–780. http://www.ncbi.nlm.nih.gov/pubmed/1548920

[21] Date H, Matsumura A, Manchester JK, *et al.* The maintenance of aerobic metabolism during lung preservation. *J Thoracic Cardiovasc Surg* 1993;105:492–501. http://www-ncbi-nlm-nih-gov.login.ezproxy.library.ualberta.ca/pubmed/?term=20.%09Date+H%2C+M.+A.+%281993%29.+The+maintenance+of+aerobic+metabolism+during+lung+preservation.+J+Thoracic+Cardiovascular+Surg%2C+492-501.

[22] Carrel A, Lindbergh CA. The culture of whole organs. *Science* 1935;81:621–623. DOI: 10.1126/science.81.2112.621

[23] Jirsch DW, Fisk RL, Couves CM. Ex vivo evaluation of stored lungs. *Ann Thorac Surg* 1970;10:163–168. http://www-ncbi-nlm-nih-gov.login.ezproxy.library.ualberta.ca/

pubmed/?term=DW%2C+F.+R.+%281970%29.+Ex+vivo+evaluation+of+stored+lungs.+Ann.+Thorac.+Surg%2C+163-168

[24] Daemen JW, Kootstra G, Wijnen RM, *et al*. Nonheart-beating donors: the Maastricht experience. *Clin Transplant* 1994:303–316. PMID:7547551

[25] Steen S, Liao Q, Wierup PN, Bolys R, *et al*. Transplantation of lungs from non-heart-beating donors after functional assessment ex vivo. *Ann Thorac Surg* 2003;76:244–252. DOI: 10.1016/S0003-4975(03)00191-7

[26] Cypel M, Yeung JC, Hirayama S, *et al*. Technique for prolonged normothermic ex vivo lung perfusion. *J Heart Lung Transplant* 2008;27:1319–1325. DOI: 10.1016/j.healun.2008.09.003

[27] Yeung JC, Cypel M, Machuca TN, *et al*. Physiologic assessment of the ex vivo donor lung for transplantation. *J Heart Lung Transplant* 2012;31:1120–1126. DOI: 10.1016/j.healun.2012.08.016

[28] MulloyDP, Stone ML, Crosby IK, *et al*. Ex vivo rehabilitation of non-heart-beating donor lungs inpreclinical porcine model:delayed perfusion results in superior lung function. *J Thorac Cardiovasc Surg* 2012;144:1208–1215. DOI: 10.1016/j.jtcvs.2012.07.056

[29] Sanchez PG, D'Ovidio F. Ex-vivo lung perfusion. *Curr Opin Organ Transplant* 2012;17:490–495. DOI: 10.1097/MOT.0b013e328357f865

[30] Warnecke G1, Moradiellos J, Tudorache I, *et al*. Normothermic perfusion of donor lungs for preservation and assessment with the Organ Care System Lungbefore bilateral transplantation: a pilot study of 12 patients. *Lancet* 2012;380:1851–1858. DOI: 10.1016/S0140-6736(12)61344-0

[31] Brandes H, Albes JM, Conzelmann A, *et al*. Comparison of pulsatile and non-pulsatile perfusion of the lung in an extracorporeal large animal model. *Eur Surg Res* 2002;34:321. DOI: 10.1159/000063067

[32] Cypel M, Keshavjee S. Strategies for safe donor expansion: donor management, donations after cardiac death, ex-vivo lung perfusion. *Curr Opin* 2013;18:512–517. DOI: 10.1097/MOT.0b013e328365191b

[33] Bozso S, Freed D, Nagendran J. Successful transplantation of extended criteria lungs after prolonged *ex vivo* lung perfusion performed on a portable device. *Transplant Int* 2015;28:248–250. DOI: 10.1111/tri.12474

[34] A study of donor ex vivo lung perfusion in lung transplantation in United Kingdom [Internet]. 2012. Available from: DOI 10.1186/ISRCTN44922411 [Accessed: 2016-01-01]

[35] Van De Wauwer C1, Munneke AJ, Engels GE, *et al*. Insitu lung perfusion is available tool to assess lungs from donation after circulatory death donors category I-II. *Transplant Int* 2013;26:485–492. DOI: 10.1111/tri.12068 485

[36] Novel Lung Trial: Normothermic Ex Vivo Lung Perfusion (EVLP) As An Assessment of Extended/Marginal Donor Lungs. 2015. Available from: https://clinicaltrials.gov/ct2/show/NCT01365429?term=NOVEL&rank=406. [Accessed: 2016-01-01]

[37] Raemdonck VD, Neyrinck A, Rega F, *et al*. Machine perfusion in organ transplantation: a tool for ex-vivo graft conditioning with mesenchymal stem cells? *Curr Opin Organ Transpl* 2013;18:24–31. DOI: 10.1097/MOT.0b013e32835c494f

[38] Cypel M, Keshavjee S. The clinical potenial of ex-vivo lung perfusion. *Expert Rev Respir Med* 2012;6:27–35. DOI: 10.1586/ers.11.93

[39] Steen S, Sjöberg T, Pierre L, *et al*. Transplantation of lungs from a non-heart-beating donor. *Lancet* 2001;357:825–829. DOI: 10.1016/S0140-6736(00)04195-7

[40] Ingemansson R, Eyjolfsson A, Mared L, *et al*. Clinical transplantation of initially rejected donor lungs after reconditioning ex-vivo. *Ann Thorac Surg* 2009;87:255–260. DOI: 10.1016/j.athoracsur.2008.09.049

[41] Lindstedt S1, Hlebowicz J, Koul B, *et al*. Comparative outcome of double lung transplantation using conventional donor lungs and non-acceptable donor lungs reconditioned ex vivo. *Interact Cardiovasc Thorac Surg* 2011;12:162–165. DOI: 10.1510/icvts.2010.244830

[42] Cypel M, Rubacha M, Yeung J, *et al*. Normothermic ex vivo perfusion prevents lung injury compared to extended cold preservation for transplantation. *Am J Transplant* 2009;9:2262–2269. DOI: 10.1111/j.1600-6143.2009.02775.x

[43] Zych B, Popov AF, Stavri G, *et al*. Early Outcomes of bilateral sequential single lung transplantation after ex-vivo lung evaluation and reconditioning. *J Heart Lung Transplant* 2012;31:274–281. DOI: 10.1016/j.healun.2011.10.008

[44] Aigner C, Slama A, Hötzenecker K, *et al*. Clinical ex-vivo lung perfusion pushing the limits. *Am J Transplant* 2012;12:1839–1847. DOI: 10.1111/j.1600-6143.2012.04027.x

[45] Popov AF, Sabashnikov A, Patil NP, *et al*. Ex vivo lung prefusion - state of the art in lung donor pool expansion. *Med Sci Monit Basic Res* 2015;21:9–14. DOI: 10.12659/MSMBR.893674

[46] Celli BR, Cote CG, Marin JM, *et al*. The body-mass index, airflow obstruction, dyspnea, and exercise capacity index in chronic obstructive pulmonary disease. *N Engl J Med* 2004;350:1005–1012. DOI: 10.1056/NEJMoa021322

[47] Vasanthan V, Nagendran J. Compliance trumps oxygenation: Prediciting quality with ex vivo lung perfusion. *J Thorac Cardiovasc Surg* 2015;150:1378–1379. DOI: 10.1016/j.jtcvs.2015.07.025

[48] Sanchez PG, Rajagopal K, Pham SM, Griffith BP. Defining quality during ex vivo lung perfusion: the University of Maryland experience. *J Thorac Cardiovasc Surg* 2015;150:1376–1377. DOI: 10.1016/j.jtcvs.2015.06.018

[49] Lowe K, Alvarez DF, King JA, Stevens T. Perivascular fluid cuffs decrease lung compliance by increasing tissue resistance. *Crit Care Med* 2010;38:1458–1466. DOI: 10.1097/CCM.0b013e3181de18f0

[50] Pomfret EA, Sung RS, Allan J, *et al*. Solving the organ shortage crisis: the 7th annual American Society of Transplant Surgeons' State-of-the-Art Winter Symposium. *Am J Transplant* 2008;8:745–752. DOI: 10.1111/j.1600-6143.2007.02146.x

Chapter 11

Mechanical Circulatory Support Devices

Sagar Kadakia, Vishnu Ambur, Sharven Taghavi,
Akira Shiose and Yoshiya Toyoda

Additional information is available at the end of the chapter

http://dx.doi.org/10.5772/62875

Abstract

Heart failure (HF) is a global public health concern that has the potential to reach epidemic proportions. The gold standard for treating end-stage HF remains heart transplantation. Unfortunately, given the scarcity of available organs, alternative means for providing cardiac support are required. Mechanical circulatory support devices (MCSDs) have the potential to treat many patients with end-stage HF. They replace some of the mechanical functions of the failing heart to improve cardiac output and organ perfusion. These include the intra-aortic balloon pump, extracorporeal membrane oxygenation, ventricular assist devices, and the total artificial heart. In this chapter, we will discuss a brief history of MCSD, available devices, indications, patient selection, surgical procedures, postoperative management, complications, and outcomes.

Keywords: heart failure, intra-aortic balloon pump, extracorporeal membrane oxygenation, ventricular assist device, total artificial heart

1. Introduction

Heart failure (HF) is a global public health concern, affecting 26 million people worldwide at an estimated cost of $108 billion in 2012. It typically affects the elderly, and both the right heart and left heart can be involved. In right HF, the right ventricle cannot effectively pump blood to the lungs. In left HF, which is more common, the left ventricle cannot effectively pump blood to meet the body's demands. In our aging world, where 22% of the population is expected to be over the age of 60 by 2050 [1], HF has the potential to reach epidemic proportions. Although medications such as beta-blockers, angiotensin-converting enzyme inhibitors, and angiotensin II receptor blockers can alleviate the symptoms of HF and improve mortality [2], the gold standard for treating end-stage HF remains heart transplantation. Unfortunately, given the scarcity of available organs, only about 4500 heart transplantations were performed worldwide in patients of all ages in 2013 [3]. The demand for heart transplantations is expected to far exceed the available supply for the foreseeable future.

Mechanical circulatory support devices (MCSDs) replace some of the mechanical functions of the failing heart to improve cardiac output and organ perfusion. They have the potential to treat many patients with end-stage HF who cannot be transplanted either due to lack of available organs or socioeconomic reasons. Between June 2006 and December 2014, 15,745 patients were implanted with ventricular assist devices (VADs) and the total artificial heart (TAH) in the United States. These numbers have been rising steadily, from approximately 1000 devices implanted in 2009 to approximately 2500 devices implanted in 2014 in the United States [4]. Besides the VAD and the TAH, other types of MCSD exist, including the intra-aortic balloon pump (IABP) and extracorporeal membrane oxygenation (ECMO). The IABP, ECMO, and VAD can be utilized as a bridge to recovery (BTR). All four types of MCSD can be utilized as a bridge to transplantation (BTT), whereas only VADs can be utilized as destination therapy (DT).

In this chapter, we will discuss a brief history of MCSD, available devices, indications, patient selection, surgical procedures, postoperative management, complications, and outcomes.

1.1. History

MCSDs trace their origin to the early days of cardiac surgery. In 1953, Dr. Gibbon successfully utilized the heart–lung machine, which he developed over the course of two decades, to repair an atrial septal defect (ASD) in an 18-year-old woman [5]. This patient did well and was discharged home. Although his subsequent efforts to utilize the heart–lung machine to close ASD were met with poor results, secondary to misdiagnosis and bleeding complications, he laid the foundation for modern-day open-heart surgery with cardiopulmonary bypass [6]. Soon afterwards, it became clear that failure to wean off cardiopulmonary bypass was a significant problem in the field of cardiac surgery. Dr. Spencer ushered in the use of mechanical support for postcardiotomy cardiac recovery in 1959. He utilized left atrial–femoral cardiopulmonary bypass to provide temporary cardiac support in postoperative patients. This early work in mechanical support set the stage for mechanical support for cardiogenic shock [7]. In 1966, Dr. DeBakey performed the first successful implantation of a VAD. He implanted a paracorporeal VAD from the left atrium to the right subclavian artery in a patient with cardiogenic shock after a double valve replacement. The patient required mechanical support for 10 days and ultimately recovered [8]. Dr. Kantrowitz was the first to successfully utilize the IABP in 1967. His patient was a 45-year-old woman who was in cardiogenic shock secondary to an acute myocardial infarction. She remained on the IABP for 7 hours and, during this time, was weaned off all vasopressors ([9]. In 1984, Dr. DeVries reported on the first clinical use of the TAH. Although the patient ultimately died after 112 days from multiorgan system failure, the TAH remained functional and uninvolved in any thrombotic or infectious processes [10].

http://dx.doi.org/10.5772/62875

Our modern era of MCSD began in 2001 with the Randomized Evaluation of Mechanical Assistance for the Treatment of Congestive Heart Failure (REMATCH) trial. This landmark study compared patients with advanced HF who underwent left ventricular assist device (LVAD) implantation versus maximal medical therapy. It showed a survival benefit of 52% in the LVAD group versus only 25% in the medical therapy group at 1 year ($p = 0.002$). Likewise, using a variety of quality-of-life questionnaires including the SF-36, Minnesota Living with HF, and Beck Depression Inventory, the patients who underwent LVAD implantation had a statistically significant improved quality of life when compared to the medically managed patients [11]. This pivotal study played a key role in the approval of the LVAD for DT in the United States in November 2002 [12].

Each of these technological advancements in mechanical support has been monumental. Equally important was the creation of a national database, the Interagency Registry for Mechanically Assisted Circulatory Support (INTERMACS), in the United States. In 2005, this was developed as a joint venture between the National Heart, Lung, and Blood Institute, the Food and Drug Administration, the Centers for Medicare and Medicaid Services, and the University of Alabama at Birmingham. This database serves as a registry for all patients who have been implanted with VAD and TAH. It collects data from the index hospitalization, follow-up appointments, and all major adverse events to improve clinical outcomes and promote research into new devices [4, 13].

2. Devices

2.1. Intra-aortic balloon pump

2.1.1. Background

The IABP is the most frequently utilized MCSD, having been in clinical practice for more than 40 years. When mechanical support is indicated, it is often the first one employed as it could be readily inserted and has a relatively low complication rate. Upwards of 70,000 patients are supported annually with the IABP in the United States [14]. It serves as a temporary MCSD that can be placed quickly at the bedside, in the interventional cardiology suite, or in the operating room to improve shock and promote organ perfusion.

2.1.2. Basic principles

The IABP results in decreased myocardial oxygen demand and an increase in myocardial oxygen supply. These physiologic effects are achieved through a reduction in the afterload and an increase in coronary perfusion [15]. The IABP functions by reducing left ventricular afterload, which leads to a decrease in left ventricular wall stress. Since wall stress is proportional to oxygen consumption, this reduction in afterload and wall stress results in decreased myocardial oxygen consumption. In addition, the IABP increases aortic diastolic pressures.

Since the coronary arteries are perfused during diastole, this increase in aortic diastolic pressures leads to increased coronary perfusion and thus myocardial oxygen supply [16, 17]. The combined physiologic effects of afterload reduction and augmented coronary perfusion lead to an improvement in cardiac output.

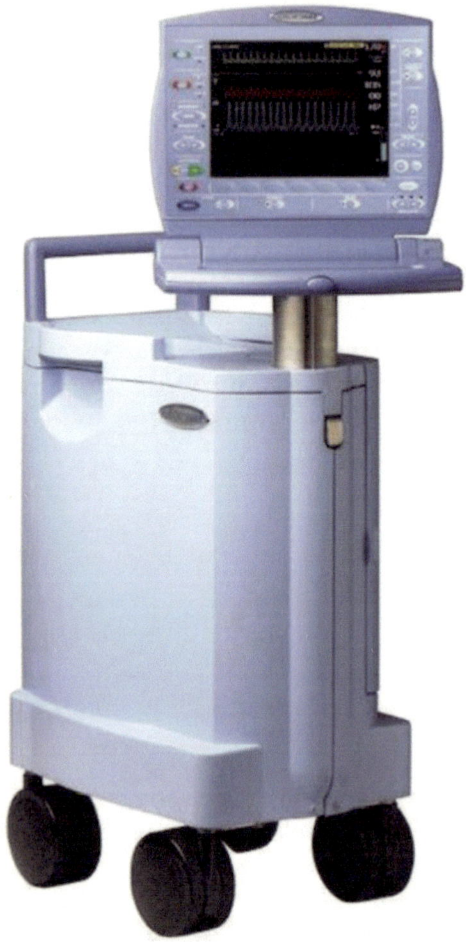

Figure 1. IABP Console (Image courtesy of Teleflex.com).

The sequential inflation and deflation of the IABP is synchronized to the electrocardiogram (EKG), pacemaker, or to the arterial pressure tracing. This results in counterpulsation and the various hemodynamic changes that are observed. IABP inflation is timed to coincide with the closure of the aortic valve. As seen on the aortic pressure tracing, this coincides with the dicrotic notch. Alternatively, it is timed to coincide with the T-wave of the EKG. With counterpulsation, the IABP rapidly inflates. This inflation increases the intra-aortic pressures and displaces a volume of blood equivalent to the volume of the balloon (usually 30–50 mL in adults, 2.5–25 mL in children) away from the balloon. This results in increased coronary perfusion.

http://dx.doi.org/10.5772/62875

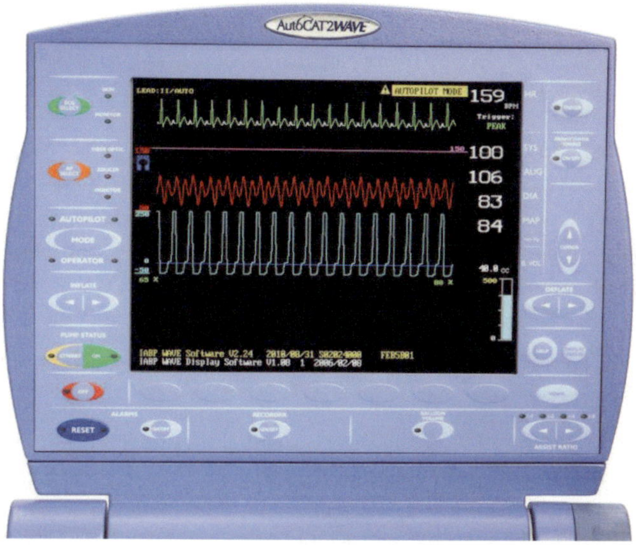

Figure 2. IABP Screen with EKG and aortic pressure tracing (Image courtesy of Teleflex.com).

The second phase of the counterpulsation occurs with deflation of the IABP. Deflation is timed to occur with the onset of the R-wave, or alternatively before the start of systole. Deflation occurs as late as possible, in order to maintain the increased aortic diastolic pressures. It is also timed to occur rapidly, which results in a vacuum effect that leads to a reduction in the afterload by movement of blood toward the balloon [18].

There are several factors that influence the efficacy of the IABP, including heart rate, rhythm, balloon volume, proximity to the aortic valve, and aortic compliance. As the heart rate increases, the amount of time the heart spends in diastole decreases. Thus, the IABP is less likely to function efficiently with tachycardia, since there would be less diastolic coronary flow augmentation. The optimal rate reported in the literature is from 80 to 110 beats/minute [19]. In addition, having a normal sinus rhythm allows for readily identifiable waves on EKG or the aortic pressure tracing, which improves the performance of the IABP. Since the balloon size is proportional to the amount of blood displaced, a larger balloon allows for increased coronary perfusion and a greater reduction in afterload. In addition, the proximity of the IABP to the aortic valve affects diastolic augmentation of coronary perfusion. There is greater diastolic augmentation when the balloon is positioned closer to the aortic valve. Finally, aortic compliance affects the function of the IABP. Increased aortic compliance, which is seen in younger patients, results in a decrease in diastolic augmentation [18, 20].

2.1.3. Components and insertion

The IABP system is composed of a dual lumen catheter, with the inner lumen serving to monitor aortic pressures and the outer lumen connected to a polyethylene balloon that inflates and deflates. It is also composed of a pump console that controls the inflation and deflation of the balloon. The catheters are available in a variety of sizes, depending on the patient's height. Helium gas is utilized to inflate the balloon, since it has a low density and rapidly transfers from the console to the balloon. In addition, helium is inert and could be rapidly absorbed into the blood stream in the event the balloon ruptures.

The IABP can be placed via both percutaneous and open surgical techniques. In the percutaneous technique, the common femoral artery is punctured with an introducer needle. Using the modified Seldinger technique, a guidewire is inserted and then the IABP catheter is inserted over the wire. The catheter is then positioned about 1–2 cm distal to the left subclavian artery and confirmed with fluoroscopy or chest roentgenogram [18]. Care has to be exercised to prevent obstruction of the left subclavian artery and left carotid artery by a highly placed IABP. Care also has to be exercised to avoid placing the IABP too low, as it could occlude mesenteric and the renal arteries.

Alternatively, the IABP can be placed via open surgical techniques. This is typically reserved for patients with severe peripheral vascular disease (PVD) affecting the distal aorta, iliac arteries, or femoral arteries. In such cases, placement of an IABP can lead to critical limb ischemia. For these patients, the IABP can be inserted into the ascending aorta, aortic arch, common iliac artery, subclavian artery, axillary artery, and brachial artery [21].

2.1.4. Indications and contraindications

The indications for the IABP include postcardiotomy syndrome, prophylactic support for high-risk percutaneous coronary interventions, myocardial infarction or its mechanical complications, unstable angina, cardiogenic shock, and as a bridge to heart transplantation. The Benchmark Registry, a multi-institutional study with nearly 17,000 patients, investigated the patient demographics, outcomes, and complications of the IABP. They found that the indications for the IABP were most frequently hemodynamic support during or after cardiac catheterization (21%), cardiogenic shock (19%), and weaning from cardiopulmonary bypass (16%) [22].

There are several important contraindications to using the IABP. These include aortic regurgitation, since the IABP would result in increased regurgitation during diastolic augmentation. In addition, severe aortic diseases, such as aneurysm or aortic dissection, are a contraindication. In this setting, the placement of an IABP could result in aortic rupture or extension of the dissection. Placing them in the femoral region is contraindicated in patients with known severe PVD [18, 23].

The authors believe the IABP should be the first MCSD that should be placed for typical cardiogenic shock, when no obvious contraindications exist. Despite the interpretation of the controversial IABP-Shock II trial, which showed that the IABP did not lead to a reduction in 12-month all-cause mortality in patients undergoing early revascularization for myocardial infarction complicated by cardiogenic shock [24], we believe the IABP should be the first to be placed for cardiogenic shock. We believe this for a number of reasons, including its availability at most hospitals, the ability to initiate its use quickly, and the ability to upgrade it to a more advanced MCSD if the cardiogenic shock remains poorly addressed.

2.1.5. Weaning and removal

Little data exists on how to wean patients off the IABP with minimal hemodynamic consequences. Generally, weaning is performed in one of two ways: rate reduction or volume deflation. In the first method, the ventricular assist rate is gradually reduced from full support of every beat (1:1) to cardiac support every other beat (1:2) to finally cardiac support every three beats (1:3). Once the patient demonstrates that he can tolerate this wean, the IABP is discontinued. The IABP can also be weaned by maintaining a ventricular rate of 1:1 and deflating the balloon over several hours. This leads to a decrease in the counterpulsation and a decrease in diastolic augmentation [25, 26]. There are limited studies in the literature that have assessed which weaning method is superior. Onorati et al. [26] showed that weaning using volume deflation led to improved hemodynamic and metabolic parameters in their study.

Once the patient has demonstrated that he can tolerate being weaned, the IABP is removed. The removal of percutaneously placed IABP can be performed at the bedside. After prepping the femoral artery entry site, the balloon catheter is disconnected from the console. It is then completely deflated and the catheter is removed. Retrograde bleeding is first allowed, which enables blood clots to flush into the wound. This potentially prevents distal embolization of blood clots. After this, antegrade flushing is allowed, to once again prevent distal embolization of blood clots. Finally, the puncture site in the femoral artery is compressed and pressure is maintained for about 30 minutes. Inadvertent placement of the IABP above the inguinal ligament can result in a retroperitoneal bleed, while poor technique at the time of removal can result in a femoral artery pseudoaneurysm and distal embolization with leg ischemia.

2.1.6. Complications

The overall complication rate has been reported to be low. The Benchmark Registry found that the incidence of all complications to be 7%. This study found that severe complications occurred in 2.8% of the patients. Severe complications were defined as severe bleeding (with hemodynamic instability requiring transfusions or surgical interventions), major limb ischemia (with loss of pulse or sensation or the presence of pallor), balloon rupture, or in-hospital mortality related to the IABP. Multivariate logistic regression analysis identified several predictors of major complication, including female gender, PVD, body surface area $<1.65\ m^2$, and age >75 years [22].

Additional complications include renal artery occlusion and renal failure if the IABP is placed too distally. By manipulating the aorta with the guidewire and catheter, there is always the possibility of distal embolism, resulting in bowel ischemia or lower extremity ischemia.

In the Benchmark Registry, the incidence of balloon rupture was found to be 1% [22]. Balloon rupture usually could be detected by the presence of blood either in the IABP driveline or in console alarms. Balloon rupture is thought to occur secondary to abrasive contact between the balloon and atherosclerotic plaque in the aorta. It necessitates the immediate removal of the IABP to prevent thrombus formation around the balloon and distal embolization.

2.2. Extracorporeal membrane oxygenation

2.2.1. Background

Veno-arterial extracorporeal membrane oxygenation (VA-ECMO) is another modality for short-term mechanical support in patients with HF refractory to medical management. Initial reports of its success were described by Baffes et al. in the 1970s in the pediatric population [27]. Since that time, its applications have been broadened to include adult patients with reversible cardiogenic shock and as a bridge to VAD implantation or transplantation. It can also serve as rescue therapy in patients with cardiopulmonary arrest [28]. Chen et al. showed that VA-ECMO could be utilized in patients in cardiopulmonary arrest after 10 minutes of unsuccessful advanced cardiovascular life support. It was shown that VA-ECMO could extend the duration of cardiopulmonary resuscitation (CPR) with 50% survival with acceptable neurologic status at 30 minutes [29]. A recent meta-analysis showed ECMO in adult patients in cardiac arrest had statistically significant improved outcomes if they were younger (age 17–41) and had a shorter duration of ECMO support (0.9–2.3 days) [30].

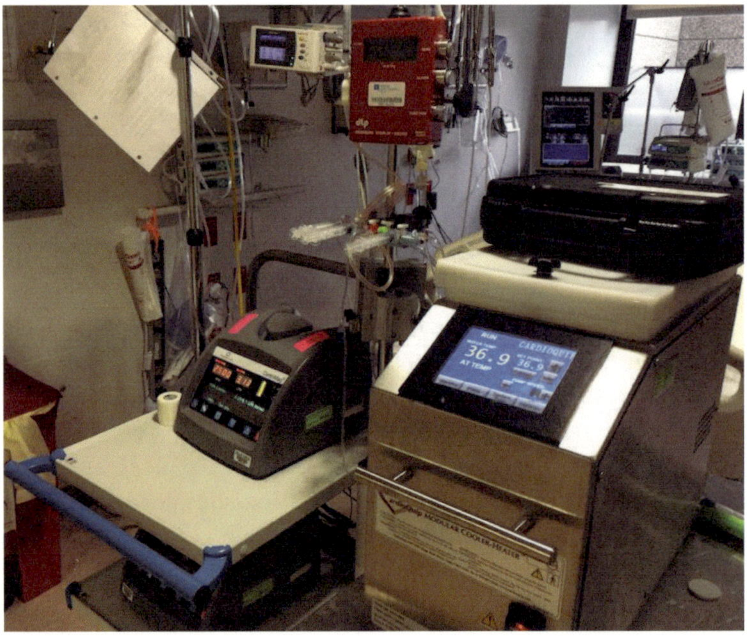

Figure 3. ECMO circuit with pump and heater.

2.2.2. Basic principles

VA-ECMO is a form of advanced cardiopulmonary life support which functions essentially like cardiopulmonary bypass. Blood is drained from a central vein, circulated in the ECMO circuit, and then returned to the arterial system. In neonates and children, the carotid artery is

http://dx.doi.org/10.5772/62875

typically accessed for arterial cannulation. In adults, arterial cannulation is obtained via the femoral, axillary, or carotid artery. Venous access is obtained via the femoral or internal jugular vein. It provides cardiac support by augmenting cardiac output and respiratory support by assisting in gas exchange. VA-ECMO can be utilized for a period of days to weeks [31].

2.2.3. Components and insertion

The ECMO circuit consists of a blood pump and membrane oxygenator with a heat exchanger connected to the VA-ECMO cannulas. The membrane oxygenator has a membrane that readily allows diffusion of oxygen and carbon dioxide across it. Oxygen can be added to the system by increasing the amount of oxygen supplied to the oxygenator. Carbon dioxide can be adjusted by changing the gas flow rate or the "sweep." The heat exchange helps maintain normothermia, as heat is readily lost through the circuit.

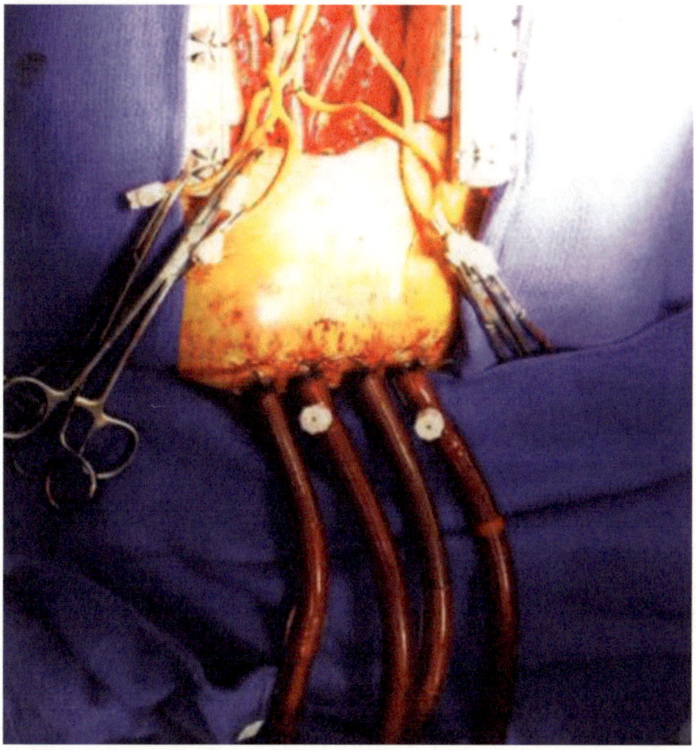

Figure 4. Biventricular assist devices (Centrimag).

Cannulation insertion techniques include both percutaneous and open surgical approaches. Percutaneous cannulas are inserted using the Seldinger technique and can be placed readily at the bedside. After gaining access, the vessels are serially dilated and the cannula is then placed over the guidewire. The patient requires full anticoagulation with heparin. The femoral vessels are most commonly used in the adult. For adults, the arterial cannula size ranges between 12 French (Fr) and 22 Fr and the venous cannula size ranges between 18 Fr and 28 Fr. An arterial perfusion cannula (typically 5–8 Fr) can also be added to perfuse the lower extremity, as lower extremity ischemia is a source of significant morbidity and mortality. A similar venous drainage line can be placed to drain blood from the lower extremity, as venous outflow obstruction too can lead to lower extremity ischemia [32].

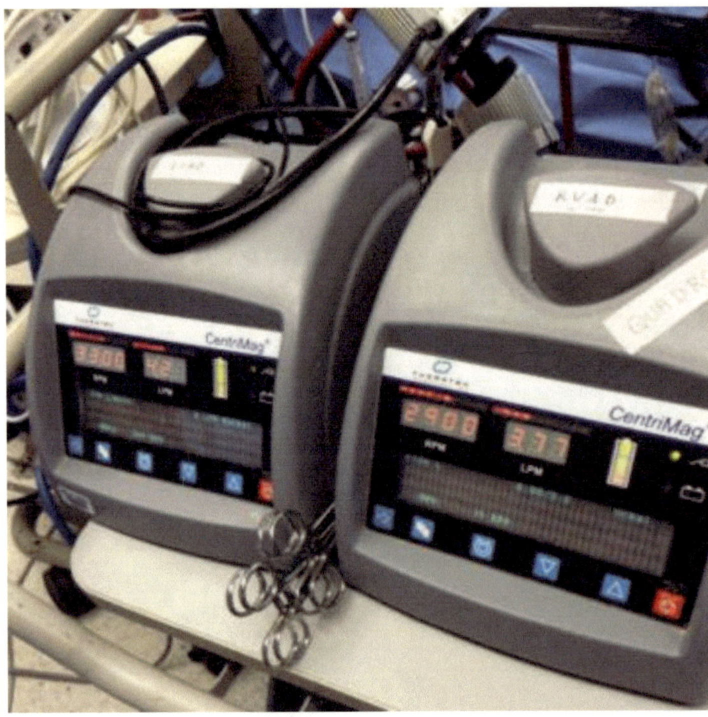

Figure 5. Biventricular assist devices (Centrimag).

Our institutional practice has been to use a 15 Fr arterial cannula placed via the Seldinger technique for patients who need modest support. This allows us to decannulate the patient at bedside without needing to perform a cutdown. When patients require more robust cardiac support, we use larger cannulas, typically 17–21 Fr. We prefer to perform open insertion when these larger cannulas are required. It also requires decannulation in the operating room. We prefer to initiate VA-ECMO in the operating room whenever possible, provided the patient is stable enough to tolerate transport and waiting for operating room availability. Distal perfusion cannulas should be routinely placed. If they are not utilized, the lower extremity has to be monitored for ischemia. There has to be a low threshold for insertion of a distal perfusion cannula, as the morbidity and mortality of an ischemic limb in a patient on VA-ECMO can be catastrophic. We perform central VA-ECMO on our patients who have postcardiotomy cardiogenic shock or in patients who need robust support. We usually use 18–22 Fr arterial cannulas placed in the ascending aorta and 31–40 Fr venous cannulas placed in the right atrium.

http://dx.doi.org/10.5772/62875

2.2.4. *Indications and contraindications*

The indications for VA-ECMO in adult patients are cardiogenic shock from a variety of causes including acute myocardial infarction, myocarditis, drug toxicity, and pulmonary embolism. It also includes peripartum cardiomyopathy, decompensated chronic HF, postcardiotomy shock, and as a bridge to VAD implantation or heart transplantation. Typically, patients have low cardiac index (<2 L/min/m^2) and hypotension (systolic blood pressure <90 mmHg) despite inotropic agents, IABP, and adequate volume resuscitation [33]. Advantages of VA-ECMO over temporary VAD include ease of insertion bedside and not needing to transport a hemodynamically unstable patient to the operating room.

Absolute contraindications to ECMO include patients who are not candidates for transplantation or VAD implantation, disseminated malignancy, unwitnessed cardiac arrest, end-stage organ dysfunction, non-compliance, and patients with prolonged CPR without adequate tissue perfusion. Relative contraindications include advanced age, obesity, and contraindications to anticoagulation [33, 34].

2.2.5. *Management*

There are no randomized trials to date that have validated management guidelines. However, there are general management strategies that are implemented at most institutions. Such strategy is geared toward minimizing multiorgan system dysfunction. The complex management of a patient on VA-ECMO requires coordination and communication between the cardiothoracic surgeon, critical care intensivist, perfusionist, nurses, and ancillary staff.

For the respiratory system, successful management requires aggressive pulmonary toileting. This necessitates frequent endotracheal suctioning and possible bronchoscopy, positional changes, nebulizers, and chest roentgenogram. The fraction of inspired oxygen (FIO_2) is minimized in order to lessen oxygen toxicity. In order to lessen atelectasis, increased positive end-expiratory pressures (PEEPs) is often implemented [33]. Schmidt et al. showed that higher PEEP during the first 3 days on ECMO led to improved survival [35].

Successful cardiovascular support requires maintaining perfusion and aggressive volume resuscitation during the first few days on ECMO. Since ECMO promotes release of cytokines and a generalized systemic inflammatory response syndrome, adequate volume resuscitation with crystalloid or colloid is paramount. In addition, inotropic support is often required as the heart recovers.

The management of the renal system is often complex in the ECMO patient. Nearly 70–85% of patients on ECMO develop acute kidney injury (AKI) [36]. The first 2 days on ECMO usually require aggressive fluid resuscitation and is associated with oliguria. The diuretic phase usually begins after 2 days. Frequently, diuretics are utilized to improve mobilization of extravascular fluid. If AKI does not improve, renal replacement therapy often becomes indicated. However, the requirement for dialysis carries a significant mortality risk. Kielstein et al. showed that patients on ECMO who required dialysis had a 3-month survival rate of 17% while those on ECMO who did not required dialysis had a 3-month survival rate of 53% (p = 0.001). They also showed that duration of dialysis was associated with increased mortality [37].

Management of the gastrointestinal system and nutrition focuses on maintaining the integrity of the gastrointestinal mucosa, in order to lessen translocation of bacteria. This is accomplished with proton pump inhibitors or histamine blockers and enteral nutrition when possible [38]. However, parenteral nutrition is often required to supplement nutrition, as enteral nutrition is often interrupted. A recent study by Ridley et al. showed that enteral nutrition was interrupted for a median of 8 hours on 53% of the days. This was secondary to high gastric residual volume or fasting for a procedure or diagnostic test [39].

Neurologic complications are very common with ECMO and the clinician needs to have a low threshold to pursue imaging to rule out intracranial hemorrhage and acute stroke. Recently, all patients who received ECMO between 2001 and 2011 were selected from the Nationwide Inpatient Sample. Neurologic complications included acute ischemic stroke, intracranial hemorrhage, and seizures were evaluated. Of the 23,951 patients included in the study, 10.9% of patients suffered seizures, 4.1% suffered strokes, and 3.6% suffered intracranial hemorrhage. Patients who suffered intracranial hemorrhage were found to have a higher mortality rate, length of stay, and discharge to a long-term facility than those who did not have intracranial hemorrhage. Similarly, patients who suffered acute ischemic stroke had higher rates of discharge to long-term facilities and length of stay than patients who did not have an acute ischemic stroke. No difference in outcomes was found between those who had seizures and those who did not [40].

2.2.6. Weaning

Currently, there is a lack of established guidelines on weaning patients from VA-ECMO. Generally, patients have to demonstrate hemodynamic stability, recovery of organ dysfunction, resolution of pulmonary edema, and be in a euvolemic state. Echocardiogram is an invaluable tool for assessing cardiac recovery. Different institutions utilize different weaning parameters. Generally, weaning is accomplished once echocardiogram shows improvement of cardiac function. ECMO support is then gradually weaned, with flows reduced to 50% and then 25%. If the patient tolerates this, the circuit is then clamped between 30 minutes to 4 hours. The cannulas must be flushed with heparinized saline frequently to prevent thrombosis. Once the patient tolerates this, decannulation can be performed at bedside or in the operating room for large cannulas [41].

2.2.7. Complications

The most common complications in patients on VA-ECMO are bleeding and thrombosis. Bleeding requiring surgical treatment has been reported to occur in nearly 34% of patients on VA-ECMO [42]. It is a major concern for patients on VA-ECMO since the patients are anticoagulated with heparin and have platelet consumption and dysfunction [33]. Anticoagulation is a critical component to prevent circuit thrombosis, although there are no clear guidelines for standardized goals. However, most institutions use heparin with an activated partial thromboplastin time (aPTT) of 60–80 seconds. There is also an increased risk of disseminated intravascular coagulation (DIC) and heparin-induced thrombocytopenia (HIT). HIT mandates anticoagulation with a non-heparin-based agent. Available medications include bivalirudin and argatroban. Additional complications include infection, neurological complications, and limb ischemia. Limb ischemia is a function of cannula size and positioning in relation to the patient's vasculature. Reperfusion cannulas to perfuse distal to the entry site have decreased the risk of this complication [32, 43].

2.3. Ventricular assist devices

2.3.1. Background

VAD technology has advanced rapidly since the landmark REMATCH trial, which demonstrated survival and quality of life improvement in patients who underwent implantation of an LVAD compared to patients receiving maximal medical therapy. It also highlighted several limitations of pulsatile devices, namely device failure and thromboembolism [11]. Advancement in technology has led to the development of continuous-flow devices. These devices have been associated with significantly improved survival free from stroke and device failure at 2 years, when compared to pulsatile devices [44]. Overall survival with the current continuous-flow VADS in use today is reported to be 80% at 1 year and 70% at 2 years post implantation [4].

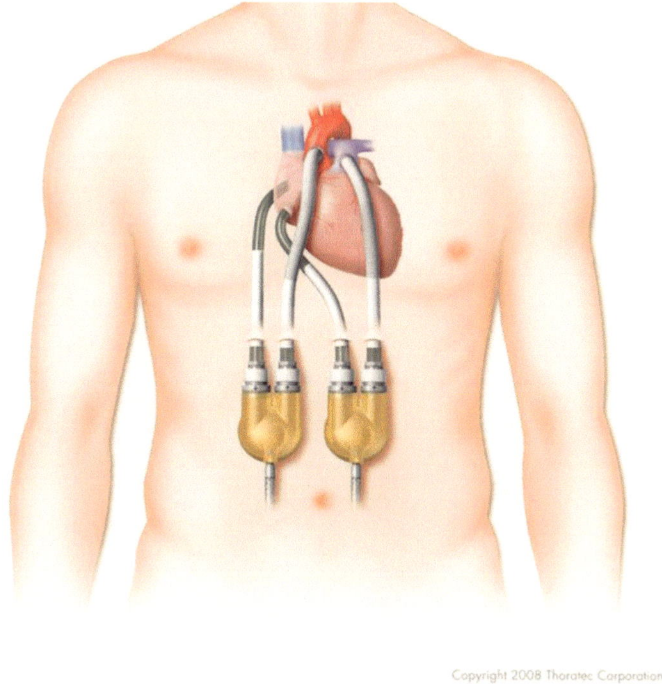

Figure 6. Paracorporeal ventricular assist devices (Reprinted with the permission of Thoratec Corporation).

Most frequently, VADs are implanted to assist the left ventricle. The inflow cannula is inserted into the left ventricle and the outflow cannula is inserted into the ascending or descending aorta. They can also provide right ventricular and biventricular support. In a right ventricular assist device (RVAD), the inflow cannula is inserted into the right atrium or right ventricle and the outflow cannula is inserted into the pulmonary artery.

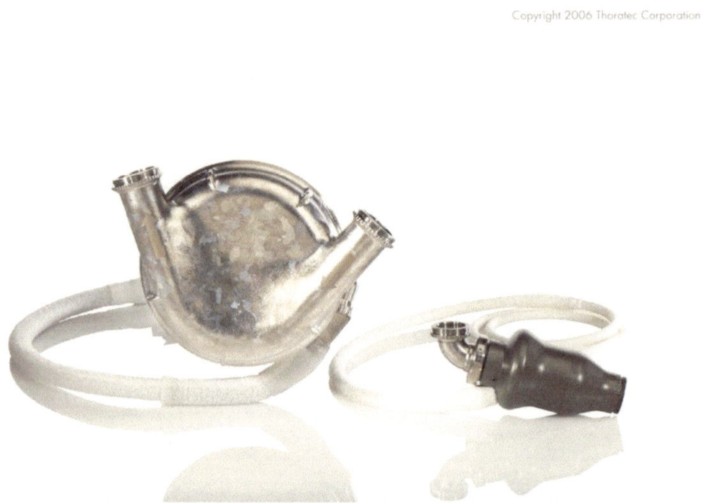

Figure 7. HeartMate XVE (left) and HeartMate II (right) (Reprinted with the permission of Thoratec Corporation).

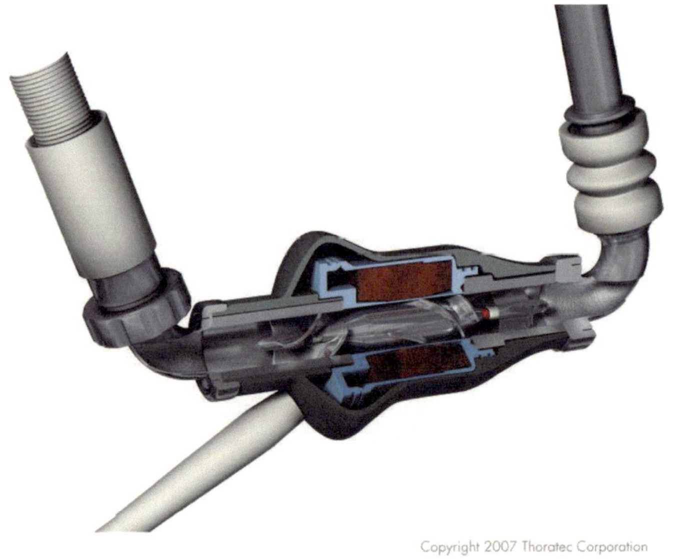

Figure 8. HeartMate II cross-section view with internal rotor (Reprinted with the permission of Thoratec Corporation).

VADs can be classified based on how they function mechanically. The first-generation VADs rely on pulsatile-flow technology. These VADs contain one-way valves and a flexible pumping chamber, which is compressed by an electric motor or pneumatic pressure. This forces blood

http://dx.doi.org/10.5772/62875

into the circulation. These patients will have a palpable pulse and a measurable blood pressure. The second-generation VADs are continuous axial flow devices while the third-generation VADs are continuous, centrifugal flow devices. These nonpulsatile, continuous-flow devices have internal rotors, which propel blood continuously. These patients have either weak, irregular pulses or non-palpable pulses.

In addition, VADs can provide both short-term and long-term circulatory support. Those designed for short-term circulatory support serve to restore organ perfusion quickly to relieve organ ischemia. They are used for BTR and BTT. These are non-implantable and provide support for days to weeks. Long-term VADs are implantable and are used for DT or BTT. The majority of VAD are implanted surgically. However, there are devices currently available that can be placed percutaneously.

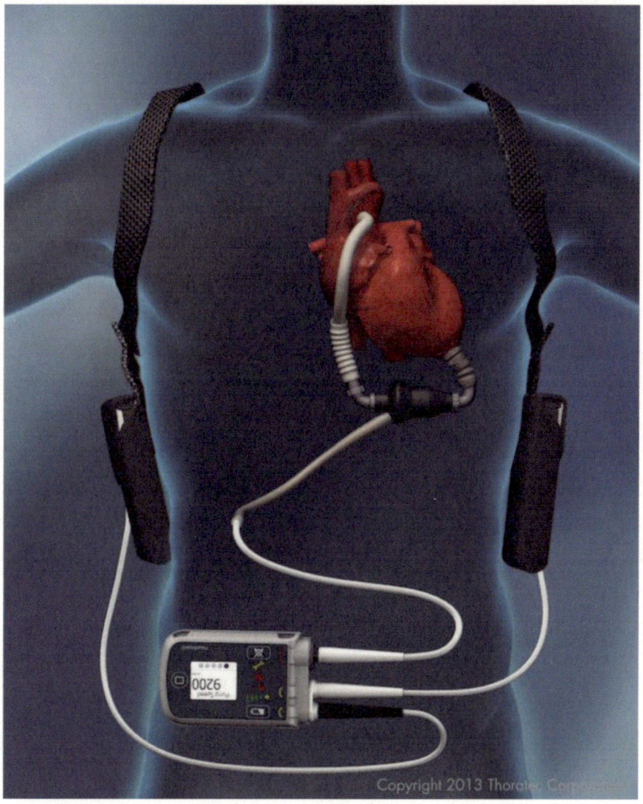

Figure 9. HeartMate II (Reprinted with the permission of Thoratec Corporation).

VADS are preload dependent and afterload sensitive. They can function independently of the EKG and most require anticoagulation. Generally, these devices are prone to infection, bleeding, hemolysis, thrombosis, cerebrovascular accidents, and mechanical malfunction. In addition, right ventricular dysfunction is a known complication of LVAD insertion, as the right ventricle has to increase its output to match the left heart and LVAD.

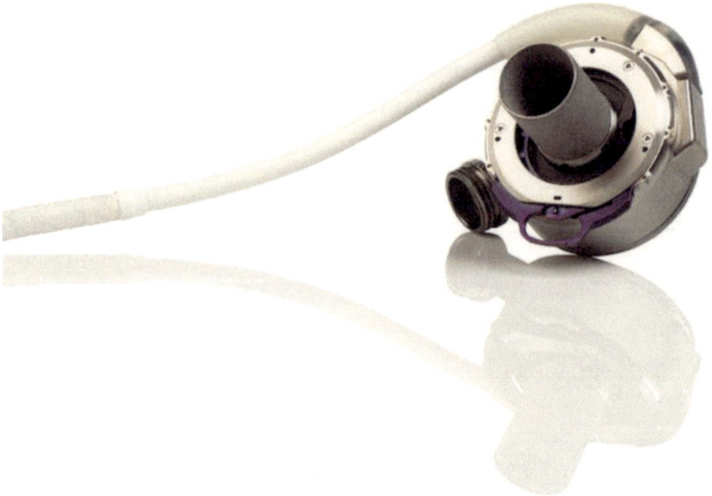

Figure 10. HeartMate 3 (Reprinted with the permission of Thoratec Corporation).

2.3.2. Indications for VAD

As mentioned earlier, indications for VAD can be divided into three main groups: BTR, BTT, and DT. Mechanical support with a VAD is used as a BTR in patients with acute decompensated HF. These patients typically have reversible causes of HF, such as postcardiotomy syndrome, medicine-induced cardiomyopathy, postpartum cardiomyopathy, and viral myocarditis. A retrospective study showed that patients who have acute fulminant myocarditis that progressed rapidly (median of 7 days from onset of symptoms to VAD implantation) had a greater likelihood of recovery of cardiac function and VAD explantation than patients who had a more indolent presentation (median of 22 days between onset of symptoms to VAD implantation). Those with a more indolent presentation were more likely to progress to needing a heart transplantation [45].

BTT remains the most common indication for MCSD. The Seventh INTERMACS report showed that implantation of VADs as BTT was about 51% in 2014 [4]. VADs allow patients with advanced HF to become healthier while awaiting heart transplantation. It has been shown that patients who receive a VAD as a BTT have improved functional capacity and quality of life [46].

DT refers to the use of VAD as definitive treatment for patients who do not qualify for heart transplantation. The Seventh INTERMACS report showed that implantation of VADs as DT has been steadily rising. In the year 2014, 45.7% of all VADs implanted in the United States have been for DT, up from 43.6% in 2013. This is in stark contrast to the 2008–2011 time period, when only 28.6% of all VADs implanted were for DT [4].

A fourth group, bridge to decision (BTD), is a new designation for those patients whose candidacy for heart transplantation or permanent VAD is still not determined, either due to medical or socioeconomic reasons. A recent study investigating the CentriMag VAD, an external continuous-flow device, as BTD therapy in patients with refractory cardiogenic shock demonstrated survival of 69.2% at 30 days and survival of 48.6% at 1 year. This study showed that 30% of patients had sufficient myocardial recovery to allow explantation of the VAD. Another 15% of patients progressed to needing a permanent VAD and 18% of patients required heart transplantations [47].

2.3.3. *Short-term VADs*

Short-term VADs are available as pulsatile and nonpulsatile devices. The short-term pulsatile device includes the first-generation Abiomed BVS 5000 and the second-generation Abiomed AB 5000, which allows the patient to be more mobile. These are paracorporeal devices that can provide left ventricular, right ventricular, or biventricular support for several weeks. In a retrospective single institution review, the Abiomed BVS 5000 was inserted for precardiotomy cardiogenic shock in 18 patients and for postcardiotomy cardiogenic shock in 53 patients. Of these, 62% of the patients survived, with 41% of patients being successfully weaned after myocardial recovery, 11% receiving a long-term LVAD, and 10% receiving a heart transplantation [48]. Similar to other VADs, patients require anticoagulation while being supported by this device.

Nonpulsatile short-term devices that could provide univentricular and biventricular support include the Impella and TandemHeart. These devices require anticoagulation and could be readily placed in the interventional cardiology suite for acute HF. The Impella LP 2.5 is a catheter-based VAD that is inserted via the femoral artery. It is passed into the aorta, through the aortic valve, and into the left ventricle. The catheter has an inlet at its tip and an outlet more proximally. This device functions by pumping blood through the inlet located in the left ventricle and into the outlet located in the ascending aorta. This lessens the amount of work the left ventricle has to perform and augments cardiac output. The Impella LP 5.0 works similarly but is larger and requires a formal aortotomy or femoral artery cutdown.

However, the TandemHeart consists of a centrifugal pump and a cannula placed through the femoral vein and guided into the right atrium. From there, the cannula is placed transeptally into the left atrium. A femoral artery cannula is also placed and blood from the left atrium is passed into the femoral artery, thereby bypassing the left ventricle [49]. In the largest study of its kind, Patel et al. showed that percutaneous VADs such as the TandemHeart and Impella led to a statistically significant reduction in mortality when compared to the IABP in patients undergoing percutaneous coronary intervention [50].

2.3.4. *Long-term VADs*

Long-term VADS can be divided into three generations. The first-generation VADs rely on pulsatile flow technology. It includes the HeartMate XVE, a VAD that has been extensively studied. In fact, it was this device that was studied in the seminal REMATCH trial. It has a textured inner surface, which promotes pseudoneointimal lining formation throughout the pump. Consequently, anticoagulation is not necessary and these patients often only receive antiplatelet therapy in the form of aspirin. The incidence of neurologic events remains low with this device. A small retrospective study with 21 patients showed no strokes or transient ischemic attacks during the average of 531 days of LVAD support. Only two of these patients developed metabolic encephalopathy, which resolved [51]. Major limitations of this device include increased incidence of infection, device malfunction, and its large size, which makes implantation into patients of a body surface area of less than 1.5 m^2 not feasible. Other first-generation devices include the Novacor, EXCOR, Thoratec IVAD, and Thoratec PVAD.

The second-generation VAD rely on a rotatory axial pump design. These are typically much smaller than the first-generation VADs because of the nonpulsatile flow design. By eliminating pulsatile flow, the need for having valves and chambers was eliminated. In addition, there are less moving parts leading to less hardware dysfunction. They also require less energy consumption. This group includes the HeartMate II, MicroMed DeBakey (now ReliantHeart), and Jarvik 2000. The HeartMate II has been extensively studied and has revolutionized the field of VAD. It was investigated against the HeartMate XVE by Slaughter et al. In their study, they showed that continuous flow LVAD had a statistically significant improved probability of survival free from stroke and device failure, when compared to pulsatile devices. In addition, the HeartMate II had actuarial survival rates of 68% at 1 year, compared to 55% for the HeartMate XVE. The survival benefit extended to 2 years, with 58% survival in the HearMate II cohort and 24% in the HeartMate XVE cohort [44].

The third-generation VAD also relies on continuous flow technology. However, instead of having a rotor in contact with blood, which results in hemolysis, there is a hydrodynamic or magnetic levitation component, which eliminates contact with blood. These include the DuraHeart, HeartMate 3, HeartWare, Evaheart, and INCOR. These remain investigational and in clinical trials in the United States. In Europe, several studies have already been conducted. A retrospective study from Italy reviewed the INCOR VAD in 42 patients. In their cohort, Iacovoni et al. showed survival of 74% at 1 year and 60% at 2 years. The most frequent adverse events included driveline infection, stroke, sepsis, and right HF. No episodes of pump thrombosis or gastrointestinal bleeding occurred [52].

2.3.5. Operative technique

Typically, VADs are placed via a median sternotomy and require cardiopulmonary bypass. A preperitoneal pocket is created to implant the device. Meticulous hemostasis is necessary since postoperative hematomas in the device pocket can predispose to infections. Alternatively, with the increasing miniaturization of the VADs, they can be placed within the pericardium.

With some of the newer models, implantation is possible via a thoracotomy incision and without cardiopulmonary bypass [53, 54].

2.3.6. Postoperative management

Postoperative care after VAD implantation requires a multidisciplinary approach to care. However, special attention has to be paid to blood pressure monitoring, anticoagulation, and right ventricular function. While arterial lines are in place, blood pressure can be titrated to mean arterial pressure (MAP) of 70–80 mmHg. Once invasive lines are discontinued, a Doppler probe and sphygmomanometer can be utilized to measure blood pressure. Antiplatelet therapy and anticoagulation is started within a few days postoperatively, once risks of bleeding and coagulopathy have subsided. Antiplatelet therapy is started with aspirin. Anticoagulation is started with a heparin drip and the transitioned to oral warfarin. Alternatively, starting warfarin without a heparin bridge has been reported. It has been shown that such management reduces the need for blood transfusions without increasing risks for short-term thrombosis or thromboembolic events [55]. The right ventricle is supported with the use of inotropes and pulmonary vasodilators such as nitric oxide, prostaglandins, and milrinone. Despite maximal medical therapy, if central venous pressures remain consistently above 20 mmHg and the cardiac index remains below 2 L/min/m^2, implantation with a temporary RVAD may be indicated.

2.4. Total artificial heart

2.4.1. Background

The TAH is a mechanical support device, which has not yet gained widespread acceptance. Only 66 were implanted in the United States in 2013 [4]. It provides pulsatile biventricular support and is pneumatically powered. With this device, the right and left ventricle and all the heart valves are removed. The removal of the native ventricles and valves eliminates many of the problems seen with LVAD or biventricular support, namely right HF, valvular regurgitation, and arrhythmias. The TAH is connected directly to the atria. It is currently approved

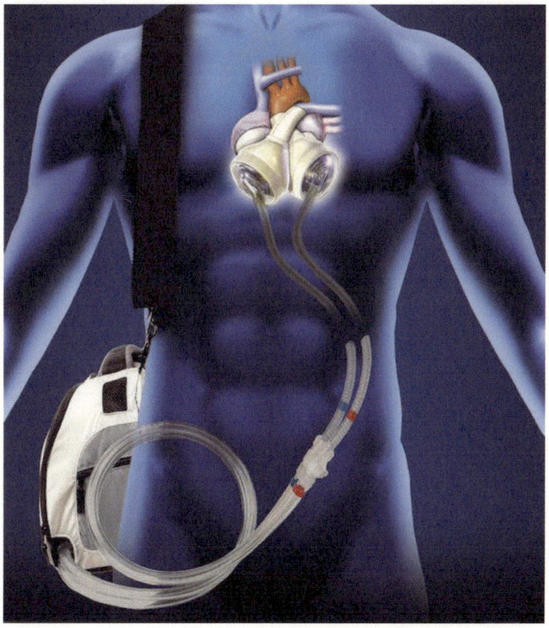

Figure 11. Total Artificial Heart with battery pack (Image courtesy of Syncardia.com).

for support for biventricular HF as a BTT [56]. It is available as the SynCardia TAH and AbioCor.

2.4.2. Indications

The main indication for the TAH is as a BTT for biventricular failure. It can be used in patients who have contraindications to LVAD and biventricular assist devices implantation. Such patients include those infiltrative or restrictive cardiomyopathies, aortic regurgitation, severe cardiac arrhythmias, and left ventricular thrombus.

In a study by Copeland et al., 81 patients were implanted with the TAH as a BTT. Of these, the rate of survival to transplantation was 79%. The overall 1-year survival for patients implanted with the TAH was 70%. In those patients who received heart transplantation after a TAH, the 1-year survival was 86% and the 5-year survival was 64% [57].

2.4.3. Limitations and complications

Major limitations to its use include its large size, requiring the patient to have a body surface area of at least 1.7 m^2. It also requires extensive surgery to remove both of the ventricles and all the valves. It is also fraught with complications including infection, postoperative bleeding, and thromboembolic events [58].

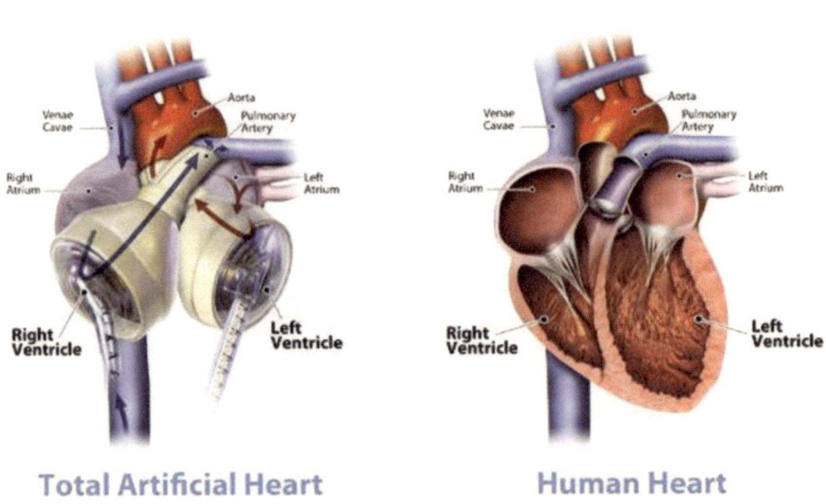

Figure 12. Total Artificial Heart (Image courtesy of Syncardia.com).

3. Conclusion

With the increase in HF and the lack of available hearts for transplantation, MCSDs will continue to play a greater role as a BTR, BTT, or DT.

http://dx.doi.org/10.5772/62875

Author details

Sagar Kadakia[1], Vishnu Ambur[1], Sharven Taghavi[2], Akira Shiose[3] and Yoshiya Toyoda[3*]

*Address all correspondence to: yoshiya.toyoda@tuhs.temple.edu

1 Department of Surgery, Temple University School of Medicine, Philadelphia, PA, USA

2 Department of Surgery, Division of Cardiothoracic Surgery, Washington University School of Medicine, St. Louis, MO, USA

3 Department of Cardiac Surgery, Temple University School of Medicine, Philadelphia, PA, USA

References

[1] Ageing | UNFPA. United Nations Population Fund [Internet]. [Cited 2015 Dec 19]. Available from: http://www.unfpa.org/ageing

[2] Esper SA, Subramaniam K. Heart failure and mechanical circulatory support. Best Pract Res Clin Anaesthesiol. 2012 Jun;26(2):91–104.

[3] Lund LH, Edwards LB, Kucheryavaya AY, Benden C, Dipchand AI, Goldfarb S, et al. The Registry of the International Society for Heart and Lung Transplantation: thirty-second official adult heart transplantation report—2015; focus theme: early graft failure. J Heart Lung Transplant. 2015 Oct;34(10):1244–54.

[4] Kirklin JK, Naftel DC, Pagani FD, Kormos RL, Stevenson LW, Blume ED, et al. Seventh INTERMACS annual report: 15,000 patients and counting. J Heart Lung Transplant. 2015 Dec;34(12):1495–504.

[5] Gibbon JH. Application of a mechanical heart and lung apparatus to cardiac surgery. Minn Med. 1954 Mar;37(3):171–85; passim.

[6] Cohn LH. Fifty years of open-heart surgery. Circulation. 2003 May 6;107(17):2168–70.

[7] Spencer FC, Eiseman B, Trinkle JK, Rossi NP. Assisted circulation for cardiac failure following intracardiac surgery with cardiopulmonary bypass. J Thorac Cardiovasc Surg. 1965 Jan;49:56–73.

[8] DeBakey ME. Left ventricular bypass pump for cardiac assistance. Am J Cardiol. 1971 Jan 1;27(1):3–11.

[9] Kantrowitz A, Tjønneland S, Freed PS, Phillips SJ, Butner AN, Sherman JL, et al. Initial clinical experience with intraaortic balloon pumping in cardiogenic shock. JAMA. 1968 Jan 8;203(2):113–8.

[10] DeVries WC, Anderson JL, Joyce LD, Anderson FL, Hammond EH, Jarvik RK, et al. Clinical use of the total artificial heart. N Engl J Med. 1984 Feb 2;310(5):273–8.

[11] Rose EA, Gelijns AC, Moskowitz AJ, Heitjan DF, Stevenson LW, Dembitsky W, et al. Long-term use of a left ventricular assist device for end-stage heart failure. N Engl J Med. 2001 Nov 15;345(20):1435–43.

[12] Rector TS, Taylor BC, Greer N, Rutks I, Wilt TJ. Use of left ventricular assist devices as destination therapy in end-stage congestive heart failure: a systemic review. 2012 May [cited 2015 Dec 24]. Available from: http://www.ncbi.nlm.nih.gov/books/NBK99056/

[13] Kirklin JK, Naftel DC. Mechanical circulatory support registering a therapy in evolution. Circ Heart Fail. 2008 Sep 1;1(3):200–5.

[14] Parissis H, Leotsinidis M, Akbar MT, Apostolakis E, Dougenis D. The need for intra aortic balloon pump support following open heart surgery: risk analysis and outcome. J Cardiothorac Surg. 2010 Apr 5;5:20.

[15] Powell WJ, Daggett WM, Magro AE, Bianco JA, Buckley MJ, Sanders CA, et al. Effects of intra-aortic balloon counterpulsation on cardiac performance, oxygen consumption, and coronary blood flow in dogs. Circ Res. 1970 Jun;26(6):753–64.

[16] Katz ES, Tunick PA, Kronzon I. Observations of coronary flow augmentation and balloon function during intraaortic balloon counterpulsation using transesophageal echocardiography. Am J Cardiol. 1992 Jun 15;69(19):1635–9.

[17] Dunkman WB, Leinbach RC, Buckley MJ, Mundth ED, Kantrowitz AR, Austen WG, et al. Clinical and hemodynamic results of intraaortic balloon pumping and surgery for cardiogenic shock. Circulation. 1972 Sep;46(3):465–77.

[18] Papaioannou TG, Stefanadis C. Basic principles of the intraaortic balloon pump and mechanisms affecting its performance. ASAIO J. 2005 May;51(3):296–300.

[19] Papaioannou TG, Terrovitis J, Kanakakis J, Stamatelopoulos KS, Protogerou AD, Lekakis JP, et al. Heart rate effect on hemodynamics during mechanical assistance by the intra-aortic balloon pump. Int J Artif Organs. 2002 Dec;25(12):1160–5.

[20] Weber KT, Janicki JS, Walker AA. Intra-aortic balloon pumping: an analysis of several variables affecting balloon performance. Trans Am Soc Artif Intern Organs. 1972;18(0): 486–92.

[21] Sarıkaya S, Adademir T, Özen Y, Aydın E, Başaran EK, Şahin M, et al. Alternative non-femoral accesses for intra-aortic balloon pumping. Perfusion. 2015 Nov 1;30(8):629–35.

[22] Ferguson III JJ, Cohen M, Freedman Jr RJ, Stone GW, Miller MF, Joseph DL, et al. The current practice of intra-aortic balloon counterpulsation: results from the Benchmark Registry. J Am Coll Cardiol. 2001 Nov 1;38(5):1456–62.

[23] White JM, Ruygrok PN. Intra-aortic balloon counterpulsation in contemporary practice —where are we? Heart Lung Circ. 2015 Apr;24(4):335–41.

[24] Thiele H, Zeymer U, Neumann F-J, Ferenc M, Olbrich H-G, Hausleiter J, et al. Intra-aortic balloon counterpulsation in acute myocardial infarction complicated by cardiogenic shock (IABP-SHOCK II): final 12 month results of a randomised, open-label trial. Lancet Lond Engl. 2013 Nov 16;382(9905):1638–45.

[25] Manohar VA, Levin RN, Karadolian SS, Usmani A, Timmis RM, Dery ME, et al. The impact of intra-aortic balloon pump weaning protocols on in-hospital clinical outcomes. J Intervent Cardiol. 2012 Apr;25(2):140–6.

[26] Onorati F, Santini F, Amoncelli E, Campanella F, Chiominto B, Faggian G, et al. How should I wean my next intra-aortic balloon pump? Differences between progressive volume weaning and rate weaning. J Thorac Cardiovasc Surg. 2013 May;145(5):1214–21.

[27] Baffes TG, Fridman JL, Bicoff JP, Whitehill JL. Extracorporeal circulation for support of palliative cardiac surgery in infants. Ann Thorac Surg. 1970 Oct;10(4):354–63.

[28] Tramm R, Ilic D, Davies AR, Pellegrino VA, Romero L, Hodgson C. Extracorporeal membrane oxygenation for critically ill adults. Cochrane Database Syst Rev. 2015;1:CD010381.

[29] Chen Y-S, Yu H-Y, Huang S-C, Lin J-W, Chi N-H, Wang C-H, et al. Extracorporeal membrane oxygenation support can extend the duration of cardiopulmonary resuscitation. Crit Care Med. 2008 Sep;36(9):2529–35.

[30] Cardarelli MG, Young AJ, Griffith B. Use of extracorporeal membrane oxygenation for adults in cardiac arrest (E-CPR): a meta-analysis of observational studies. ASAIO J Am Soc Artif Intern Organs 1992. 2009 Dec;55(6):581–6.

[31] Turner DA, Cheifetz IM. Extracorporeal membrane oxygenation for adult respiratory failure. Respir Care. 2013 Jun 1;58(6):1038–52.

[32] Russo CF, Cannata A, Vitali E, Lanfranconi M. Prevention of limb ischemia and edema during peripheral venoarterial extracorporeal membrane oxygenation in adults. J Card Surg. 2009 Apr;24(2):185–7.

[33] Makdisi G, Wang IW. Extra corporeal membrane oxygenation (ECMO) review of a lifesaving technology. J Thorac Dis. 2015 Jul 22;7(7):E166–76.

[34] Indications and Complications for VA-ECMO for Cardiac Failure [Internet]. American College of Cardiology. [cited 2016 Jan 18]. Available from: http://www.acc.org/latest-in-cardiology/articles/2015/07/14/09/27/indications-and-complications-for-va-ecmo-for-cardiac-failure

[35] Schmidt M, Stewart C, Bailey M, Nieszkowska A, Kelly J, Murphy L, et al. Mechanical ventilation management during extracorporeal membrane oxygenation for acute respiratory distress syndrome: a retrospective international multicenter study. Crit Care Med. 2015 Mar;43(3):654–64.

[36] Askenazi DJ, Selewski DT, Paden ML, Cooper DS, Bridges BC, Zappitelli M, et al. Renal replacement therapy in critically ill patients receiving extracorporeal membrane oxygenation. Clin J Am Soc Nephrol. 2012 Aug 1;7(8):1328–36.

[37] Kielstein JT, Heiden AM, Beutel G, Gottlieb J, Wiesner O, Hafer C, et al. Renal function and survival in 200 patients undergoing ECMO therapy. Nephrol Dial Transplant Off Publ Eur Dial Transpl Assoc—Eur Ren Assoc. 2013 Jan;28(1):86–90.

[38] Sen A, Callisen H, Alwardt C, Larson J, Lowell A, Libricz S, et al. Adult venovenous extracorporeal membrane oxygenation for severe respiratory failure: current status and future perspectives. Ann Card Anaesth. 2016;19(1):97.

[39] Ridley EJ, Davies AR, Robins EJ, Lukas G, Bailey MJ, Fraser JF. Nutrition therapy in adult patients receiving extracorporeal membrane oxygenation: a prospective, multi-centre, observational study. Crit Care Resusc J Australas Acad Crit Care Med. 2015 Sep; 17(3):183–9.

[40] Nasr DM, Rabinstein AA. Neurologic complications of extracorporeal membrane oxygenation. J Clin Neurol Seoul Korea. 2015 Oct;11(4):383–9.

[41] ELSO Guidelines [Internet]. [cited 2016 Jan 22]. Available from: http://www.elso.org/Portals/0/IGD/Archive/FileManager/e76ef78eabcusersshyerdocumentselsoguidelinesforadultcardiacfailure1.3.pdf

[42] Aubron C, Cheng AC, Pilcher D, Leong T, Magrin G, Cooper DJ, et al. Factors associated with outcomes of patients on extracorporeal membrane oxygenation support: a 5-year cohort study. Crit Care Lond Engl. 2013;17(2):R73.

[43] Jackson KW, Timpa J, McIlwain RB, O'Meara C, Kirklin JK, Borasino S, et al. Side-arm grafts for femoral extracorporeal membrane oxygenation cannulation. Ann Thorac Surg. 2012 Nov;94(5):e111–2.

[44] Slaughter MS, Rogers JG, Milano CA, Russell SD, Conte JV, Feldman D, et al. Advanced heart failure treated with continuous-flow left ventricular assist device. N Engl J Med. 2009 Dec 3;361(23):2241–51.

[45] Atluri P, Ullery BW, MacArthur JW, Goldstone AB, Fairman AS, Hiesinger W, et al. Rapid onset of fulminant myocarditis portends a favourable prognosis and the ability to bridge mechanical circulatory support to recovery. Eur J Cardio-Thorac Surg Off J Eur Assoc Cardio-Thorac Surg. 2013 Feb;43(2):379–82.

[46] Rogers JG, Aaronson KD, Boyle AJ, Russell SD, Milano CA, Pagani FD, et al. Continuous flow left ventricular assist device improves functional capacity and quality of life of advanced heart failure patients. J Am Coll Cardiol. 2010 Apr 27;55(17):1826–34.

[47] Takayama H, Soni L, Kalesan B, Truby LK, Ota T, Cedola S, et al. Bridge-to-decision therapy with a continuous-flow external ventricular assist device in refractory cardiogenic shock of various causes. Circ Heart Fail. 2014 Sep 1;7(5):799–806.

[48] Morgan JA, Stewart AS, Lee BJ, Oz MC, Naka Y. Role of the Abiomed BVS 5000 device for short-term support and bridge to transplantation. ASAIO J Am Soc Artif Intern Organs 1992. 2004 Aug;50(4):360–3.

[49] Gilotra NA, Stevens GR. Temporary mechanical circulatory support: a review of the options, indications, and outcomes. Clin Med Insights Cardiol. 2014;8(Suppl 1):75–85.

[50] Patel NJ, Singh V, Patel SV, Savani C, Patel N, Panaich S, et al. Percutaneous coronary interventions and hemodynamic support in the USA: a 5 year experience. J Intervent Cardiol. 2015 Dec;28(6):563–73.

[51] Slaughter MS, Sobieski MA, Gallagher C, Dia M, Silver MA. Low incidence of neurologic events during long-term support with the HeartMate® XVE left ventricular assist device. Tex Heart Inst J. 2008;35(3):245–9.

[52] Iacovoni A, Centofanti P, Attisani M, Verde A, Terzi A, Senni M, et al. Low incidence of gastrointestinal bleeding and pump thrombosis in patients receiving the INCOR LVAD system in the long-term follow-up. Int J Artif Organs. 2015 Nov 10;38(10):542–7.

[53] Hetzer R, Potapov EV, Weng Y, Sinawski H, Knollmann F, Komoda T, et al. Implantation of MicroMed DeBakey VAD through left thoracotomy after previous median sternotomy operations. Ann Thorac Surg. 2004 Jan;77(1):347–50.

[54] Haneya A, Philipp A, Puehler T, Ried M, Hilker M, Zink W, et al. Ventricular assist device implantation in patients on percutaneous extracorporeal life support without switching to conventional cardiopulmonary bypass system. Eur J Cardio-Thorac Surg Off J Eur Assoc Cardio-Thorac Surg. 2012 Jun;41(6):1366–70.

[55] Slaughter MS, Naka Y, John R, Boyle A, Conte JV, Russell SD, et al. Post-operative heparin may not be required for transitioning patients with a HeartMate II left ventricular assist system to long-term warfarin therapy. J Heart Lung Transplant Off Publ Int Soc Heart Transplant. 2010 Jun;29(6):616–24.

[56] Cook JA, Shah KB, Quader MA, Cooke RH, Kasirajan V, Rao KK, et al. The total artificial heart. J Thorac Dis. 2015 Dec;7(12):2172–80.

[57] Copeland JG, Smith RG, Arabia FA, Nolan PE, Sethi GK, Tsau PH, et al. Cardiac replacement with a total artificial heart as a bridge to transplantation. N Engl J Med. 2004 Aug 26;351(9):859–67.

[58] Gerosa G, Scuri S, Iop L, Torregrossa G. Present and future perspectives on total artificial hearts. Ann Cardiothorac Surg. 2014 Nov;3(6):595–602.

Section 5

Kidney Transplantation

Chapter 12

ABO-Incompatible Kidney Transplantation

Masayuki Tasaki, Kazuhide Saito, Yuki Nakagawa,
Yoshihiko Tomita and Kota Takahashi

Additional information is available at the end of the chapter

http://dx.doi.org/10.5772/62399

Abstract

Previously, ABO-incompatible kidney transplantation (KTx) was believed to be a "taboo" for immunological reasons. In Japan, the Tokyo Women's Medical University reported the first successful case of such transplantation, performed on January 19, 1989. Since then, we have been striving to improve the outcome of ABO-incompatible transplantation for a quarter of a century.

At Niigata University, ABO-incompatible KTx was performed in April 1996, with 80 patients being operated by 2013. The graft survival rates for those patients were 92.5%, 92.5%, 68.6%, and 61.0% for the 1st, 5th, 10th, and 15th years after transplantation, respectively. In September 2004, we were the first medical institution in Japan to introduce desensitization therapy into our clinical practice, which involved the use of rituximab and did not include splenectomy. The graft survival rate dramatically improved after 2004: 96.7% at 1 year, 96.7% at 5 years, and 87.9% at 10 years after transplantation, respectively. Our department initiated translational research on structural analysis and immune response of ABO histo-blood group carbohydrate antigens. Based on our experimental and clinical results, desensitization therapy before transplantation was more effective to inhibit B-cell immunity than multiple antibody removal.

Keywords: ABO blood group antigen, ABO-incompatible kidney transplantation, accommodation, antibody-mediated rejection, ABO kidney transplantation

1. Introduction

Since Karl Landsteiner discovered the human ABO blood groups in 1901 [1], ABO-incompatible transplantation has been considered as an immunological contraindication because of the risk of forming antibodies against ABO blood group antigens in the grafts, leading to hyperacute rejection followed by the loss of the kidney graft function. In Japan, kidney transplantation (KTx) using deceased donors is uncommon because the number of organ donations is very low. However, the number of end-stage renal disease (ESRD) patients who require a transplant is high. This situation required us to broaden the indications for living-donor KTx.

To expand the use of living-donor transplantation, ABO-incompatible KTx has been performed in Japan since 1989. In recent years, the outcome of ABO-incompatible KTx has improved to the point that it is now in no way inferior to ABO-compatible KTx. The number of cases using incompatible transplants per year now exceeds that using deceased-donor transplants, and incompatible KTx accounts for approximately 30% of all living-donor KTx. As of 2014, more than 3500 patients have been saved by this treatment in Japan.

In this chapter, we review ABO-incompatible transplantation and describe a strategy to overcome antibody-mediated rejection (AMR) after ABO-incompatible KTx.

2. History of ABO-incompatible KTx

The first ABO-incompatible KTx was performed by Yu Yu Voronoy in Ukraine in 1933 on a 26-year-old acute renal failure patient. The recipient with type O blood group received a blood type B kidney graft from a 64-year-old male donor. One of the donor's kidneys was harvested within 6 h of his death and grafted into the recipient's femoral region, but the patient died 2 days after transplantation. In this case, the failure of the graft to function was probably due to prolonged ischemic time rather than incompatibility [2]. Thereafter, some cases of ABO-incompatible KTx achieved long graft survival [3,4]. However, in 1967, Gleason and Murray [5] compiled the statistics on KTx, applied statistical analysis to ABO-incompatible cases, and reported very discouraging results.

Some years later, in 1981, Slapak et al. [6] of the University of Portsmouth, UK, published the remarkable finding that plasma exchange effectively reduced acute AMR in a transplant from a deceased donor when, because of a procedural error, the donor and recipient were of incompatible blood types. This was the first report that clearly showed the effectiveness of plasma exchange to remove antibody for ABO-incompatible KTx.

Alexandre et al. [7–10] from Belgium were the first to design a transplantation procedure using plasma exchange for pretransplantation removal of anti-A and -B antibodies. They also strongly emphasized the importance of splenectomy in achieving long-term graft survival. However, at that time, deceased-donor KTx was the mainstream procedure in Europe, and the techniques outlined in Alexandre et al.'s study were not widespread.

In Japan, the number of deceased-donor kidney donations has always been extremely low. KTx is an absolute indication for children with chronic renal insufficiency because of their need for healthy growth and development. Thus, to broaden the indications for living-donor KTx, ABO-incompatible KTx has mainly been developed in Japan since 1989 [11–21].

http://dx.doi.org/10.5772/62399

3. AMR

Anti-A and/or -B antibodies are present in the recipients, and ABO histo-blood group antigens are expressed on endothelial cells of kidney grafts [22]. In ABO-incompatible transplantation, these antibodies react to ABO histo-blood group antigens followed by complement activation. Bleeding and thrombosis develop, which eventually lead to graft loss [23,24] (**Figure 1**). As observed in 441 cases of ABO-incompatible KTx from Japan [15], no incidence of hyperacute rejection occurred within 48 h of transplantation [24] (**Figure 2**). Many cases of acute AMR occurred during the first 2–7 days after transplantation. After this period, the incidence of AMR decreased, and rejection ceased to occur 1 month after transplantation. Based on the results of this study, we divided the posttransplantation clinical course into three periods: a 48-h "silent period" with no sign of hyperacute rejection, an 18-day "critical period" from days 2 to 19 (average, day 7) when acute AMR is most likely to develop, and a subsequent "stable period" during which acute AMR no longer occurs because transplant accommodation has been established [24]. Accommodation is defined as a phenomenon in which no clinical grafted organ injury occurs despite the presence of antibodies in the recipient's body against the ABO histo-blood group antigens of the graft [15].

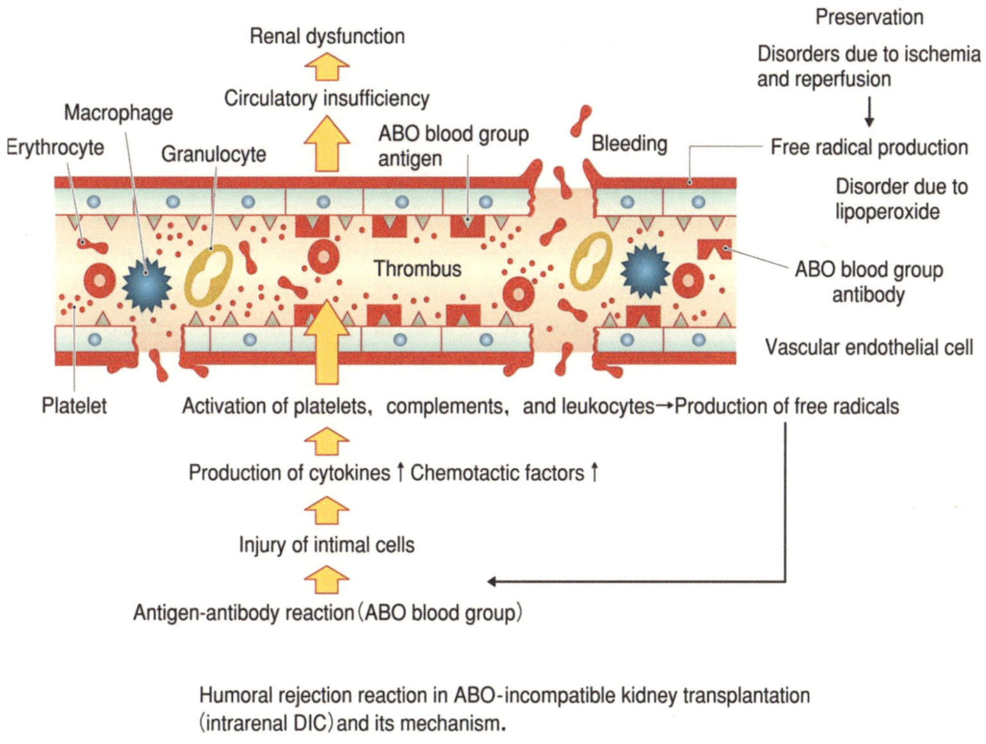

Figure 1. Acute AMR in ABO-incompatible KTx and its mechanism [23].

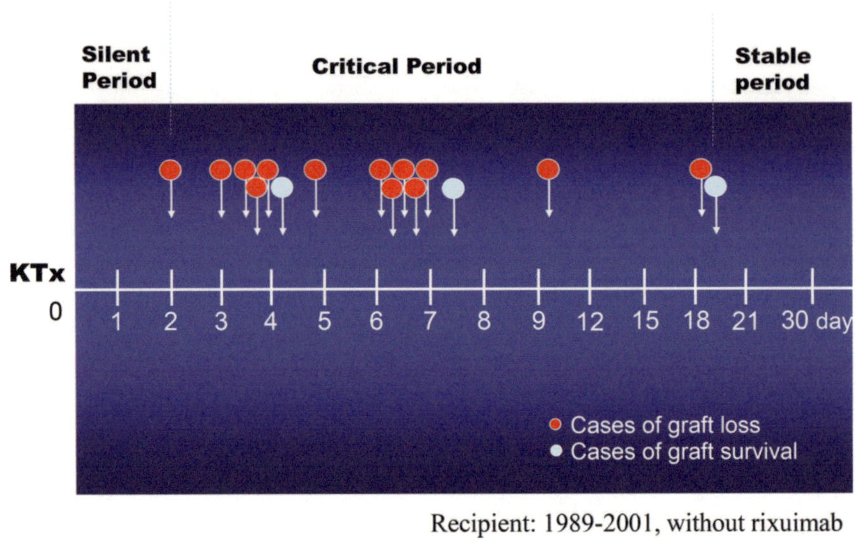

Figure 2. Onset of acute AMR [15,24].

AMR in ABO-incompatible KTx is classified into two types based on antigen stimulation and the immunological response to such stimulation [25] (**Table 1**). Type I acute AMR is caused by resensitization due to ABO histo-blood group antigens on the endothelial cells of the kidney graft. In patients at high immunological risk with high antibody titer, ABO histo-blood group antigens of the grafts can directly stimulate immunological responses, resulting in the explosive production of antibodies and leading to acute AMR. Typically, IgG antibody titers increase, accompanied by a parallel increase in IgM antibody titers. Once rejection develops, its course is dramatic, with no response to currently available therapy and ultimately leading to graft loss. Because serum IgG antibody titers are generally high before transplantation and a "rebound" in antibody production often occurs after pretransplantation antibody removal, desensitization therapy, including the suppression of memory cells, should be administered before transplantation (detailed in a later section).

	Type I	**Type II**
Occurrence of critical period	Early phase	Late phase
Recipient	Immunologically high-risk host	Immunocompromised host
Immunosuppression	Inadequate	Possible immunosuppression
Antigens	ABO histo-blood group antigens	ABO blood group-associated antigens
Sensitization	Resensitization	Primary sensitization
Response	Secondary and severe	Primary and less than type I
Antibody production	Explosive	Slow
Antibody titer	IgG↑> IgM↑	IgG→ IgM↑

http://dx.doi.org/10.5772/62399

	Type I	Type II
Treatment	Unresponsive	Responsive in early period
Prophylaxis	Desensitization	Prevention of infection
Prognosis	Graft loss	Possible graft survival

Table 1. Classification of acute AMR due to ABO blood group antigens in ABO-incompatible KTx [23].

Type II AMR is caused by a primary sensitization by ABO blood group-associated antigens. In response to bacterial infections, such as sepsis, ABO antigen-like substances on the surface of bacterial cells act as cross-reacting antigens, causing sensitization and antibody production. Type II AMR usually progresses more slowly and is less severe than type I AMR [25]. A major difference from type I rejection is the elevation of IgM antibody titers. Type II AMR also has a greater chance of responding to currently available treatment. Antibody removal and anticoagulation therapy should therefore be promptly administered.

4. Development of desensitization therapy for ABO-incompatible KTx

In this section, we summarize the history of ABO-incompatible KTx performed at our institute, Niigata University, focusing on the transition of immunosuppressive therapy as well as on the development and implementation of desensitization therapy [21].

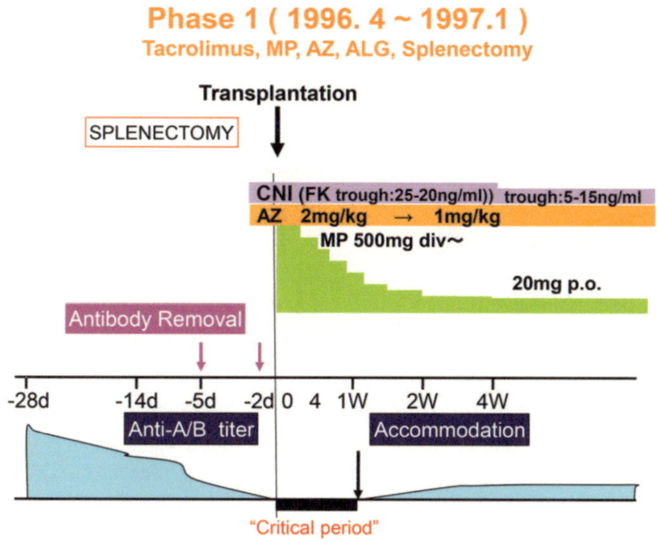

Figure 3. Immunosuppression protocol, early phase, period 1, extending from April 1996 to January 1997. Antibody removal with DFPP started from 5 to 7 days before transplantation, without any immunosuppression. FK506 and AZ were started 2 days before transplantation and splenectomy was "routinely" performed at the time of transplantation. MP, methylprednisolone.

In 1996, tacrolimus (FK506), azathioprine (AZ), steroids, and antilymphocyte globulin (ALG) were used for ABO-incompatible KTx (**Figure 3**). FK506 and AZ were initiated 2 days before surgery, splenectomy was performed at the time of transplantation, and ALG was administered for 14 days after KTx. For antibody removal therapy, double-filtration plasmapheresis (DFPP) or plasma exchange was performed. The target anti-A and -B titer immediately before KTx was set at eightfold or less, and the antibody removal protocol was repeated until the target titer was reached because high pretransplantation antibody titer against donor blood type has been reported to correlate with acute AMR [26–30].

In patients whose antibody titer rebounded after antibody removal therapies, acute AMR occurred in some cases with the increase in posttransplantation antibody titer. To avoid this, cyclophosphamide (CPA) treatment, which inhibits B cells, has been initiated along with low-dose steroids 10–14 days before transplantation since 1997 (**Figure 4**). Antibody removal, FK506, and splenectomy were performed in a conventional manner.

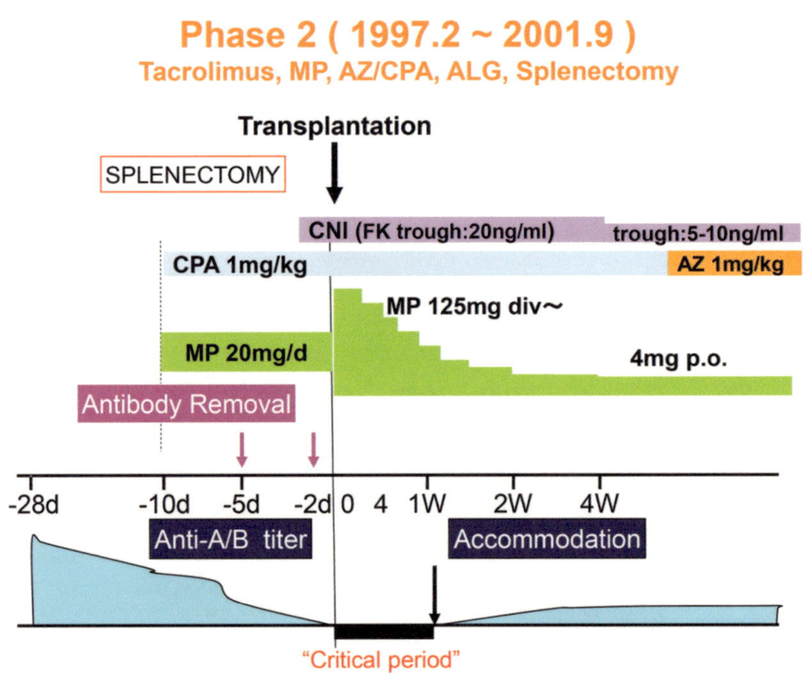

Figure 4. Immunosuppression protocol, early phase, period 2, extending from February 1997 to September 2001. CPA, a low steroid dose, and AZ were administered starting 10 days before transplantation, at the beginning of antibody removal.

However, the new protocol seemed to be less than fully adequate because two patients lost their grafts due to AMR during this period. Mycophenolate mofetil (MMF) and basiliximab have been included since 2001. To avoid AMR, MMF and steroids were started 14–28 days before the transplantation surgery (**Figure 5**). Antibody removal, FK506, and splenectomy were performed in a conventional manner.

http://dx.doi.org/10.5772/62399

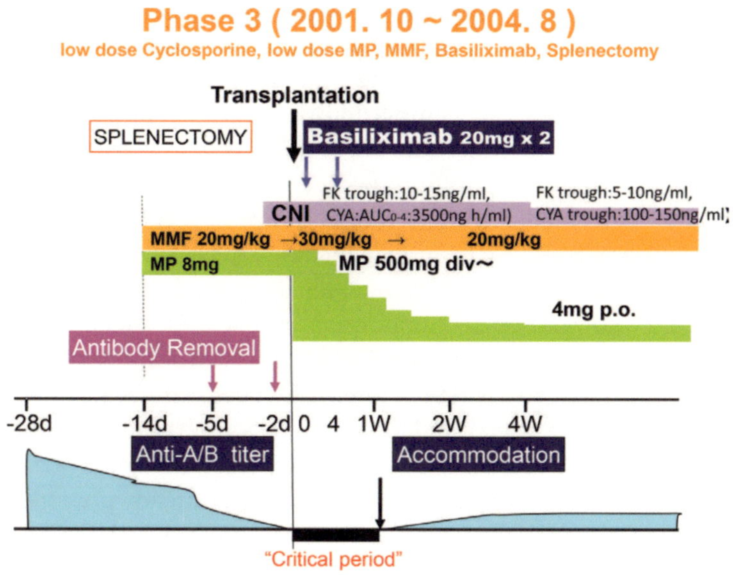

Figure 5. Immunosuppression protocol, early phase, period 3, extending from October 2001 to August 2004, using MMF and basiliximab. MMF and a low-dose steroid were started 2–4 weeks before transplantation. The concept of B-cell desensitization was adopted. AUC, area under the curve; CYA, cyclosporine.

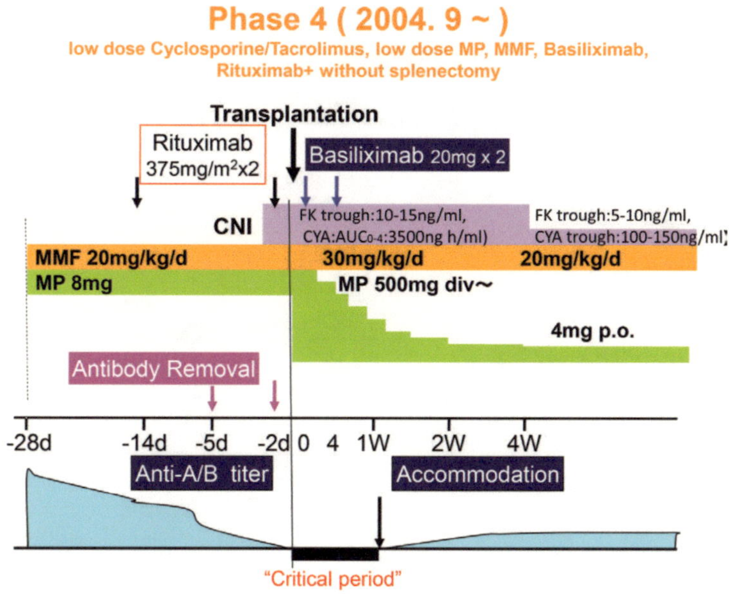

Figure 6. Late phase (September 2004–). Desensitization protocol with two doses of rituximab, MMF, a steroid, and antibody removal without splenectomy. The concept of "desensitization therapy" for ABO-incompatible KTx was introduced. MMF and a low-dose steroid were started 4 weeks before transplantation, and two doses of rituximab and a minimum antibody removal session followed. Splenectomy was completely abandoned in this phase.

Splenectomy has been considered a prerequisite for a successful outcome of ABO-incompatible KTx [31] because the spleen has a specific structure for entrapping extrinsic antigens and contains the largest pools of memory B cells and antibody-producing plasma cells in the body. However, splenectomy can lead to complications, including postoperative hemorrhage, pancreatic injury, and leakage of pancreatic juices [32]. Furthermore, the assumed immunological benefits of splenectomy are doubtful because severe AMR can still occur sometimes [26]. In such patients, extrasplenic memory B cells and plasma cells are activated to produce anti-A and -B antibodies in response to antigen loading after KTx. Strategies for preoperative immunosuppression must therefore be reconsidered. Instead of splenectomy, 375 mg/m^2 rituximab (a chimeric mouse-human monoclonal antibody formulation directed to CD20 antigens expressed on premature and mature B cells) has been administered twice since 2004: once 2 weeks before and once on the day before ABO-incompatible KTx [33] (**Figure 6**). The major goal of treatment with rituximab and MMF is to suppress the induction of differentiation from memory B cells into antibody-secreting plasma cells. Antibody removal was mainly intended for the physical removal of anti-A and -B antibodies already present in the circulating blood and also to aid in assessing the suppressive effects on the B cell line by determining the extent of antibody rebound after removal. Thus, antibody removal was considered to be a form of auxiliary therapy. As a general rule, antibody removal was limited to two times because of the serious concerns regarding the side effects of antibody removal, such as allergic reactions,

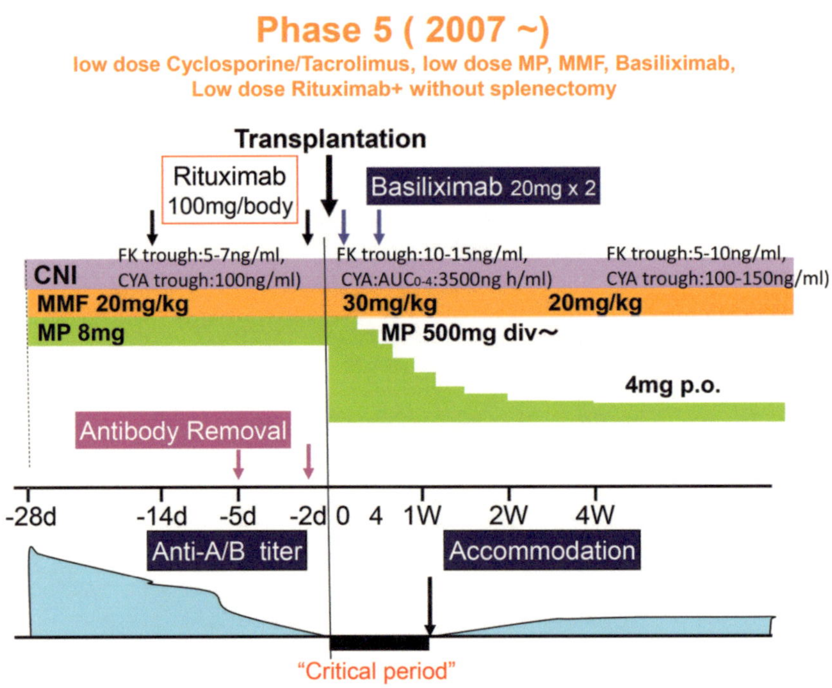

Figure 7. Late phase, modified desensitization protocol (2007–). Starting in 2007, a CNI was added 4 weeks before transplantation and one dose of rituximab was reduced to 100 mg/body. Antibody removal was limited to a minimum, and splenectomy was completely avoided.

hemorrhagic tendency due to decreased anticoagulant factors, and decreased colloid osmotic pressure and intravascular volume depletion due to hypoalbuminemia. Calcineurin inhibitors (CNI) suppressed the differentiation of B-0 cells to B-1a cells, which would otherwise progress to be anti-A and -B antibody-producing B cells [34]. Taking this point into account, CNI was started 28 days before KTx with MMF and steroids. To avoid over-immunosuppression, the dose of rituximab was eventually reduced to 100 mg/body (**Figure 7**). The number of peripheral B cells was well suppressed with this strategy for approximately 6 months after ABO-incompatible KTx (data not shown).

5. Outcomes of ABO-incompatible KTx in Niigata University

We show our clinical results divided into two periods, before and after 2004. As mentioned above, MMF and rituximab were used as a desensitization therapy without splenectomy since 2004. **Table 2** shows the characteristics of the patients who underwent ABO-incompatible KTx in Niigata University [21].

	1996–2004.5 (*n*=20)	2004.9–2013 (*n*=60)	*P*
Recipient age	33.5±11.3	44.9±13.3	0.069
Donor age	57.5±6.3	55.2±9.1	0.224
Male recipient (%)	75	72	0.555
Male donor (%)	50	28	0.037
Graft weight (g)	165.1±27.1	173.4±31.3	0.581
HLA MM	2.6±1.6	3.2±1.3	0.391
HD duration (months)	46.9±39.7	36.4±48.7	0.774
TIT (min)	63.3±27.6	82.8±28.0	0.644
WIT (min)	6.0±1.6	4.1±2.1	0.092
TAC for CNI (%)	85	50	0.000
Preemptive KTx (%)	0	20.3	0.000

Table 2. Characteristics of the patients who received ABO-incompatible KTx in Niigata University.

5.1. Patient survival rate

Patient survival rates are shown in **Figure 8** [21]. Before 2004, the patient survival rate was 95% for the first year, 90% for the first 5, 7, and 10 years, and 80% for the first 15 years after transplantation. After 2004, the patient survival rate was 100% for all available study periods (1, 5, 7, and 10 years) after transplantation. A statistically significant difference in patient survival rate was observed between the late and early phases (Kaplan-Meier analysis, *P*=0.03).

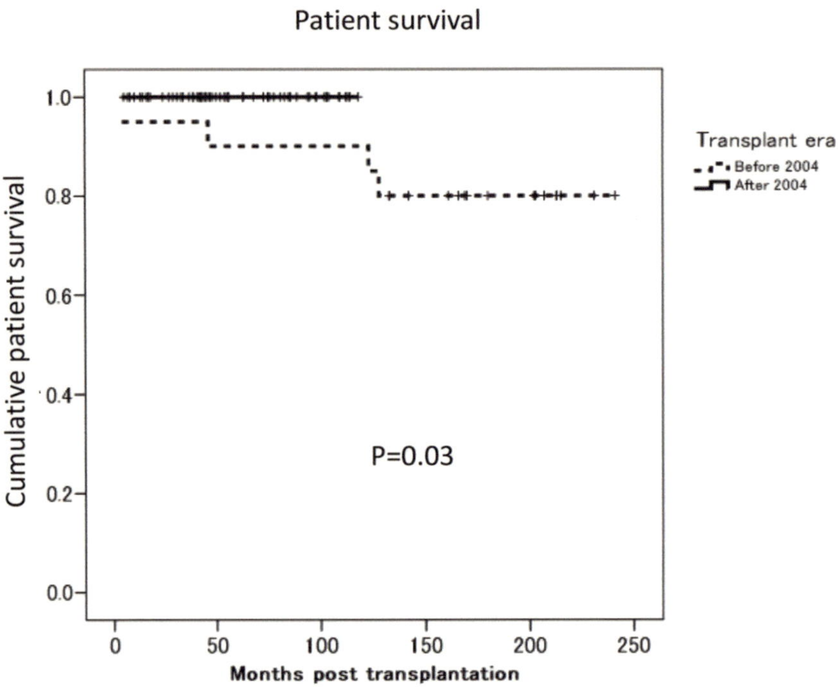

	1 year	5 years	7 years	10 years	15 years
Before 2004	95%	90%	90%	90%	80%
After 2004	100%	100%	100%	100%	N.A.

Figure 8. Patient survival before and after 2004 in ABO-incompatible KTx (Kaplan-Meier analysis). Patient survival rate of cases after 2004 was significantly improved compared to that of cases before 2004 (log-rank, P=0.03). N.A., not yet available.

5.2. Cause of death

Four patients died after transplantation, with their causes of death (time of death) being sepsis due to pleuritis (at 4 months after transplantation), sepsis (46 months), sepsis due to gastro-intestinal perforation (123 months), and brain tumor (123 months). Three of these deaths (two due to sepsis and one due to brain tumor) were deaths with functioning graft (DWFG).

5.3. Graft survival rate

Graft survival rates are shown in **Figure 9** [21]. Before 2004, the death-censored graft survival rate was 80% at 1 year, 80% at 5 years, 68.6% at 7 years, 51.4% at 10 years, and 45.7% at 15 years after transplantation. After 2004, the death-censored graft survival rate was 96.7% at 1 year, 96.7% at 5 years, 96.7% at 7 years, and 87.9% at 10 years after transplantation. A statistically significant difference in graft survival rate was observed between the late and early phases (Kaplan-Meier analysis, P=0.006).

http://dx.doi.org/10.5772/62399

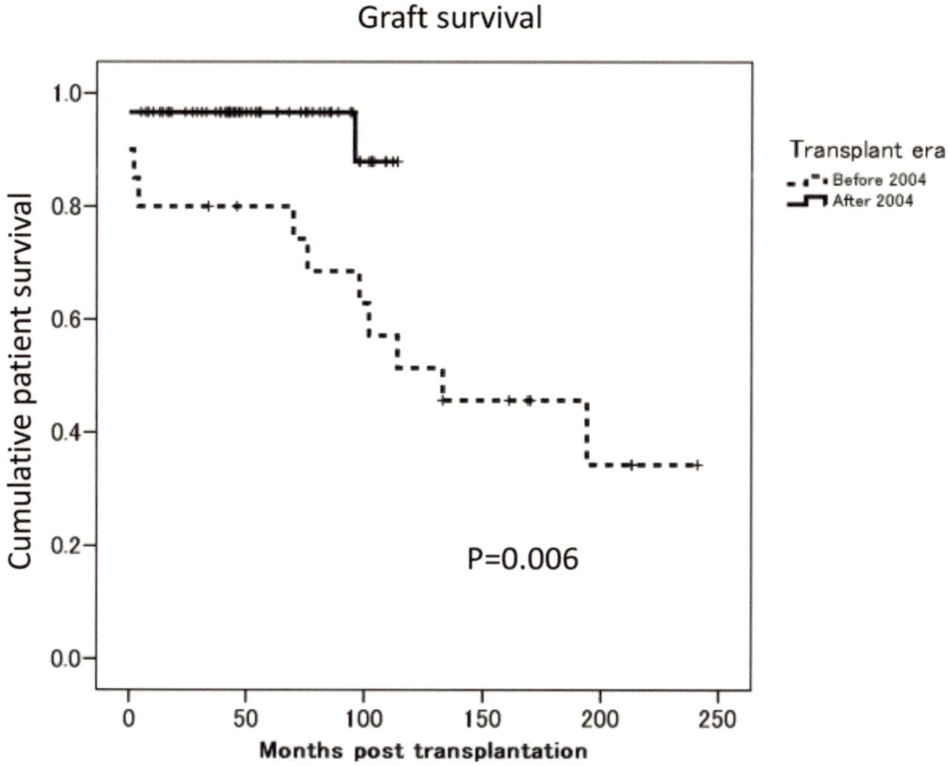

	1 year	5 years	7 years	10 years	15 years
Before 2004	80%	80%	68.6%	51.4%	45.7%
After 2004	96.7%	96.7%	96.7%	87.9%	N.A.

Figure 9. Graft survival before and after 2004 in ABO-incompatible KTx (Kaplan-Meier analysis). Graft survival in cases after 2004 was significantly improved compared to that of cases before 2004 (log-rank, *P*=0.006).

5.4. Cause of graft loss

Table 3 shows the cause of graft loss [21]. The graft was lost in 17 patients. The causes of graft loss were chronic allograft nephropathy in five cases (70, 98, 194, 133, and 102 months after transplantation), acute AMR in three cases (10, 10, and 9 days after transplantation), thrombotic microangiopathy (TMA) in one case (1 day after transplantation), acute rejection in one case (4 months after transplantation), recurrent membranoproliferative glomerulonephritis (MPGN) in one case (114 months after transplantation), recurrent IgA glomerulonephritis (IgAGN) in one case (114 months after transplantation), drug-induced nephropathy in one case (2 months after transplantation), graftectomy/total nephroureter/ectomy/cystectomy due to urothelial tumor in one case (76 months after transplantation), and patient death in three cases.

Cause of graft loss	n	Posttransplantation duration
Chronic allograft nephropathy	5	194, 133, 102, 98, and 70 months
Death with function	3	123, 46, and 4 months
AMR	3	10, 10, and 9 days
TMA	1	1 day
Acute rejection	1	4 months
Recurrent MPGN	1	114 months
Recurrent IgAGN	1	114 months

AMR: antibody mediated rejection, TMA: thrombotic microangiopathy, MPGN: membranoproliferative glomerulonephritis, IgAGN: IgA glomerulonephritis.

Table 3. Cause of graft loss in ABO-incompatible KTx.

6. Acute AMR by de novo antibody

In our studies, the indicator for acute AMR, C4d in peritubular capillaries (PTCs), was observed by graft biopsy over time, at 0-h, 1-h, or 1-month protocol biopsy or by episode biopsy. The positive rate for C4d in PTCs at 1-h biopsy was only 16.1% [24,35]. The positive rate increased to 70.9% for the 1-month protocol or episode biopsy. Biopsy was negative at 1 h in all four cases in which acute AMR developed due to anti-A and -B antibodies after ABO-incompatible KTx in our institute but was positive 1 month later. Among the cases that turned positive after negative results, no acute AMR developed except in these four cases. Considering this fact, we made the following hypotheses: (1) preexisting anti-A and -B natural antibodies do not always bind to histo-blood group antigens on the graft vascular endothelial cells and subsequently activate complement, (2) it is likely that antibodies with high affinity to the kidney allograft are newly formed postoperatively and deposited, and (3) not all antibodies produced postoperatively elicit acute AMR, and accommodation is induced and established in cases where the graft survives [22,24,35]. The important matter is that titration of anti-A and -B antibodies is most widely performed by isohemagglutinin using red blood cells (RBCs) in ABO-incompatible KTx. Our observations also suggested the diversity of anti-A and -B antibodies and antibody-producing clones and indicated that it is more important to control postoperatively produced anti-A and -B antibodies that injure target graft vascular endothelial cells (not RBCs) than to mechanically remove preformed antibodies. Finally, we previously reported that there were differences regarding the presentation of ABO blood group antigens between RBCs and endothelial cells of the kidney [22]. According to our results, we have recently excluded, on a trial basis, antibody removal before ABO-incompatible KTx in patients with antibody titers below 64-fold [36]. In 14 patients who did not receive antibody removal, the patient and graft survival after 1 year were each 100% [36].

http://dx.doi.org/10.5772/62399

7. Strategies for ABO-incompatible KTx

1. In ABO-incompatible KTx, tissue-destroying acute AMR is elicited by an extensive antibody production. This drastic antibody elevation occurs because memory B cells and plasma cells having immunological memory are inadequately suppressed and thus can react to histo-blood group carbohydrate antigens introduced by the graft, producing a second set phenomenon (type I AMR).

2. Acute AMR can be elicited by anti-A and -B antibody production that has been made possible because of a prior exposure to blood group-associated carbohydrate antigens due to certain bacterial infections (type II AMR).

3. Effective desensitization therapy should be performed by suppressing B-cell immunity rather than by several sessions of mechanical antibody removal. The effective method to protect from AMR is a pretransplantation procedure with a combination of rituximab and MMF/CNI, which blocks the induction of B-cell differentiation. The most important consideration is to inhibit B-cell immunity to a sufficient extent before ABO-incompatible KTx and potential new antibody production in the critical period. Accommodation has been established after ABO-incompatible KTx, and the recipient's posttransplantation antibody titer becomes less relevant.

Author details

Masayuki Tasaki, Kazuhide Saito, Yuki Nakagawa, Yoshihiko Tomita and Kota Takahashi*

*Address all correspondence to: takahashi-kouta@image.ocn.ne.jp

Division of Urology, Department of Regenerative & Transplant Medicine, Niigata Graduate School of Medical and Dental Sciences, Niigata, Japan

References

[1] Tagareli A. Karl Landsteiner: a hundred year later. Transplantation 2001;72:3.

[2] Barry JM, Murray JE. The first human renal transplants. J Urol 2006;176:888–890.

[3] Starzl TE, Marchioro TL, HolmesJH, HermannG, BrittainRS, StoningtonOH, TalmageDW, WaddellWR. Renal homografts in patients with major donor recipient blood group incompatibilities. Surgery 1964;55:195–200.

[4] Starzl TE, Tzakis A, Makowka L, Banner B, Demetrius A, Ramsey G, Duquesnoy R, Griffin M. The definition of ABO factors in transplantation: relation of other humoral antibody states. Transplant Proc 1987;19:4492–4497.

[5] Gleason RE, Murray JE. Report from kidney transplant registry: analysis of variables in the function of human kidney transplants. Transplantation 1967;52:343–359.

[6] Slapak M, Naik RB, Lee HA. Renal transplant in a patient with major donor-recipient blood group incompatibility: reversal of acute rejection by the use of modified plasmapheresis. Transplantation 1981;31:4–7.

[7] Alexandre GP, De Bruyere M, Squifflet JP, Moriau M, Latinne D, Pirson Y. Human ABO incompatible living donor renal homografts. Neth J Med 1985;28:231–234.

[8] Alexandre GPJ, Squifflet JP, De Bruyere M, Latinne D, Moriau M, Carlier M, Pirson Y, Lecomte Ch. ABO-incompatible related and unrelated living donor renal allografts. Transplant Proc 1986;18:452–455.

[9] Alexandre GP, Squifflet JP, De Bruyère M, Latinne D, Reding R, Gianello P, Carlier M, Pirson Y. Present experience in a series of 26 ABO incompatible living donor renal allografts. Transplant Proc 1987;19:4538–4542.

[10] Alexandre GPJ, Latinne D, Gianello P, Squifflet JP. Preformed cytotoxic antibodies and ABO-incompatible grafts. Clin Transplant 1991;5:583–594.

[11] Takahashi K, Agishi T, Ota K, et al. Extracorporeal plasma treatment for extending indication of kidney transplantation: ABO-incompatible and preformed antibody-positive kidney transplantation. In: Therapeutic Plasmapheresis IX. ICAOT Press, Cleveland, 1991; pp. 116–122.

[12] Takahashi K, Tanabe K, Ooba S, Yagisawa T, Nakazawa H, Teraoka S, Hayasaka Y, Kawaguchi H, Ito K, Toma H. Prophylactic use of a new immunosuppressive agent, deoxyspergualin, in patients with kidney transplantation from ABO-incompatible or preformed antibody positive donors. Transplant Proc 1991;23:1078–1082.

[13] Toma H. ABO-incompatible renal transplantation. Urol Clin N Am 1994;21:299–310.

[14] Tanabe K, Takahashi K, Sonda K, Tokumoto T, Ishikawa N, Kawai T, Fuchinoue S, Oshima T, Yagisawa T, Nakazawa H, Goya N, Koga S, Kawaguchi H, Ito K, Toma H, Agishi T, Ota K. Long-term results of ABO-incompatible living kidney transplantation: a single center experience. Transplantation 1998;65:224–228.

[15] Takahashi K, Saito K, Takahara S, Okuyama A, Tanabe K, Toma H, Uchida K, Hasegawa A, Yoshimura N, Kamiryo Y; Japanese ABO-Incompatible Kidney Transplantation Committee. The Japanese ABO-Incompatible Kidney Transplantation Committee. Excellent long-term outcome of ABO-incompatible living donor kidney transplantation in Japan. Am J Transplant 2004;4:1089–1096.

[16] Takahashi K. ABO-Incompatible Kidney Transplantation. Elsevier, Amsterdam, 2001; pp. 73–86.

[17] Takahashi K. Accommodation in ABO-Incompatible Kidney Transplantation. Elsevier, Amsterdam, 2004: pp. 111–124.

[18] Takahashi K. ABO-Incompatible Kidney Transplantation—Establishing a Scientific Framework. Elsevier, Amsterdam, 2007; pp. 53–72.

[19] Takahashi K. ABO-Incompatible Kidney Transplantation—Why Is Hyperacute Rejection Absent? Elsevier, Amsterdam, 2011; pp. 83–107.

[20] Takahashi K. ABO-Incompatible Kidney Transplantation—Overcoming Hyperacute Rejection and Establishing Clinical Strategies. Elsevier, Amsterdam, 2013; p. 32.

[21] Takahashi K, Saito K, Nakagawa Y, Tasaki M. ABO-Incompatible Kidney Transplantation—Moving Toward a Comprehensive and Sound Approach to Kidney Transplantation. Elsevier, Amsterdam, 2015; pp. 49–65.

[22] Tasaki M, Yoshida Y, Miyamoto M, Nameta M, Cuellar LM, Xu B, Zhang Y, Yaoita E, Nakagawa Y, Saito K, Yamamoto T, Takahashi K. Identification and characterization of major proteins carrying ABO blood group antigens in the human kidney transplantation. Transplantation 2009;87:1125–1133.

[23] Takahashi K. A new concept of accommodation in ABO-incompatible kidney transplantation. Clin Transplant. 2005;19 Suppl 14:76–85.

[24] Takahashi K, Saito K, Nakagawa Y, Tasaki M. ABO-Incompatible Kidney Transplantation—Moving Toward a Comprehensive and Sound Approach to Kidney Transplantation. Elsevier, Amsterdam, 2015; pp. 11–45.

[25] Takahashi K. Recent findings in ABO-incompatible kidney transplantation: classification and therapeutic strategy for acute antibody-mediated rejection due to ABO-blood-group-related antigens during the critical period preceding the establishment of accommodation. Clin Exp Nephrol 2007;11:128–141.

[26] Ishida H, Koyama I, Sawada T, Utsumi K, Murakami T, Sannomiya A, Tsuji K, Yoshimura N, Tojimbara T, Nakajima I, Tanabe K, Yamaguchi Y, Fuchinoue S, Takahashi K, Teraoka S, Ito K, Toma H, Agishi T. Anti-AB titer changes in patients with ABO incompatibility after living related kidney transplantations: survey of 101 cases to determine whether splenectomies are necessary for successful transplantation. Transplantation 2000;70:681–685.

[27] Chung BH, Lim JU, Kim Y, Kim JI, Moon IS, Choi BS, Park CW, Kim YS, Yang CW. Impact of the baseline anti-A/B antibody titer on the clinical outcome in ABO-incompatible kidney transplantation. Nephron Clin Pract 2013;124:79–88.

[28] Toki D, Ishida H, Setoguchi K, Shimizu T, Omoto K, Shirakawa H, Iida S, Horita S, Furusawa M, Ishizuka T, Yamaguchi Y, Tanabe K. Acute antibody-mediated rejection in living ABO-incompatible kidney transplantation: long-term impact and risk factors. Am J Transplant 2009;9:567–577.

[29] Sivakumaran P, Vo AA, Villicana R, Peng A, Jordan SC, Pepkowitz SH, Klapper EB. Therapeutic plasma exchange for desensitization prior to transplantation in ABO incompatible renal allografts. J Clin Apheresis 2009;24:155–160.

[30] Gloor JM, Lager DJ, Moore SB, Pineda AA, Fidler ME, Larson TS, Grande JP, Schwab TR, Griffin MD, Prieto M, Nyberg SL, Velosa JA, Textor SC, Platt JL, Stegall MD. ABO-incompatible kidney transplantation using both A2 and non-A2 living donors. Transplantation 2003;75:971–977.

[31] Alexander JW. Splenectomy as a prerequisite for successful human ABO incompatible renal transplantation. Transplant Proc 1985;17:138.

[32] Alexander JW, First MR, Majeski JA, Munda R, Fidler JP, Morris MJ, Suttman MP. The late adverse effect of splenectomy on patient survival following cadaveric renal transplantation. Transplantation 1984;37:467–470.

[33] Saito K, Nakagawa Y, Suwa M, Kumagai N, Tanikawa T, Nishiyama T, Ueno M, Gejyo F, Nishi S, Takahashi K. Pinpoint targeted immunosuppression: anti-CD20/MMF desensitization with anti-CD25 in successful ABO-incompatible kidney transplantation without splenectomy. Xenotransplantation 2006;13:111–117.

[34] Irei T, Ohdan H, Zhou W, Ishiyama K, Tanaka Y, Ide K, Asahara T. The persistent elimination of B cells responding to blood group A carbohydrates by synthetic group A carbohydrates and B-1 cell differentiation blockade: novel concept in preventing antibody-mediated rejection in ABO-incompatible transplantation. Blood 2007;110:4567–4575.

[35] Takahashi K, Saito K, Nakagawa Y, Tasaki M, Hara N, Imai N. Mechanism of acute antibody-mediated rejection in ABO-incompatible kidney transplantation: which anti-A/anti-B antibodies are responsible, natural or de novo? Transplantation 2010;89:635–637.

[36] Takahashi K, Saito K, Nakagawa Y, Tasaki M. ABO-Incompatible Kidney Transplantation—Moving Toward a Comprehensive and Sound Approach to Kidney Transplantation. Elsevier, Amsterdam, 2015; pp. 67–75.